Globalization, Health and the Global South
A Critical Approach

Globalization is a form of social change, reshaping the socio-spatial milieu in which humans strive, and in which health and disease are managed and controlled. And yet the effects of globalization are distributed unevenly, with opportunities open for some but not for all.

Globalization, Health and the Global South is an important textbook for any student of this fascinating area. Examining the dynamics of globalization through the lens of the Global South, it highlights risks and vulnerabilities that affect different regions and contexts, exacerbating inequalities despite the continuing speed of global processes. The book takes a critical approach to the topic, offering readers a deep understanding of health discourses and discusses a range of key topics, including migrant health, the role of politics and diplomacy and the Coronavirus pandemic.

Including further reading and end of chapter discussion questions, this essential textbook will be important reading for students across the health sciences and social sciences.

Jimoh Amzat is a full Professor at the Department of Sociology, Usmanu Danfodiyo University, Sokoto (UDUS), Nigeria, and Senior Research Associate at the Department of Sociology, University of Johannesburg, South Africa. He was a recipient of Erasmus Mundus scholarships (both as a graduate student and a visiting scholar) and Alexander von Humboldt postdoctoral fellowship (Germany). His research work focuses on the African context of various health issues. Amzat has published books and numerous papers in peer-reviewed journals.

Oliver Razum is full Professor and Dean of the School of Public Health, Bielefeld University, Germany, where he also heads the Department of Epidemiology and International Public Health. His main research field is social epidemiology, with a particular focus on the health of immigrants, and on the role of contextual factors in the production of health inequalities. He has published over 200 scientific papers and numerous book chapters.

Globalization, Health and the Global South

A Critical Approach

Jimoh Amzat and Oliver Razum

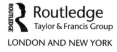 Routledge
Taylor & Francis Group

LONDON AND NEW YORK

First published 2022
by Routledge
2 Park Square, Milton Park, Abingdon, Oxon OX14 4RN

and by Routledge
605 Third Avenue, New York, NY 10158

Routledge is an imprint of the Taylor & Francis Group, an informa business

British Library Cataloguing-in-Publication Data
A catalogue record for this book is available from the British Library

Library of Congress Cataloging-in-Publication Data
Names: Amzat, Jimoh, author. | Razum, Oliver, author.
Title: Globalization, health and the global south : a critical approach /
Jimoh Amzat and Oliver Razum.
Description: Abingdon, Oxon; New York, NY: Routledge, 2022. |
Includes bibliographical references and index. |
Summary: "Globalization is a form of social change, reshaping the
socio-spatial milieu in which human strive, and in which health and
disease are managed and controlled. And yet the effects of globalization
are distributed unevenly, with opportunities open for some but not for all.
Including further reading and end of chapter discussion questions, this
essential textbook will be important reading for students across the health
social sciences"–Provided by publisher.
Identifiers: LCCN 2021032331 (print) | LCCN 2021032332 (ebook) |
ISBN 9781032162980 (hbk) | ISBN 9781032126654 (pbk) |
ISBN 9781003247975 (ebk)
Subjects: LCSH: Social medicine. | Globalization–Social aspects.
Classification: LCC RA418 .A635 2022 (print) | LCC RA418 (ebook) |
DDC 362.1–dc23
LC record available at https://lccn.loc.gov/2021032331
LC ebook record available at https://lccn.loc.gov/2021032332

ISBN: 978-1-032-16298-0 (hbk)
ISBN: 978-1-032-12665-4 (pbk)
ISBN: 978-1-003-24797-5 (ebk)

DOI: 10.4324/9781003247975

Typeset in Times New Roman
By Deanta Global Publishing Services, Chennai, India

Contents

Figures

Tables

Preface

Globalization is intricately connected to population health. Invariably, there is a need to continually interrogate the dynamics of this connectedness in various contexts/settings. This book, *Globalization, Health and the Global South: A Critical Approach*, projects some critical and macro analytical standpoints to describe, analyze and understand the relationship between globalization and health. Globalization is about the instantaneous exchange of information, ideas, goods and virtual and primary proximity (global village) among different parts of the world. Globalization presents some intense dynamic forces penetrating all spheres of life. It is a constant and persistent process that exacts immeasurable influence on human life. Globalization is now like the air we breathe, abundant but with varying quality from place to place. It is complex and boundless. It is multifactorial: Political, economic, cultural, social, religious and technological—with multiplier effects on health. Globalization is a form of social change, i.e., reshaping the socio-spatial milieu in which humans strive to produce and reproduce health and control diseases. The existing relationship is also reciprocal: Globalization affects health, and health affects globalization. Risks increasingly bound the world, so even the global efforts to curtail several pandemics are affected. Unfortunately, globalization in an un-equalizing process—with context-specific opportunities, uncertainties and adverse effects—all of which reflect in global health inequalities between the Global North and South.

Globalization, Health and the Global South: A Critical Approach examines the global health situation and impacts of globalization on health through the lens of the Global South. The book is spread over 11 chapters. Chapter 1 conceptualizes globalization and health, examines Ritzer's globalization of *nothing* and *something*, the confluence of health and globalization, then projects critical and analytical standpoints to describe, analyze and understand the relationship between globalization and health. The first major question addressed is: Why the focus on the globalization of health? The chapter examines the mutual characters of globalization and health as both responsive, transitional, measuring, reflexive, multidimensional and with differential effects in different regions, especially between the divide of North and South. The chapter also hints at the narrow conception of global health from a securitization agenda, while neglecting the manufactured epidemics and related global concerns. Chapter 2 discusses some definitions of global health and examines the many faces of globalization of health. The chapter then examines the various manifestations of the impacts of the globalization of health. Such manifestations include globalization of health risks/vulnerabilities; globalization of lifestyle diseases; globalization of healthcare; globalization of health technology; globalization of health indicators and targets; globalization of health policies and partnerships; globalization of medicalization; and globalization of health rights. The third chapter examines how the un-equalizing process of globalization manifests in the poor social determinants and the exploitative global determinants of health. The chapter examines social determinants, which explain the uneven distribution of diseases among individuals and countries, global determinants of health, which operate to accentuate some health crises in the South. The main argument is that some global processes are consequential for the local health condition.

Chapter 4 situates the discourse of globalization and health within some theoretical precepts. A structuralist approach derived from Giddens' structuration theory examines levels of responsibilities, and how structural arrangement influences population health. The chapter explores the risk society theory with some in-depth reflection on the notions and characters of risk society. The last perspective is the political economy of globalized health, adapting Wallerstein's theory described as global health systems. Both risk society and political economy perspectives reiterate that, due to global relations, more profound adverse health consequences are felt in the less developed regions. Chapter 5 examines the rise of noncommunicable diseases (NCDs) concerning the increasing modernization and globalization. This chapter also discusses the behavioral factors in NCDs, with a focus on how globalization accounts for the proliferation of the risk factors (in recent times), which double-burdens the weak health systems of most countries of the Global South. The argument is situated within McDonaldization theory, that the digital world has not merely McDonaldized food but also other *marketables* or *commodifiables*, especially in the realm of risk goods (including tobacco and alcohol). The focus of Chapter 6 is on infectious diseases in the Global South. Most parts of the Global South are still confronted with traditional risks, i.e., the risk of infectious diseases, while also facing the rising threat of noncommunicable diseases. This chapter examines global health emergencies, using Zika and Ebola as examples. The development tragedies occasioned by exploitative global relations reflect in the prevalence of infectious diseases. The declaration of global health "emergencies" shows the narrow conception (through securitization) of global health.

The book further examines the Coronavirus disease of 2019 (COVID-19) which became a pandemic and overwhelmed the world (see Chapter 7). The spread of COVID-19 is a manifestation of a risk society, fueled by globalization, or specifically, human mobility. The chapter examines the state of COVID-19, especially in the Global South. It looks at the series of delays, insufficient preparedness, "complicity" of China and the World Health Organization which accelerate the spread of the virus. The chapter also looks at the global control efforts, socioeconomic shocks of COVID-19 and how global health politics plays out as nations struggle to contain the virus.

Chapter 8 examines the political health issues involved in the control of diseases and how to ensure functional health for all. Global health is also a domain of power relations exercised among global health actors. The chapter examines the context of global health politics, including differential concern and priorities, differential capacity and resources, trickle-down science and weak health governance and political will. Lastly, this chapter examines the fundamental frames, including global health security, global health rights and ethics, among others, that shape global health politics and policies. Chapter 9 examines migration patterns necessitated by globalization and how they have become a public or global health issue and, therefore, how they are also responsible for various health challenges. The chapter examines the most worrisome dimension of migration of global health importance, which is called forced migration. The dimension includes human smuggling, trafficking and displacement with their accompanying severe humanitarian and health crises. The main concern of the chapter is the migration–health nexus. The push factors in the South, especially conflict and development tragedies, have a lot to do with globalization through the economic interests and military activities of the North. The potential impacts of migration on health in terms of the health consequences and vulnerabilities are essential issues, which necessitate the research efforts on migration and health. Chapter 10 examines the historical health targets from "Health for All by the Year 2000", then health aspects of the millennium development goals to the third goal of sustainable development goals (SDGs). All the SDGs are intricately connected to the realization of the set health targets. The last aspect of the chapter examines the situation of healthcare in the Global South with a macro analytic lens. Chapter 11 draws on some critical lessons from various efforts to improve population health in the Global South through Global Health Initiatives (GHIs). Several challenges embedded in their modes of operation (of the GHIs) limit global health goals. There is available finance within the global financial system, but it is not channeled at the scale required to achieve global development needs. The initiatives have emerged with powerful structures coercive of national structures, most times undermining the overall national health strategies and goals for fragmented or disease-specific funding, responsible for poor harmonization and community engagement. The methods of the GHIs also brew mistrust and medical conspiracies concerning suspected malevolent goals, either intended or unintended, in the Global South.

Globalization, Health and the Global South: A Critical Approach critically examines the various aforementioned issues. This book is a globally relevant reference text for understanding the impacts of globalization on health, especially in the Global South. The target audience includes students (at various levels of study), professionals, researchers, policy-makers and others interested in the various health discourses relating to globalization. The book is macro analytical and critical in its approach with adequate illustrations and objective points. The multidisciplinary character of globalization and health explains the relevance of this book across various disciplines, including but not limited to health social sciences (e.g., medical sociology, medical anthropology, health psychology, medical demography, medical geography and health economics) and health sciences (e.g., medicine, public health, epidemiology, bioethics and medical humanities). The book is conceived as a teaching text for global health but with significant relevance beyond the classroom for professionals, researchers, policy-makers and others interested in the various health concerns relating to globalization.

Acknowledgments

This is to acknowledge the Alexander von Humboldt Foundation, Germany for providing a special renewed research fellowship to Jimoh Amzat through which this book was written, and the host institution, University of Bielefeld, School of Public Health, for providing a supportive academic environment.

1 Conceptualizing Globalization and Health

1.1 Introduction

Entering into any discussion about globalization is challenging because of the complexity of the subject and the process of globalization. Such complexity is informed in the globalization of "everything" and as "everything" is globalizing. Globalization is a force penetrating nearly every aspect of human endeavor, and therefore, almost every human endeavor can be explained in terms of the intricacies of globalization. That we are living in a truly global world is incontrovertible, but the rate at which different regions are globalizing and if these regions reap the benefits of globalization is open to debate. Globalization is a process with differential effects in different regions. Globalization can also be observed from various positions or perspectives and could be region-specific. The primary focus of this chapter is to examine the meaning and intricacies of globalization and health. The interconnectedness between globalization and health is continuously being examined, because their combined implications, on the epidemiology of diseases, strengths of the healthcare system and access to healthcare, are still unfolding.

Globalization is also perpetually under investigation because it is an unstoppable force in human evolution and it facilitates increasing interdependence. In the mid-1970s, Wallenstein (1976, 2004) explained the world as a capitalist system, thereby demonstrating the differential socio-economic and political positions of the regions. Wallenstein expressed the unequal trends of the global connectedness (of the regions) in terms of globalization of capitalism or economic "cooperation". Wallenstein (1976, 2004) observed that globalization is historical, and it is a reality that every society has to contend with. Again, globalization, as an evolutionary force, continues to infiltrate every aspect of human life. Health is not an exception. The evolution of globalization is enabled partly by increasing technologization, which is facilitating diverse trajectories, possibilities and challenges.

Globalization is a ubiquitous process: No region is exempted from it. It is a trend, a process and it is probably irresistible. The remotest part of the world is also beckoning for a global connectedness or experiencing the trend in some ways. Such a remotest place that is considered disadvantaged because of the limited waves of globalization is a source of concern. The limited experiences of the indices of globalization define certain places as remote and therefore hold specific implications for their social existence, including health conditions. One process enhancing globalization is transportation technology, which is creating boundless boundaries, thereby also ensuring conglomeration of ideas and diffusion of cultures. The world is characterized by shared ideas, values, cooperation, unprecedented growth and, more importantly, a common destiny in every sphere of life. The "common destiny" is also expressed in population health. Before venturing into some specific matters of globalization and health, it is essential to make some conceptual clarifications to lay a clear foundation for subsequent polemics in subsequent sections and chapters.

DOI: 10.4324/9781003247975-1

1.2 How to Define Globalization and Health

Both globalization and health are complex processes, but deeply interrelated. As it will later be seen (see Section 1.3), there are fundamental justifications to discuss globalization and health. The first critical question is, how do we define globalization and health?

1.2.1 What Is Globalization?

Globalization is not entirely a new concept; it has always been with us. It has featured in previous writings of great philosophers, including Friedrich Hegel, Auguste Comte and Karl Marx (see Eriksen, 2007). Eriksen (2007) asserted that Hegel (1770–1831) speculated about globalization when he observed the notion of consciousness of connections between disparate places. Hegel foresaw a world-spirit (*Weltgeist*), a global community or village. Comte's idea of the science of human society can also be likened to the notion of globalization. Comte was particular about social statics, what holds that society together; and social dynamics, what changes society (Amzat and Omololu, 2012). Globalization has, to some extent, been both a factor of social statics and dynamics. Comte espoused that the last stage of social development is an industrial or scientific stage, which is one of the hallmarks of the globalized era. Karl Marx and Friedrich Engels (2012 [originally published 1848]) also discussed the world capitalist system, which can be correlated with a global adventure. Marx and Engels (2012) envisaged a global expansion of the world capitalist system to increase the accumulation of capital. Marx explained the idea of historical materialism, which starts with the material production activities of human beings (Shirong, 2016). The extensive material production is a significant impetus explaining the social transition from regional history to world history (Shirong, 2016). The first manifestation of globalization is economic globalization, which is a result of the global expansion of capitalism. Overproduction leads to the spread of capitalism, basically in search of new market, which propels economic globalization. Marx and Engels advanced a grand narrative predicting a world situation with many contradictions, including capital accumulation, pauperization, alienation and exploitation.

Most grand narratives are ambitious by viewing human society as a single entity, thereby projecting "global" theories of society (Amzat et al., 2015; Amzat and Maigari, 2020). It can, thus, be argued that industrialization or the industrial revolution of the 18th century set the pace for globalization. Colonialism and the expansion of capitalist projects also prelude the development of globalization. The concept of division of labor in the work of Ibn Khaldun and later Emile Durkheim was also a historical antecedent of globalization. Durkheim was more interested in the societal division of labor, which necessitates and ensures mutually interdependent or symbiotic relationships, thereby ensuring integration and interaction, which are the defining issues in globalization. Durkheim identified some elementary forms of globality, including the extent of constrictive geographical boundaries, the degree of political centralization, the degree of consensus over cultural symbols, the intensity and ease of communication and transportation—all of which contribute to greater moral and material density of the globalized era (Hirsch et al., 2009).

Globalization is a gradual process but only became a significant discourse in the 1980s. Before, there was westernization, which in the Global South is often described as neo-colonialism or imperialism. Globalization is sometimes regarded as an instrument of neo-colonialism, which creates apprehensions in many quarters. There is always the tendency to reduce the entire process of globalization to cultural globalization (Javed, 2014). Although colonialism had been abolished, globalization is its technical extension, which involves a means of domination in terms of education, economy and politics (Javed, 2014). Such domination dovetails into all cultural practices, including eating habits and value orientation. Westernization is often used to connote the imposition of western cultures on the rest of the world. The expansion of western culture is evident around the globe, and such expansion is simply a minute aspect of globalization. Therefore, westernization is not synonymous with globalization (Eriksen, 2007). Westernization is one-directional, but globalization involves a multi-directional flow of ideas—globalization advocates for harmony in heterogeneity, not homogenization. Events or ideas from a Global South may become global. For instance, there is a global fight against any gender violence irrespective of place.

Irrespective of how globalization is conceived, it is close to three of the central concepts in sociology: Society, solidarity and conflict. The notion of a global village equates to a unified society with intense connectedness or unified heterogeneity. Some social precepts are global, including solidarity, universal healthcare and happiness. It is often difficult to act blind to the enormous social problems of infant mortality, famine and conflict around the world because their projection is often on a global scale (see Luhmann, 1997). There is often much to achieve with solidarity or globalization. The preceding is not without caution to the internationalization of health risk and conflict or terrorism, which now occur also on a global scale. This kind of physical conflict is not even the only conception of conflict in sociology. The main conflict is between groups (for instance, South and North) with different interests and ideologies, which set the regions in constant rivalry. Hence, the conception of globalization is different across regions, and the yardsticks of measuring also vary accordingly.

Globalization is about increasing socio-political and economic scales and influences across several boundaries. The dissipating boundaries can be observed in every sphere of life with the instantaneous speed in social change (in all forms) and the exchange of information. Globalization is a process resulting in the complex, yet simple, nexus of all regions of the world's affairs. "Globalization is a social change, increased connectivity among societies and their elements due to transculturation; the explosive evolution of transport and communication technologies to facilitate international cultural and economic exchange" (Ernest, 2007, p. 20). Globalization is the instantaneous exchange of information, ideas, goods and virtual primary proximity (as a single society) among different parts of the world. The world is now in the era of global relationships, with both positive and negative impacts, that break the barrier of distance and a drive toward a common "destiny".

In addition, globalization means "an unprecedented compression of time and space reflected in the intensification of social, political, economic, and cultural interconnection, interdependency and the transformation of human society" (Anonymous, 2019). In other words, globalization facilitates interaction and integration among the people and various component institutions (political, economic, religious and educational), which have become so intense, dynamic and boundless. To Lechner (2005, p. 331), "globalization refers to the worldwide diffusion of practices, expansion of relations across continents, organization of social life on a global scale, and growth of a shared global consciousness" (see Table 1.1). Globalization signifies the compression of the world as a single society, which gives rise to a widespread intensification of socio-political and economic interaction and shared consciousness. Communication technologies have always been seriously implicated as a significant force driving globalization. The information and communication technologies have facilitated the multiple webs of interaction and the increasing integration of various global components. The ease of communication explains the limitless interaction patterns beyond physical contact. The embrace of virtual realities is the basis for a new form of communication without any form of "deep" social interrogation. Identities are now virtually represented, reified and accepted as real persons with whom communication or transaction is enabled. The new trend of machine-driven communication has set the world closer than ever before. The most exciting aspect is the high acceptability, i.e., trust in technology in the representation of identities and realities. It is a (global) world of virtual connectivity.

Table 1.1 Definitions of globalization

Lechner (2005)	Globalization refers to the worldwide diffusion of practices, expansion of relations across continents, organization of social life on a global scale and growth of a shared global consciousness.
Ernest (2007)	Globalization is a social change, increased connectivity among societies and their elements due to transculturation and the explosive evolution of transport and communication technologies to facilitate international cultural and economic exchange.
Authors'	Globalization is the instantaneous exchange of information, ideas, goods, virtual and primary proximity (as a single society) among different parts of the world.

Globalization manifests in some intense dynamic and persistent forces responsible for social change or transformation. The forces include transportation, communication technology, social media and trade. For example, the advancement in transportation is limiting the space and distance across boundaries. The boundaries are disappearing bit by bit; the world regions are closer than ever before, and the gradual dissipation of the boundaries is still on. While this is highly expedient, it can also be facilitative of the outbreak of infectious diseases (such as the Coronavirus and Ebola virus diseases). Social media is another driving force, which is responsible for social connectedness across the globe. Social media facilitates the technology-driven exchange of information, ideas and interests.

From the foregoing, it is evident that globalization exhibits some basic features. First, it standardizes, deterritorializes and modernizes (Eriksen, 2007). For instance, the pharmaceutical industries exhibit some form of conformity with prevailing standards in drug manufacturing and prescriptions. Treatments/therapies are being standardized across the globe. Standardization demonstrates how organizations and industries are connected and implement standard terms and practices irrespective of place. The world of products and services is globally standardized. Globalization also deterritorializes (compression of space and time); the world is becoming borderless despite movement restrictions imposed by various governments against some social groups, especially people coming from the Global South. Globalization also modernizes. The major trend in healthcare in the Global South is the adoption of a modern healthcare system. Even though ensuring total coverage is still a struggle, the drive continues.

Furthermore, globalization, beyond the driving forces, may be understood from three components: Social, political and economic components. The socio-cultural dimension is gradually harmonizing the differential cultures. It creates an avenue for the exchange of cultural material and products. The media, in general, and social media, in particular, facilitate the process of cultural flow from various regions of the world. However, the reality of the emerged and emerging globalization-driven inequality is always a dominant debate. Eriksen (2007, p. 14) also affirmed that

> globalization creates a shared grammar for talking about differences and inequalities. Humans everywhere are increasingly entering the same playing field, yet they do not participate in similar ways, and thus, frictions and conflicts are an integral part of globalizing processes.

The main problem is that the advantaged group might not see the imbalance in the system. This is why Eriksen (2007) observed that global players often assume that it is a single and equal playing field. The inequality is expanding the Global North and South divide in terms of power and prosperity (Eriksen, 2007). The divide between the Global North and South is glaring in terms of population health and access to healthcare, with the South bearing the greater brunt of both communicable and noncommunicable diseases and, unfortunately, with limited access to healthcare. The previous assertion is not meant to completely undermine the benefits in terms of healthcare aids that globalization has also facilitated; it shows that there is still a wide gap in terms of the differential burden of disease and access to care. The enormous burden rivals the benefits in resource-constrained settings.

Another related concept that is worth defining is globalism. Nye (2002) described globalism as a way of explaining a world characterized by networks of socio-spatial connectivity. Globalism is an ideology of globalization. It is a product of globalization. Ideas are now taking a global stance, and many people believe that globalization should be expanding and reinventing the world. The world should be meaningful globally. Nye (2002) asserted that a dimension of globalism is socio-cultural, which involves the movement of ideas, information and images, and of people who carry the information.

In short, globalization has created an avenue for acculturation, and to some extent, social tolerance and intersection of ideas. People are now more susceptible to the ideas of "strangers". The Internet is facilitating socio-cultural globalism, mainly the exchange of information and ideas. People are exposed to ideas and places which otherwise might not be accessible without globalization. There is an unprecedented flow of students and labor, and consequently, more profits for the Global North, which returns more from the flow. Another vital benefit is the transfer of technology, which is enhancing the progress of some otherwise remote communities. Modernists have always advocated for the transfer and acceptability of modern technology as an effective panacea to development. Therefore, globalization is also expediting the modernist agenda. Globalization facilitates an increasing spread of medical devices, biotech and healthcare services. There is a gradual development of telemedicine, artificial body parts and even rapid diagnostic tools. The Global South must be susceptible to the transfer of modern technologies to keep pace in health welfare and social protection.

Globalization also comes with some uncertainties; in fact, sometimes overwhelming uncertainties. The unpredictability of the process of globalization, imbalanced power relations and the ensuing inequalities between and within societies are major global concerns. The uncertainty is about social and economic development and certain speculative and real by-products, including uncertainty in the labor market, uneven risk accumulation between and within groups, cybercrime, epidemics as a result of human movement, among others. Beyond the definitions of globalization, it is crucial to further conceptualize it with reference to Ritzer's conception of globalization of *nothing* and *something*.

1.2.2 *Globalization of* Nothing *and* Something

A significant contribution to the globalization debate comes from Ritzer (2003, 2004), called "globalization of *nothing*". It was an attempt to conceptualize globalization or query its understanding further. Ritzer defined *nothing* as events that are distinctively empty in forms (in all its dimensions, including social forms) but centrally conceived and controlled. Ritzer defined *something* in terms of distinctive contents. The definition of globalization as *nothing* is significant, irrespective of the distinction between *nothing* and *something*. It is *nothing* that facilitates *something*. Ritzer observed that it is easier to export empty forms (*nothing*) than loaded content (*something*) throughout the globe. Ritzer and Ryan (2002, p. 52) further broke down the concept of *nothing* into four subtypes, including *non-places* (empty settings), *non-things* (such as credit), *non-people* (e.g., e-customer care) and *non-services* (e.g., dispensing machine operated by customers). The central deduction is that the primary drivers of globalization are non-physical materials. Globalization is the flow of enchantments, ideas or abstractions and symbols transmittable in their virtual forms. The Internet, for instance, is a primary means or facilitator of the flow. Most globalized products that individuals see everywhere are *something* carried by *nothing*. "Places" are not movable but can be visualized or imagined and represented. Also, individuals interact with machines (a kind of dehumanization), make electronic payments and play electronic games.

In general, the empty forms are easily acceptable since they are genuinely *nothing*; they merely facilitate *somethings*. It is easy to accept the Internet but to reject some transmittable contents. *Nothing* can easily be replicated across the globe, perhaps, with different contents. *Something*, in general, is antithetical to *nothing* and can be broken down into four categories: *Places* (or settings), *things* (mostly materials) *people*, and *services* (Ritzer, 2003). Therefore, there is the globalization of *nothing* and *something* at the same time. *Somethings* are forms that are rich in content (Ritzer, 2003). Unlike *nothing*, *something* can easily be perceived, could create anxiety and come in conflict with local norms. Globalization facilitates the worldwide spread of nothingness, the global proliferation of lack of unique content, the generic, lack of local ties, timelessness and dehumanization (Ritzer, 2003). The critical caution is that both *something* and *nothing* mutually coexist and are interdependent. *Something* must drift with the flow of *nothing*.

Ritzer further unpacked globalization through the use of two related concepts: Glocalization and grobalization. Glocalization is a blend of local and global (Robertson, 2001). It is about thinking and acting both locally and globally. It is essential to examine the local context of disease prevalence, think of global best practices and policies and explore how the solution will be customized for local benefits. Grobalization is a conception of globalization as the imperialistic instrument focusing on the growth of capitalism, westernization and modernization. The capitalistic aspect of healthcare is the commodification of health and profit motives in health-related services both at local and global levels. The westernization aspect of health starts with the spread of modern/western healthcare itself and the denigration and displacement of alternative healthcare. McDonaldization, a key aspect of the modernization drive, is the spread of principles of fast-food sufficiency, calculability, predictability and control which dominate the world (see Section 5.4). While the principles appear favorable, a critical assessment reveals that the principles help in the spread of fast-food culture implicated in the spread of some non-communicable diseases (including obesity, hypertension and heart diseases) responsible for a considerable high global death burden. The principles also aid the manufacturing of modern risks (see Sections 1.4.1.1, 2.3.1 and 4.3), thereby generating a risky society of health concerns and related uncertainties.

Figure 1.1 presents the globalization of nothing concerning health. Ritzer noted the beginning of tension in the process of globalization; it is about the grobalization of nothing (e.g., medical hegemony in the form of modern medicine) at the expense of the grobalized something (e.g., modern healthcare), on the one hand, and on the other hand, glocalized nothing (e.g., healthcare) and glocalized something (e.g., primary healthcare or integrative care system). It is herein vital to summarize the "complex" conception of globalization as the nexus of nothing/something and grobal/glocal. It is about non-service and services such as online DNA testing services facilitated with information technology when samples can be sent across and results obtained within a few days revealing medical indications, some of which might require further services (medical follow-up). It is about the place, e.g., a particular pharmaceutical company, and non-place, e.g., political economy of drug production.

The compression of time and space is greatly facilitated by the grobalization of *nothing* but later accompanied by the grobalization of *something*. Ritzer (2003, p. 203) observed that the grobalization of *nothing* dominates in all spheres of life, including medicine, science, pharmaceuticals, biotechnology and education, among others. However, it should be noted that the grobalization of *something* is more important in the analysis of globalization. Grobalization is associated with the mass production of loaded contents, effects and forms.

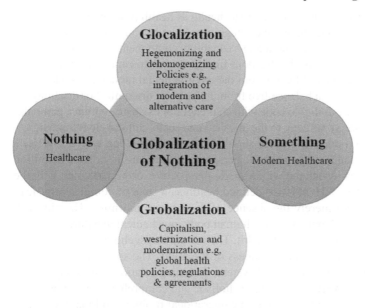

Figure 1.1 Globalization of nothing concerning health

However, there is a far higher demand for *nothing* (easily mass-produced or extended) than *something* (the substantively rich forms), but *nothing* often comes with *something* and vice-versa. The control and production of both *nothing* and *something* are not evenly distributed. The unequal-ness has been a significant debate about globalization. The argument in this respect is that the high-income countries control the production of both *nothing* and *something*. Therefore, grobalization dominate the globalization process. In order to create some balance, then emerged the concept of glocalization, to emphasize the triumph of some local contents or forms. Therefore, glocalization, developed to mitigate the "evils" of globalization, is a dehegemonizing and dehomogenizing process (Ritzer, 2003). There are local products (material and non-material) primarily from the Global South that have also permeated the North. There is also glocalization of *nothing* and *something*, through the creation of glocal forms. The critics of globalization often find solace in glocalization, although with the awareness that globalization is ubiquitous and irresistible. After globalization, the next concept is health.

1.2.3 What Is Health?

Like several concepts, the concept or notion of health is controversial not only in its measurement but also definition (see Amzat and Razum, 2014, 2018). Beyond the controversy, the idea of health implies the capacity to function in society, which signifies freedom from illness or injury. The primary issue with illness is the tendency to incapacitate individuals. Health is a state of wellness, a form of a positive state of physical, mental and social condition. Health is an ability because it is central in the day-to-day functioning in society. Such ability varies from one individual to the other depending on the state of health. Health has instrumental value: A state of health provides the capability required to carry out day-to-day tasks.

Larson (1999, p. 125) averred that health is better defined using multiple perspectives or models. Hence, Larson suggested wellness and environmental models apart from the World Health

Organization (WHO) model. The wellness model treats health as health promotion and progress toward effective functioning, comfort, energy and integration of body, mind and spirit (Larson, 1999). The model has various components, including a capability component when "functioning" and "energy" are considered. Comfort is also freedom from pain and constraints; it is a state of ease. Larson (1999) further conceived of health from the environmental model as an adaptation to physical and social surroundings—a balance free from undue pain, discomfort or disability. In this sense, health is regarded as the ability to cope with challenges of existence within a particular space. It is thus a coping or adaptive strategy to the physical and socio-cultural environment.

For Larson (1999), the two models examined should be considered along with the WHO's definition of health. The importance of the multiple perspectives is to ensure holistic definition and mitigate some controversies associated with a single perspective, or in particular, with the WHO's definition of health. The WHO (1946) defined health as a state of complete physical, mental and social well-being, not merely the absence of disease and infirmity. The physical, also physiological, is the biological makeup of the human body, mechanical in nature, and must be working correctly to ensure a good state of health. The mental or psychological is about the state of mind, i.e., a sense of coherence or soundness of the mind. The social aspect is about the degree of role performance within the social system, including relationships, cooperation, and integration with others. The WHO's definition is holistic and comprehensive, although not without some criticisms. The criticisms are about the operational problem and that the definition does not cater for those living with chronic diseases (see Amzat and Razum, 2014). It was due to the criticism that there have been some alternative definitions and, perhaps, the main reason why Larson proposed multiple models in defining health.

Parsons (1972) was particular about the social model of health, which the WHO portrayed in the social well-being component of its definition. The individual is supposed to interact with others and perform essential roles in society. As earlier mentioned, health in this sense is in terms of the capability of an individual's role performance. Society is made up of essential roles of the component units (either individuals or groups). The ability to imbibe societal traits and exhibit the capabilities acquired as a member of society in various situations signifies a state of being healthy. The crucial aspect of this social model is the consideration of the contribution of the social factors to population health. Health is a function of particular social factors or conditions, which are greatly influenced by global precepts. Another significant aspect of the social model of health is the acquisition of "risks" through "risk behavior" within a "risky context". Global forces shape the "risky context" in terms of the magnitude and mitigation measures available to individuals in society. The social model advances the discussion of health beyond the reductionism of the germ theory of disease, mostly focusing on pathology to the varying socio-contexts of health and illness.

Table 1.2 shows some definitions of health, including alternative definitions to the WHO's. Frankish et al. (2001) defined health using the capability or capacity approach and proposed an alternative definition that would cater for most health conditions deviating from the absoluteness of the WHO's definition. Frankish et al. (2001) defined health as the capacity of people to adapt to, respond to, or control life's challenges and changes. Like, Frankish et al., Bircher (2005) was particular about the fluctuation of capability across the life course and, more importantly, about those living with chronic diseases (not curable but manageable) (see Table 1.2). The attainment of potentials commensurate to different age and society also define health. Bircher's definition is similar to that of Huber et al.'s (2011), who advanced that health is the ability to self-manage in the face of social, physical and emotional challenges. The glaring tendency in their definition is about coping with situations. A wheelchair-bound person who can move around is healthy. He/she only faces constraints when society is not sensitive to the needs of people living with disability.

Table 1.2 Definitions of health

World Health Organization [WHO] (1946)	State of complete physical, mental and social well-being and not merely the absence of disease or infirmity.
Talcott Parsons (1972)	The state of optimum capacity of an individual for the effective performance of the roles and tasks for which the individual has been socialized.
Frankish et al. (2001)	Health is the capacity of people to adapt to, respond to or control life's challenges and changes.
Bircher (2005)	A dynamic state of well-being characterized by physical and mental potential, which satisfies the demands of life commensurate with age, culture and personal responsibility.
Huber et al. (2011)	The ability to adapt and self-manage in the face of social, physical and emotional challenges.

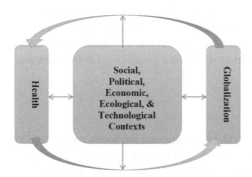

Figure 1.2 Confluence of health and globalization

The main concern of this chapter is not to dabble into the various controversies surrounding the definition of health but to situate the meaning of health within the global context. Health is highly contextual or circumstantial; it is a function of socio-spatial, political and economic conditions, and globalization invariably affects the context—the first simple model, as presented in Figure 1.2, shows the confluence of health and globalization. The confluence depicts reciprocal relationships: Globalization predicts and modifies the contexts, which affect health. Invariably, health also affects the contexts, which also have profound implications for globalization. Some specific contextual factors will be examined in the subsequent chapters.

Within this discussion of the confluence of health and globalization comes another concept called global health (see Chapter 2), which lays credence to the argument about a "common destiny" about health. Global health is also a concept, which conveniently merges globalization and health. The health condition of a village in the Global South might affect a city or countryside in the Global North and vice-versa (see discussion on noncommunicable and infectious diseases in relation to globalization in Chapters 5 and 6). Again, health is defined by global trends, increasing reciprocated interdependence and vulnerabilities over vast distances. Health is, thus, a global phenomenon. The next section will examine some concrete basis for the focus on globalization and health.

1.3 Globalization and Health: The Basic Links

Globalization is intricately connected to population health (see Murray and Smith, 2001; Collins, 2003; Huynen et al., 2005). However, there is a need to continually interrogate the dynamics of

Table 1.3 Why globalization and health

Globalization is social change	Health is responsive to social change
Globalization impacts need a measurement	Health is a significant barometer of globalization
Globalization is on a ubiquitous scale	Health risk and care are ubiquitous
Globalization is multifactorial	Health exhibits similar multifactorial dimensions (to globalization)
Experience of globalization is differential	Health inequalities are a function of the differential experience of globalization

this connectedness in various contexts/settings. Globalization is a fundamental health determinant. It is thus a worthwhile endeavor to project critical and analytical standpoints to describe, analyze, and understand the relationship between globalization and health. The first question is: Why the focus on the globalization of health? It is crucial to justify this focus with specific points further. In the maiden edition of the journal, *Globalization and Health*, Martin (2005) observed three significant points on the need to focus on globalization and health. Two additional points (making five points) are examined, which justify the focus on globalization and health (see Table 1.3).

1.3.1 Health Is Responsive to the Globalizing Social Change

Globalization is a form of social change (Martin, 2005). It is reshaping the socio-spatial milieu in which humans strive to produce and reproduce health and control diseases. The social geography is wide open to constant transformation in the name of globalization, which seems irresistible and serves as a vital determinant of health. Globalization is now part of what in sociology is referred to as social dynamics. It is responsible for social fluctuation or alteration. The succession of alteration within the social milieu is most times inevitable and more significantly affects all spheres of life, including health, health risks or vulnerability and healthcare.

More than ever, and continuously, the world is becoming global. Figure 1.1 shows the various contexts of globalization. ILO (2003) reiterated that globalization brings societies and individuals closer together. The glaring consequence of globalization is that it exacts impacts on social life, work and work environment, play and leisure. For the ILO, the primary concern is about the impact of globalization on employment, working conditions, income and social protection. The ILO also acknowledged the sphere of the impact of globalization beyond the world of work to security, culture, identity, the cohesiveness of families and communities. Globalization comes with enormous opportunities in various sectors of society and uncertainties as well (mostly expressed in the concern about unemployment, inequality and poverty). Globalization is reshaping social structures, institutions and human agency across the globe. The compression of space and intensification of cooperation and interdependency are the hallmark social changes which globalization occasioned.

Again, the central argument is that globalization is a factor of social change or transition, and health is responsive to social change. Social transition is intricately connected to epidemiological and demographical transition. Epidemiologic transition is about the complicated change in patterns of health and disease and on the interactions between the pattern and contextual factors, including demographic, economic and sociologic determinants and consequences (Omran, 2005). While the assertion might not be entirely accurate for the Global South, to some extent, there have been increasing shifts in the pattern from infectious to chronic diseases; the world is confronted with lifestyle and degenerative diseases as the primary causes of morbidity and mortality (Omran, 2005). There is a complex and changing pattern of mortalities and morbidities greatly influenced by globalization. Demographic transition is also about the changing pattern of population dynamics and growth, especially from high to low mortality and birth rates. One profound implication of these epidemiological and demographical transitions is also the changing patterns of healthcare needs of the population (Brodsky and Clafield, 2017). For instance, Lifestyle diseases are mostly chronic, thereby requiring long-term care and social support.

In general, how are changes in society affecting health, healthcare, health institutions and health practices? Wadsworth (1997) observed that changing social factors hold tremendous implications for health both at individual and societal levels. There are varying ways to also examine social change: In terms of stability and disorganization or disruption. Globalization brings both positive and negative health social implications. As the world is modernizing (with traditional institutions giving away for a progressive transformation or transition to more organized and sophisticated forms), so is healthcare in most parts of the world modernizing. There is a gradual expansion of modern healthcare as the mainstay in healthcare in the Global South. A central concern about healthcare is mostly about how to ensure universal coverage of modern healthcare. Multilateral supports in healthcare often focus on the challenges of modern healthcare in the respective states. In the last five decades, there have been unprecedented changes in the modernization of healthcare, including pharmaceuticals and emerging health technologies. Previous areas not touched by modern healthcare are realizing the need to adopt and expand the modern healthcare system. There has been the development of many drugs, including modern contraceptives for family planning.

Over the years, the world has witnessed historical materialist epidemiology i.e., the connection of human health, healthcare and distribution of diseases to the prevailing economic and political systems (see Krieger, 2001; Holtz et al., 2006; Navarro, 2009). Globalization expands the world capitalist system, which has been implicated in the health inequalities around the world (Holtz et al., 2006; Navarro, 2009). With the incorporation into the world capitalist system, the Third World is also on the move to improve "western" or modern medicine, thereby relegating ethnomedicine as complementary or alternative medicine. With the growth of modern medicine, The world has witnessed the expansion of child immunization to cut down the rate of childhood diseases. There have been remarkable improvements in child health across the globe, although there is still a need for more improvement in the Global South, which incidentally still lags in achieving some previously set health goals such as health for all by the year 2000.

In relation to infectious diseases, health condition is always a function of trilateral factors: The host, agent and environment (i.e., epidemiologic triangle). The host now operates within a global terrain, embedded with far and near forces, shaping individual immunity or vulnerability milieu. The forces are sometimes overwhelming and could be global in their dimensions. The agent also exists within a particular setting, which either inhibits or promotes its existence. The environment seems to be an increasingly complicated context. It is ecological, but also economic, political and social: All combined account for a complicated domain of host existential realities.

1.3.2 Health as an Indicator of Globalization

The second point is that it is essential to measure the process called globalization continually. Incidentally, health is one of the significant benchmarks or barometers from which the effects of globalization can be measured or operationalized. The measure of the various effects of globalization on health provides a yardstick for determining whether globalization is positive or negative (see Martin, 2005). It has been argued that globalization is consequential for all aspects of life. The globalization pessimists and optimists will rely on the various effects to strike a point on the nature of globalization. "It [Health] is a marker of social infrastructure and social welfare and as such can be used to either sound an alarm or give a victory cheer as our interconnectedness hurts and heals the populations we serve" (Martin, 2005).

The current tendency is to describe population health as global health. The interconnectedness of local and global spheres is like a wellspring from which flow, to a large extent, common consequences for health. Since globalization is often regarded as a fundamental determinant of health, measuring the various sides of the consequences on health is inevitable to determine the direction of events. The envisaged possibility is that globalization can be functional or dysfunctional for health. Both the functions and dysfunctions of globalization must be monitored: To promote the functions and mitigate the dysfunctions. Beyond the apparent negative consequences, some unintended (or latent) consequences could still be apparent.

There are two faces of the measurement task about globalization and health assessing and mitigating the impacts. Responding to such consequences at both national, community and individual levels is a challenging mission. Woodward et al. (2001, p. 875) observed that "there is no consensus either on the pathways and mechanisms through which globalization affects the health of populations or on the appropriate policy responses". It is essential to acknowledge that there is hidden or now growing tension about the unequal impacts of globalization on health. Due to the tension, there are controversies about how different countries should protect or promote health in the face of globalization (Woodward et al., 2001). For instance, for the high-income countries, the primary concern is about the importation of various diseases from low-income countries such as tuberculosis (TB), Ebola virus disease and Coronavirus disease. It is crucial to examine the realities of such concerns, which is a cause of many discriminatory practices, including medical screening as one of the visa requirements (which is now eradicated in some embassies). On the other hand, the low-income countries develop a welcoming attitude for migrants/tourists from the high-income areas, thereby neglecting the feasibility of health risk transfer. It is, therefore, important to measure or assess the globalization of risk transfer, among others.

Objectively, globalization also holds promise as a common good, and of course, without neglecting the possibility of latent consequences and dysfunctions. For instance, regarding the common good, globalization has been facilitating the "spread" of modern healthcare and medicines. In some instances, the thought about globalization is often that of optimism, which is in line with the humanitarian view of social processes. "Globalization" is often portrayed in favorable terms, and therefore, to subdue the skepticism, globalization must be checked against the series of expectations.

Martens et al. (2010) used an index of globalization to assess some health indicators. The researcher observed that more globalized countries are better in terms of infant, under-five and adult mortality rates. The research stipulated that globalization is a typical disequalizing process as some benefit while some lose. Therefore, the research outcome signaled that the positive outcome observed might not be enough to conclude that globalization is mostly good for human health. As earlier argued, health and healthcare have become fundamental indicators of assessing the consequences of globalization.

1.3.3 *Reflexive Relationship between Globalization and Health*

The third point is that of reflexivity, a kind of bi-directional relationship between globalization and health. The existing relationship is reciprocal: Globalization affects health, and health affects globalization. The relationship is not one-way-directional. This is another point why the study of globalization and health is highly challenging and sometimes elusive to grasp. There is always the tendency to focus on the impact of globalization on health and not vice-versa. Health enhances all the socio-economic and political drivers of globalization. Health could also be contextual for globalization, or in the other way, the need for health could also enhance the process of globalization. Then, it is possible to discuss health as a driver of globalization. Therefore, health is affecting globalization trends and patterns in many ramifications.

Martin (2005) put this reflexive relation succinctly when he observed that health and disease affect globalization as typified by the enactment of quarantine laws and the devastating economic effects of the AIDS pandemic, especially in the low-income countries. Pandemics and other public health disasters often affect the gains and trends of globalization. Diseases affect international trade and tourism; it limits the so-called social connectivity and economic cooperation. The effects of health and disease on globalization are manifold. Such effects also manifest in the declaration of global health emergencies in cases of certain health conditions that have the potential to escalate globally (such as severe acute respiratory syndrome [SARS] and Ebola virus disease).

Figure 1.1 also depicts this bi-directional relationship between health and globalization. The confluence is about similar contextual issues driving both events. The confluence accounts for increasing internationalization of health risks and control strategies (see Pang and Guindon, 2004). The world is increasingly bound by risks, and so there are global efforts to curtail pandemics. The world faces the era of global partnership to control risk and diseases: The synergy is imperative and sacrosanct. It is a global village, with virtual proximity that can almost explain instantaneous risk spreading, sharing and control which affects patterns of social existence, including globalization.

1.3.4 Multidimensional Globalization and Health

The fourth point is the multifaceted nature of the process of globalization and health. It is multifactorial: Political, economic, cultural, social, religious and technological—with multiplier trends on health. Health is also multifactorial, especially in terms of the social determinants of health. Globalization is a contextual factor for health: The multifactorial factors of globalization affect health. For instance, globalization is a political event; it has a lot to do with politics and policies. Globalization emanates from political decisions and choices. The same political events also determine population health. Globalization involves economic liberations, trade flow, capital mobility, trade competition and increasing income. Globalization is about economic development, employment opportunities, the spread of technical knowledge and new consumer values. All these dimensions and factors interplay to account for what is called globalization.

Health is also a contextual factor for globalization. Health regulations are typically political decisions. Choices in healthcare and regulations of health markets are also political. Health can be seen as a form of politics: Health is political because responses to health problems depend upon political decisions regarding the allocation of appropriate resources. Motivation and remuneration of health workers also depend on political decisions. Likewise, the working condition, including the provision of vital equipment, depends on the allocation of resources. The location of a health facility is generally a political decision. Health condition also largely depends on economic development. Maintaining population health requires substantial economic resources both at the national and community levels. Primarily, the economic condition of a state mirrors the health condition and vice-versa.

The two concepts are complex and multidimensional. The interconnectedness of the two concepts also demands a multidimensional approach in terms of assessment. There have also been measurement issues regarding globalization and health. Dissecting the complex forces or drivers in time and space, and their antecedents and aftermaths have always been a complicated task. The operationalization of health is also challenging. The discussion of globalization and health becomes a cesspool of complexities requiring a great deal of empirical and ontological dissection to institute indices of the two concepts. Therefore, the multidimensional complexities also inform the study of the impacts of globalization on health.

1.3.5 Differential Effects of Globalization on Health

Martin (2005) averred that the

> effects of globalization on health and health systems are neither universally good nor bad, but rather context-specific. The extent to which individual states can engage the process of globalization on their terms differs widely from one country to the next.

The veracity of the preceding statement reflects in differential experiences of globalization, and ultimately concerning population health, explains global health inequalities, variation in health systems and access to care. The critical questions are thus: Where does the Global South stand regarding healthcare and disease burden? What global determinants of health operate in the Global South and why? What are the current global efforts, and how effective are they? How are health risks globally attracted or transmitted across regions? How can global preventive strategies be useful in the Global South? How are health and illness behavior shaped within the local context by global currents? Does higher experience of globalization equal better health conditions or vice-versa? There are many critical questions regarding the differential experience of globalization and how it accounts for human health.

Cornia (2001) envisaged certain preconditions, including strong institutions and appropriate social protection and safety nets, to enhance the positive impacts of globalization. Cornia further observed that the health gain in some Asian countries (including China and Viet Nam) could be linked to global market liberalization and transfer of technology. It is, however, observed that for many countries in the Global South, globalization has little impact on improving domestic conditions; therefore, the result is "a slow, unstable and unequal pattern of growth and stagnation in health indicators" (Cornia, 2001, p. 834). De Vogli (2011) also noted that the financial crisis resulting from the neoliberal globalization policies emanating from high-income countries have also produced unfavorable health effects. Tausch (2015) focused on Arab countries and observed the increasing globalization but with a resultant growth in inequalities, which adversely affect health gains.

The perception of globalization as a disequalizing process is further buttressed in the various studies (Cornia, 2001; De Vogli, 2011; Tausch, 2015). The fundamental question remains: What gap exists and how wide is it between the major divide (South and North) of the world and what is the actual role of globalization in expanding or bridging the gap? It is with the view of globalization as a disequalizing process that Marten et al. (2010) recommended the analysis of health impacts of globalization in order to ensure appropriate adjustment and optimization of the process of globalization to ensure sustainable health goals for all. Martin (2005) further recommended that there should be special consideration for the disadvantaged in adjusting the direction of the process of globalization. Mostly in global health, the vulnerable groups or regions always deserve special attention. The extent to which the global partners have focused on and mitigated the health challenges of the Global South remains an important reoccurring matter, which in fact, also partly justifies the emerging Global South perspective on globalization and health.

1.4 Globalization and Health: Setting the Global South Perspective

Modern human history reflects inequalities in all of its ramifications, and some manifestations of inequalities can be traced to historical antecedents, cultural systems and relations. Some degree of inequality seems inevitable because absolute equality is utopian. Some concerns arise because inequality reflects in detrimental effects such as poor access to basic needs and infrastructure. The inequality gap is wide; there are detrimental consequences. Such consequences manifest in all spheres of life, including health. Social inequality is defined in terms of unequal power, prestige and wealth among social groups. Global history depicts unequal power and economic relations, which explain some fundamental problems confronting the world. Inequality manifests at different levels of concern, including global inequalities, which also manifest in global health inequalities. Inequalities exist within a country and among nations. Global inequality implies unequal power and wealth among nations. Some nations are regarded as high-income countries, most of the Global North, while some are regarded as low- and middle-income countries (LMICs), most of the Global South. It is justifiable to subscribe to this broad classification without unfolding some other levels of inequalities among the high-income countries or low-income countries. The implication is that further classification of upper- or lower-middle-income countries is ignored for a more general classification (see World Bank, 2019).

The Global North–South divide is a general classification, which is the major concept herein adopted. The North is predominantly the western nations of the G8 countries, the European Union, Australia and New Zealand, and some high-income countries of Asia (including Japan, Singapore and South Korea). The Global South includes nations other than the rich nations of the North; some regions and countries of Asia, including parts of China, all countries of Africa, Latin America, the Caribbean, Asia (except the aforementioned high-income Asian countries, but including the Middle East). There are other concepts, including the developing world, the Third World, LMICs, less developed countries, emerging economies and transitional economies, less industrialized countries, which have been interchangeably used with the Global South. The concepts used interchangeably with the Global North include the First World, developed and high-income countries (Pike et al., 2014). Shared phenomena concerning economic prosperity (including the national income), power (including military and economic powers), industrialism, human rights and freedom and technological advancement are the primary benchmarks in the classification of Global North and South. The South, in general, is disadvantaged in terms of the benchmarks mentioned earlier. The majority of the Global South countries also share a common history of colonial exploitation mostly by some countries of the Global North.

There are shared characteristics across the divide. For instance, the World Bank (2019) defined high-income countries of the Global North with a Gross National Income (GNI) of more than $12,736, while those with less income constitute the Global South. Within the Global South, there are countries with a meager income below $1,000, while some are still better off. The general situation in the Global South can be situated within the historical experience of colonialism and neo-colonialism. Such historical experience and resultant developmental impacts perpetually put some countries of the North at an advantage but with many countries of the South yet to recover from the historical exploitation. "History" is continuous with the extension of the relations in new forms. Therefore, unequal historical relations continue to exist in new forms, including global market regulations and other forms of neo-colonialist moves. Again, continuous unequal relations reflect not only economic relations but also global health. Before venturing into global health issues, it is essential to note that economic inequality is a fundamental frame that defines other aspects of a global system. Hence, it is not surprising that high-income countries have better health indicators. The economic position also influences the power relations, which further generate more imbalances in the global system. It is also important to reiterate that global inequality defines approaches to global issues, including global poverty and health.

1.4.1 Globalization and Health: Critical Matters Arising

Global health emerges as a distinct field and practice to address health issues that transcend nations' borders (see Section 2.2 for the conceptualization of global health). The dis-equalizing process of globalization manifests not only in research and practice but also in risk transmission and health systems. This text is not just about adding a voice to the whole debate in global health discourse but also to examine some critical realities, which if addressed, could impact considerably on the imbalance in the global health situation. The short history of global health shows precarious dominations and cruel realities, with the Global South always at a disadvantage. It is important to note the artificial character of the world order which impacts on global health. The character shows some differential perspectives and generates some crucial global health debates. While this section will examine two critical matters, some questions will also be raised, which will be addressed in other chapters of this book.

1.4.1.1 Manufactured Epidemics

The notion of manufactured epidemics is related to manufactured risks, which will later be theoretically explored (see Section 4.3). The global health situation is not a matter of natural inequality: The global relations, actions and policies woven around what is now regarded as global determinants of health are crucial issues in explaining global health inequalities. For instance, historically, noncommunicable diseases were considerably lower in the Global South, then globalization resulted in the global proliferation of obesogenic foods and western-style fast-food outlets (Fox et al., 2019) (also see Section 5.4 for McDonaldization theory). The global weight gain is a product of globalization, which also accrues enormous profits to the Global North. It is a case of double tragedy: As nations consume more western-style food, they also lose economically (capital flight).

Globalization involves socio-economic expansionism (North to South) and dependency (South on the North), which aid the massive transmission of modern risks from North to South. Fox et al. observed that the adverse health consequences of global food trade regimes may be exaggerated, but food is part of the modernization to which local economies aspire. Therefore, the economic expansion of risk products such as fatty foods and snacks, alcohol and cigarettes cannot but be emphasized. Stuckler et al. (2012) described the whole process of the spread of unhealthy global food as a manufactured epidemic, which is fast growing in the Global South with little or no further growth expected in the North. The Global South has a high population and, therefore, a significant market attraction for industrialists for all kinds of products. Stuckler et al. (2012) noted that the increasing consumption of unhealthy foods correlates strongly with higher tobacco and alcohol sales; hence, the attendant increase in the spread of modern epidemics. It is further noted that rising income is associated with the increase in such consumption patterns but subject to high foreign direct investment and free-trade agreements, which open the gate for the inflow of all sorts of goods.

The global food corporation, with enormous political and economic powers, has forced a food transition in developing countries over the years. Such food transition accounts for the increasing burden of all food-related noncommunicable diseases. The transnational food corporations also negotiate how to increase trade, most times, against the local health goals and policies. Such corporations have strong ground and power to resist local health policies that violate their trade goals (see Friel et al., 2013). Friel et al. (2013) further observed that in some trade agreements, legal instruments could be used to protect trade against the governments' public health goals. Therefore, in most trade agreements between the North and South, global/public health goals are often deemphasized (Hawkes, 2005, 2006; Stuckler et al., 2012; Baker and Friel, 2014).

Many scholars advocated for "degrowth" to curtail expansion in a way that would sustain global well-being. Economic expansion or modernization is not only in terms of the global grade but also the devastating consequences of global ecology. The Global South also bears the greater brunt of the unpleasant industrial practices of the North. It is thus a matter of growing at the expense of the other divide. The South has become a dumping site not only for industrial waste but second-hand goods, especially e-wastes, most of which are certified dangerous for the human environment but still find their way to markets in the developing world. The case of aged electronics and automobiles is a typical illustration. Millions of vehicles without roadworthiness in the North find their ways to the South with resultant air quality degeneration. Electronic wastes (e-waste), regularly electronic products at the end of their "useful life" are dumped in the South (Rodhain, 2018). Such wastes constitute a tremendous hazard to population health. Unfortunately, there is a weak political power to curtail such practice in the South. Rodhain (2018, p. 97) observed that "transport of e-waste from countries in the Global North to those in the South is completely illegal—yet 80% of the e-waste from the United States is shipped to these very countries". Most industrialized countries find solace in circumventing the laws in waste management at the detriment of the South. Such illegal practice, because it is to the benefits of the North, is not a top priority on the global health agenda. Rodhain (2018) reiterated the economic rationale behind the practice as the cost of responsible e-waste treatment is often too expensive compared to the practice of dumping them in the Global South. Rodhain (2018, p. 97) stressed that:

> Transferring [the e-waste] to the South is 10 times less expensive … Recycling is too expensive in an economy where the environmental costs related to consumption are not passed on to corporate taxation. Responsible recycling is no match for organized crime: according to the rationale of the capitalist system, good recycling behavior does not pay and offers no competitive advantage.

The global trade is often silent about global waste trade, which involves the shift of hazardous waste to the South. The situation is described as toxic colonialism: The shift of the burden of toxic wastes from the North to South as an inexpensive alternative for disposal (see Pratt, 2011). Unfortunately, the disadvantaged socio-economic and political position of the South makes it hard to resist the flow of global waste, which comes with agonizing social and health costs. The migration of global wastes and junks to the South is often embedded in neoliberal/capitalist policies; such type of migration of wastes is palatable to the North, which builds fortresses through rigid migration policies against the flow of people from South to North. The discussion on manufactured epidemics is a typical example of how globalization is impacting on global health and creates an unequal environment that puts the South at a disadvantage. Again, the major problem is that the North is often reluctant either to take responsibility for such manufactured epidemics or to reverse the trend as quickly as possible, at least if not for anything, in the name of global health.

1.4.1.2 Global Health and Securitization Agenda

Due to unequal political and economic standing, global health often reflects the agenda and interest of the North. The significant concern is that such an agenda or interest exists at the detriment of the South. Normally, the language of global health is often about how to provide health security to the North. The securitization of global health allows for selective concentration on infectious diseases, which are diseases mostly transmittable across borders (through physical contacts), and sometimes constitute what is often termed as global health "emergencies". Wenham (2019) reported that several health issues are constructed as threats to health security. The context of such security implies the protection of certain groups or interests against others. Such a conception explains the narrow understanding of global health, and what is often termed as a global health security concern. In such a narrow conception, global health security is flexible depending on the context, pathogen and who/what is at risk (Wenham, 2019).

The language of global health is often about "protection", "response", "risks", "preparedness", "outbreak", "epidemics" and "exposure" among others. Since global health is about the interplay of regions within the health context, the idea is often protecting one region from the other. Therefore, it is about activities to curtail the spread of infectious diseases. Hence, most global health activities are about Zika, Ebola, Lassa fever, TB, malaria, dengue fever, Coronavirus disease, cholera and other infectious diseases of "global security importance". Apparently, global health is highly fragmented since there are some diseases of interest and neglect or given poor attention. For instance, instead of securitization leading to a selective response to certain diseases, the health target of universal health care (UHC) is more important in the Global South. The UCH is a holistic preparedness that would help in alleviating the burden of the so-called diseases of global security threats. Another implication is that selective response leads to the displacement of priorities, which leads to focus on diseases of interest to the Global North. For global health to be global, it has to be holistic with a focus on the ideal priorities of the different regions. More importantly, preparedness in healthcare is better comprehensive than fragmented.

Most of the countries of the Global South need sector-wide intervention more than fragmented intervention. In most instances, priorities are donor-driven, thereby forcing a focus on diseases that might not be of immediate priority. It is much easier to mobilize a global response for Ebola than diarrhea or pneumonia. For Ebola, response and structure are only maintained as far as the outbreak lasts. This signifies periodic response or assistance, unlike in the case of more prevailing conditions that require a continuous response. Global health will be better with a holistic preventive response rather than a reactive one.

In sum, globalization is a cursor for global health. The process of globalization further reinforces specific political and economic imbalances, which in turn impact on global health. The dominant character of the North continues to raise more questions about the motive of some policies and practices. Many questions still require answers and ingenuity in addressing them. What are the dominant frames in setting the global health agenda? Charity, responsibility or security? Who sets the global health agenda and why? Is global health about the extension of economic and political dominance? How holistic is the global health agenda? Does the global health agenda conform to the priorities of the disadvantaged regions? What are the crucial manifestations of the effects of globalization on health? What global forces are driving the increase in many communicable and noncommunicable diseases? How effective are global health initiatives in addressing global health challenges? These are some of the critical questions that will be addressed in subsequent chapters.

1.5 Summary

- Globalization is a complex process, as there is the globalization of "everything" and as "everything" is globalizing. Globalization is an unprecedented compression of time and space and intensification of interconnections and interdependency on a global scale.
- Globalization manifests in some intense dynamic and persistent forces, especially in transportation, communication, social media and trade, responsible for social change or

transformation. Hence, globalization exhibits some basic features: It standardizes, deterritorializes and modernizes.

- George Ritzer is a sociological theorist who conceptualizes globalization as the flow of *nothing* and *something*. Ritzer defined *nothing* as events that are distinctively empty in forms (in all its dimensions, including social forms) but centrally conceived and controlled. Ritzer defined *something* in terms of distinctive contents.
- Ritzer further unpacked globalization through the use of two related concepts: Glocalization and grobalization. Glocalization is a blend of local and global: Thinking and acting both locally and globally. Grobalization is a conception of globalization as the imperialistic instrument focusing on the growth of capitalism, westernization and modernization.
- Health is a significant domain where globalization has an enormous impact. Globalization and health are interconnected, in terms of the epidemiology of diseases, healthcare systems and access to healthcare.
- There is a mutual character of globalization and health as both are responsive, transitional, measuring, reflexive, multidimensional and with differential effects in different regions, especially between the Global North and South.
- Globalization is a disequalizing process in all ramifications, including global health. The process of globalization further reinforces specific political and economic imbalances, which in turn impact on global health. Hence, there is the narrow conception of global health from the securitization agenda while neglecting the manufactured epidemics and related global concerns.
- Globalization involves socio-economic expansionism (North to South) and dependency (South on the North), which aid the massive bi-directional flow of modern and traditional health risks from North to South and South to North, respectively.
- Globalization involves a massive transmission of modern risks from North to South. There is the global economic expansion of risk products (such as fatty foods and snacks, alcohol, cigarettes), which has been described as manufactured epidemic with adverse health consequences.
- The Global South also bears the greater brunt of the unpleasant industrial practices of the North. The South is a dumping site not only for industrial waste but second-hand goods, especially electronic waste (e-wastes) that are dangerous for human environment and population health.
- The securitization of global health allows for selective concentration on infectious diseases, including Zika, Ebola, Lassa fever, TB, malaria, dengue fever, Coronavirus and cholera, among others, mostly transmittable across borders (through physical contacts), and sometimes constitute what are often termed as global health "emergencies".
- For global health to be global, it has to be holistic with a focus on the ideal priorities of the different regions. More importantly, preparedness in healthcare is better comprehensive than fragmented.

Critical Thinking Questions

- How can globalization and health be defined? In what ways do you think globalization and health are intertwined? Why is it important to examine the impacts of globalization on health?
- In what ways do you think the concepts of grobalization and glocalization can be analyzed in connection with global health?
- How is globalization disequalizing concerning health, especially between the Global North and South?

- Health–security nexus is a dominant narrative in global health. Do you think such securitization of health is enough to improve global health in the different world regions? If so, or not, give some cogent reasons.
- What mechanisms or measures could help in balancing the disequalizing tendencies of globalization of health?
- What should be the priorities of the Global South in harnessing the opportunities of globalization to improve population health in the region?

Suggested Readings

- Amzat, J. and Razum, O. (2014). Sociology and Health. In: *Medical Sociology in Africa.* Cham, Switzerland: Springer International Publishing. doi 10.1007/978-3-319-03986-2_1. The chapter describes the conception and understanding of health from a sociological perspective.
- Cornia, G. A. (2001). Globalization and health: Results and options. *Bulletin of the World Health Organization, 79*(9), 834–841. A good historical article on the disequalizing process of globalization and its impacts on health in the different regions.
- Martin, G. (2005). Editorial: Globalization and health. *Globalization and Health,* 1:1. doi:10.1186/1744-8603-1-1. A short introduction on the links between globalization and health.
- Lee, K. (2003). *Globalization and Health: An introduction.* London: Palgrave Macmillan. doi: 10.1057/9781403943828. The book presents a clear conceptual framework for understanding the various impacts of globalization on health.
- Ritzer, G. (2004). *The globalization of nothing.* California: Pine Forge Press. The book presents a theoretical and practical understanding of globalization as a sociological concept and process.
- Wenham, C. (2019). The oversecuritization of global health: Changing the terms of debate. *International Affairs, 95*(5), 1093–1110, https://doi.org/10.1093/ia/iiz170. The article assesses the health–security nexus, which has become a dominant narrative, and the ensuing path dependencies which have shifted in recent times.

References

Amzat, J., & Maigari, A. M. (2020). Micro and macro perspectives in sociology. In Olorunlana, A., Tinuloa, F. R. & Fasoranti, O. O. (Eds.), *Introduction to Sociology: African Culture, Context and Complexity* (pp. 82–91). Lagos: Apex Publishers.

Amzat, J., & Omololu, F. (2012). The basics of sociological paradigms. In Ogundiya, I. S. & Amzat, J. (Eds.), *The Basics of Social Sciences* (pp. 115–134). Lagos: Malthouse Press.

Amzat, J., & Razum, O. (2014). Sociology and health. In *Medical Sociology in Africa.* Cham, Switzerland: Springer International Publishing. doi: 10.1007/978-3-319-03986-2_1.

Amzat, J., & Razum, O. (2018). Key Concepts in Healthcare Delivery. In: *Towards a Sociology of Health Discourse in Africa.* Cham, Switzerland: Springer International Publishing. doi: 10.1007/978-3-319-61672-8_1.

Amzat, J., Omololu, F. & Abdullahi, A. A. (2015). Realists and nominalist traditions in sociology. In Ogundiya, I. S. & J. Amzat (Eds.), *Foundations of the Social Sciences* (pp. 137–147). Lagos: Malthouse Press.

Anonymous (2019). SOCI 320: Globalization and social change. https://soan.gmu.edu/courses/soci320/course_sections/27036. Accessed on July 18, 2019.

Baker, P., & Friel, S. (2014). Processed foods and the nutrition transition: Evidence from Asia. *Obesity Reviews, 15*(7), 564–577. doi: 10.1111/obr.12174.

Bircher, J. (2005). Towards a dynamic definition of health and disease. *Medicine Health Care and Philosophy*, *8*, 335–341.

Brodsky, J. A., & Clarfield, M. (2017). Long term care in health services. In *International Encyclopedia of Public Health* (pp. 459 –446, 2nd ed.). doi: 10.1016/B978-0-12-803678-5.00257-5.

Collins, T. (2003). Globalization, global health and access to health care. *International Journal of Health Planning and Management*, *18*, 97–104.

Cornia, G. A. (2001). Globalization and health: Results and options. *Bulletin of the World Health Organization*, *79*(9): 834–841.

De Vogli, R. (2011). Neoliberal globalization and health in a time of economic crisis. *Social Theory and Health*, *9*, 311–325. doi: 10.1057/sth.2011.16.

Eriksen, T. H. (2007). *Globalization: The Key Concepts*. Oxford: Berg.

Ernest, P. C. (2007). Epistemological issues in the internationalisation and globalization of mathematics education. In Atweh B., Barton, A. C., Borba, M., Gough, N., Keitel, C., Vistro-Yu, C. & Vithal, R. (Eds.), *Internationalisation and Globalisation in Mathematics and Science Education* (pp. 19–38). Springer.

Fox, A., Feng, W. & Asal, V. (2019). What is driving global obesity trends? Globalization or "modernization"? *Globalization and Health*, *15*, 32. doi: 10.1186/s12992-019-0457-y.

Frankish, C. J., Green, L. W., Ratner, P. A., Chomik, T., & Larsen, C. (2001). Health impact assessment as a tool for health promotion and population health. *WHO Regional Publications. European Series*, *92*, 405–437.

Friel, S., Gleeson, D., Thow, A. M., Labonte, R., Stuckler, D., Kay, A. & Snowdon, W. (2013). A new generation of trade policy: Potential risks to diet-related health from the trans Pacific partnership agreement. *Globalization and Health*, *9*, 46.

Hawkes, C. (2005). The role of foreign direct investment in the nutrition transition. *Public Health Nutrition*, *8*(4), 357e365.

Hawkes, C. (2006). Uneven dietary development: Linking the policies and processes of globalization with the nutrition transition, obesity and diet-related chronic diseases. *Globalization and Health*, *2*(4), 1–18.

Hirsch, P., Fiss, P. & Hoel-Green, A. (2009). A durkheimian approach to globalization. In Adler, P. (Ed.), *The Oxford Handbook of Sociology and Organization Studies: Classical foundations* (pp. 223–245). Oxford: Oxford University Press.

Holtz, T. H., Holmes, S., Stonington, S. & Eisenberg, L. (2006). Health is still social: Contemporary examples in the age of the genome. *PLoS Medicine*, *3*(10), e419. doi: 10.1371/journal.pmed.0030419.

Huber, M., Knottnerus, J. A., Green, L., van der Horst, H., Jadad, A. R., Kromhout, D., Leonard, B., Lorig, K., Loureiro, M. I., van der Meer, J. W. M., Schnabel, P., Smith, R., van Weel, C. & Smid, H. (2011). How should we define health? *BMJ 343*, d4163 doi: 10.1136/bmj.d4163.

Huynen, M. T. E, Martens, P., & Hilderink, H. B. M. (2005). The health impacts of globalisation: A conceptual framework. *Globalization and Health*, *1*,14 doi: 10.1186/1744-8603-1-14.

International Labour Oragnization (ILO) (2003). Social dimension of globalization. www.ilo.org/public/english/wcsdg/globali/globali.htm. Accessed on July 19, 2003.

Javed, N. (2014). Globalization or cultural colonialism. *International Journal of Development Research*, *4*(4), 825–827.

Krieger, N. (2001). Emerging theories for social epidemiology in the 21st century: An ecosocial perspective. *International Journal of Epidemiology*, *30*, 668–677.

Larson, J. S. (1999). The conceptualization of health. *Medical Care Research and Review*, *56*(2), 123–136.

Lechner, F. (2005). Globalization. In G. Ritzer (Ed.), *Encyclopedia of Social Theory* (Vol. 1, pp. 331–333). California: SAGE Publications, Inc.

Luhmann, N. (1997). Globalization or world society? How to conceive of modern society. *International Review of Sociology*, *7*(1) 67–79.

Martens, P., Akin, S. M., Maud, H., & Mohsin, R. (2010). Is globalization healthy: A statistical indicator analysis of the impacts of globalization on health. *Global Health*, *17*(6), 16. doi: 10.1186/1744-8603-6-16.

Martin, G. (2005). Editorial: Globalization and health. *Globalization and Health*, *1*, 1. doi: 10.1186/1744-8603-1-1.

Marx, K., & Engels, F. (2012). *The Communist Manifesto: A Modern Edition*. London: Verso.

Murray, C. J. L., & Smith, R. (2001). *Diseases of Globalisation*. London, Earthscan Publication Ltd.

Navarro, V. (2009). What we mean by social determinants of health. *Global Health Promotion, 16*(1), 5–16.

Nye, J. (2002). Globalism versus globalization. www.theglobalist.com/globalism-versus-globalization/ Accessed on July 17, 2019.

Omran, A. R. (2005). The epidemiologic transition: A theory of the epidemiology of population change. *Milbank Quarterly, 83*(4), 731–757. doi: 10.1111/j.1468-0009.2005.00398.x.

Pang, T., & Guindon, E. (2004). Globalization and risks to health. *European Molecular Biology Organization (EMBO) Reports, 5*(Spec No), S11–S16.

Parsons, T. (1972). Definition of health and illness in the light of American values and social structure. In E. G. Jaco (Ed.), *Patients, Physicians and Illness* (pp. 107–127). New York: Free Press.

Pike, A., Rodríguez-Pose, A., & Tomaney, J. (2014). Local and regional development in the Global North and South. *Progress in Development Studies, 14*(1), 21–30.

Pratt, L. A. (2011). Decreasing dirty dumping? A reevaluation of toxic waste colonialism and the global management of transboundary hazardous waste. *William and Mary Environmental Law and Policy Review, 35*(2), 581–623.

Ritzer, G. (2003). Rethinking globalization: Glocalization/grobalization and something/nothing. *Sociological Theory, 21*(3), 193–209.

Ritzer, G. (2004). *The globalization of nothing*. Thousand Oaks, CA: Pine Forge Press.

Ritzer, G., & Ryan, M. (2002). The globalization of nothing. *Social Thought and Research, 25*(1/2), 51–81.

Robertson, R. (2001). Globalization theory 2000+: Major problematics. In G. Ritzer & B. Smart (Eds.), *Handbook of Social Theory* (pp. 458–471). London: Sage.

Rodhain, F. (2018). Electronic waste dumped in the global South: Ethical issues in practices and research. In Moulin, A. M., Oupathana, B., Souphanthong, M. & Taverne, B. (Eds.), *The Paths of Ethics in Research in Laos and the Mekong Countries* (pp. 95–101). Éditions de l'IRD and L'Harmattan-Sénégal, hal-01967074.

Shirong, L. (2016). Marx's thoughts on economic globalization. *Social Sciences in China, 37*(2), 5–19. doi: 10.1080/02529203.2016.1162008.

Stuckler, D., McKee, M., Ebrahim, S. & Basu, S. (2012). Manufacturing epidemics: The role of global producers in increased consumption of unhealthy commodities including processed foods, alcohol, and tobacco. *PLoS Medicine, 9*(6), 10e10.

Tausch, A. (2015). Is globalization really good for public health? General considerations and implications for the Arab world. Munich Personal RePEc Archive (MPRA) Paper No. 64516. https://mpra.ub.uni-muenchen.de/64516/1/MPRA_paper_64516.pdf. Accessed on July 22, 2019.

Wadsworthx, M. E. J. (1997). Changing social factors and their long-term implications for health. *British Medical Bulletin, 33*(1), 198–209.

Wallerstein, I. M. (1976). *The Modern World-system: Capitalist Agriculture and the Origins of the European World-economy in the Sixteenth Century*. New York: Academic Press.

Wallerstein, I. M. (2004). *World-systems analysis: An introduction*. Durham, NC: Duke University Press.

Wenham, C. (2019). The oversecuritization of global health: Changing the terms of debate. *International Affairs, 95*(5), 1093–1110. doi: 10.1093/ia/iiz170.

Woodward, D., Drager, N., Beaglehole, R., & Lipson, D. (2001). Globalization and health: A framework for analysis and action. *Bulletin of the World Health Organization, 79*(9), 875–881.

World Bank (2019). World Bank Country and lending groups: Country classifications. https://datahelpdesk.worldbank.org/knowledgebase/articles/906519. Accessed on December 5, 2019.

World Health Organization (WHO) (1946). Preamble to the Constitution of the World Health Organization as adopted by the International Health Conference, New York, 19–22 June, 1946.

2 Many Faces of Globalization of Health

2.1 Introduction

Globalization has become another ontological reality or a social fact, which consciously or unconsciously influences the human way of life and circumstances. The world has adjusted to the reality of globalization as a process of change, and even the "constructivistically minded scholars tend to regard globalization as an undeniable and inescapable part of the contemporary experience" (Bartelson, 2000: p. 180). Although the constructionists often argue that it is not coercive of human behavior, the subjective perception also makes globalization an irrefutable process. It is not only a concept within the realist ontology; it is a kind of conceptual wave, which cuts across all epistemological divides. Therefore, globalization is a process that should always be managed and assessed. Its management involves the identification of specific indicators or indices. While globalization has been conceived in many ways, how it is felt in different quarters is of paramount importance.

Globalization has always been overwhelmingly colored with politics. It is sometimes regarded as a political event or ideology. The perspective of the Global South shows a tendency toward the conceptualization of globalization as a capitalist or imperialist ideology meant for territorial expansion of the Global North (Ferguson, 1992; Javed, 2014). The fundamental question here is how globalization is linked with health and to explain some of the significant manifestations of globalization's impacts on health. Then comes the concept of global health; in the first instance, it is a combination of globalization and health. Global health is a way of understanding population health and healthcare within a global context. It is the acknowledgment of the linkages of globalization and health. The postulation is that a holistic and comprehensive context of health will provide a better approach to alleviate health challenges around the world.

There is an increasing acceptance of this holistic view due to the globalization of health risks and the global importance of healthcare. WHO is leading the global agenda to improve healthcare worldwide. Health goals are often paramount in the global development agenda (as reflected in Millennium Development Goals). Unfortunately, most of the health goals were not met at the deadline of 2015. The struggle continues toward the attainment of some health goals included in the Sustainable Development Goals (SDGs). The (global) approach is to ensure a global commitment and strategies that would ensure universal health coverage irrespective of location. A healthy world can be achieved together through some deliberate efforts and strategies. This realization has prompted the establishment of many centers of global health around the world. Although a majority of these centers are in the Global North, the Global South has also realized the importance of such centers. The main crux of this chapter is to conceptualize global health and examine the many faces of the globalization of health.

DOI: 10.4324/9781003247975-2

2.2 Conceptualizing Global Health

Global health has emerged as a popular concept and an approach to health issues in the world. As previously argued, globalization is an irresistible force shaping human affairs in all ramifications. Health conditions have become one of the most significant aspects of these global discourses. Hence, the idea of global health serves a crucial purpose in understanding health needs and fulfilling the promise of universal healthcare. Understanding critical issues around global health reflect health measures of globalization, which would help to grasp the connection between globalization and health. The previous chapter provided some definitions of globalization (see Chapter 1). Before examining some manifestations of globalization and health, understanding global health is central. What is global health? What is global about global health? Why global health? These are fundamental questions. It is all about the global village, but can health be approached from a global perspective? Meanwhile, before the popularization of global health, there were other popular health concepts, such as international and public health.

Global health is an ambitious attempt to focus on health issues on a global scale (see Table 2.1 for some definitions). It involves all aspects of healthcare (surveillance, prevention and clinical care), with a vast scope in both focus and geographical coverage. Brown et al. (2006: p. 62) defined global health as the "consideration of the health needs of the people of the whole planet above the concerns of particular nations". Brown et al. observed that the term global health is now a significant concept in describing population health. They observed that the WHO long ago embraced the term in describing the efforts of the Global Malaria Eradication Program launched in the mid-1950s.

Kickbush and Buse (2001) defined global health as "those health issues that transcend national boundaries and governments and call for actions on the global forces that determine the health of people". Since globalization is transcendent, so are health issues, therefore they require new forms of governance that think on a global scale to address the issues. More importantly, the determinants of health are also transcendent. Hence, it is essential to initiate global actions to improve population health (Kickbush, 2006). In a more concise definition, Beaglehole and Bonita (2010) defined global health as "collaborative trans-national research and action for promoting health for all". The definition is derived from and a concise summary of Koplan et al.'s (2009) definition, which will be analyzed subsequently. The primary quality of Beaglehole and Bonita's definition is that it is short and captivating.

Koplan et al. (2009: p. 1994) defined global health as "an area for study, research, and practice that places a priority on improving health and achieving health equity for all people

Table 2.1 Definitions of global health

Kickbush and Buse (2001)	Global health signifies those health issues that transcend national boundaries and governments and call for actions on the global forces that determine the health of people.
Koplan et al. (2009)	Global health is an area for study, research and practice that places a priority on improving health and achieving equity in health for all people worldwide. Global health emphasizes transnational health issues, determinants and solutions; it involves many disciplines within and beyond the health sciences and promotes interdisciplinary collaboration, and is a synthesis of population-based prevention with individual-level clinical care.
Beaglehole and Bonita (2010)	Global health is collaborative transnational research and action for promoting health for all.
Authors'	Global health is a multidisciplinary and participatory understanding of health needs, goals, and challenges to promote population health on a global scale.

worldwide". Koplan et al. (2009: p. 1995) added that the focus of globalization is on "transnational health issues, determinants, and solutions; involves many disciplines within and beyond the health sciences and promotes interdisciplinary collaboration; and is a synthesis of population-based prevention with individual-level clinical care". It is an academic area of teaching and research that attempts to provide an "eagle-eye" approach to the understanding of health. It is a grand approach and it is holistic by exploring the global nature of the world to examine the current state of health conditions and possible threats and opportunities. It is also an area of practice that involves linkages across the globe, whether to receive or provide support in health-related matters. The general purpose is to ensure health equity, especially by focusing on health needs and interventions across the globe.

Koplan et al. (2009) defined the basic scope of global health (see Table 2.2). They observed that the common denominator of these three health concepts (global, international and public) includes priority on the general population and disease prevention. Surveillance and prevention of health risks are significant tasks in global health, as well as in public and international health. The focus is on the general population extending across boundaries. The second denominator is the focus on vulnerable and underserved populations (such as the poor). Thirdly, all are multidisciplinary and involve several stakeholders across the globe. Taylor (2018) observed that global health is typically an organizing framework for thinking and action, but that understanding the concept of global health requires a polymathic capability in order to note the various contributing perspectives and disciplines.

The definition by Koplan et al. is all-encompassing and includes all the various dimensions of global health, both as a discipline and a practice. One crucial element of note is that, according to the definition, global health encompasses what is often described as public and international health. Public health, also multidisciplinary, primarily focuses on preventive health interventions in a particular country or community and is not necessarily associated with global cooperation. In contrast, international health involves bi- or multilateral cooperation on health issues (Koplan et al., 2009). In this sense, global health provides a more all-inclusive and universal approach to health issues, therefore requiring more global cooperation or partnerships and resources. It also holds the promise of ensuring a gradual realization of global equity in healthcare and related interventions.

The fundamental polemic is not that public and international health do not focus on equity among nations or worldwide health issues. Koplan et al. argue that global health embraces more complicated connectivity between societies. The idea is not just a one-directional flow of responsibility or vulnerability; the emphasis of global health is on "the mutuality of real partnership, a pooling of experience and knowledge, and a two-way flow between developed and developing countries. Global health thus uses the resources, knowledge, and experience

Table 2.2 Scope of global health

Geographical reach	Focus on issues that directly or indirectly affect health, but that can transcend national boundaries.
Level of cooperation	Development and implementation of solutions often requires global cooperation.
Individuals or populations	Embraces both prevention in populations and clinical care of individuals.
Access to health	Health equity among nations and for all people is a primary objective.
Range of disciplines	Highly interdisciplinary and multidisciplinary within and beyond health sciences.

Source: Koplan J. P. et al. (2009, p. 1994).

of diverse societies to address health challenges throughout the world" (Koplan et al., 2009). While it is also interesting to note that the three areas sometimes overlap, the distinguishing factors for global health are the philosophy, scope, nature of partnership and the health goals (see Table 2.2).

It follows then that global health should reflect a multidisciplinary and participatory understanding of health needs, goals and challenges to promote population health on a global scale. Global health is essential because health as a public good is not equally distributed across the world. Even though health is a right, some regions only observe such rights on paper. In practice, there are several communities in sub-Saharan Africa (SSA) without modern health services. Such communities experience frequent adverse health events resulting in high morbidity and mortality. The quality of healthcare is also not equal across world regions. The Global South experiences relatively poor health services, in many instances making the population (e.g., in SSA) highly susceptible to various adverse health conditions, mainly preventable diseases such as malaria, diarrhea and cholera. In many developing countries, the health system is not adequate to cater to the health needs of the population.

Global health is also crucial because of the unequal distribution of health workers. Health professionals are grossly inadequate in many countries in the Global South. Hence, there is always the need for external aid, through the supply of health workers, to curtail certain epidemics. Where health facilities are available—in some instances, there is a lack of adequate equipment—there is a constant need for technology and capacity transfer to cater to underserved regions. Global health serves as a bridge, linking the South and North, to meet those needs. In 2011, the Director-General of the WHO discussed the increasing importance of global health (Chan, 2011). She recounted that with the advent of global health initiatives, there had been a massive improvement in the number of people (from 200,000 to 7,000,000) in the Global South receiving antiretroviral therapy for AIDS (Chan, 2011). She also acknowledged a substantial drop in the number of under-five mortality, among other milestones. She attributed the achievements to global collaborations.

When viewing it positively, globalization is a blessing to healthcare because it is reshaping the landscape of healthcare around the world. The world is witnessing the unprecedented flow of pharmaceuticals, which has helped in numerous ways to meet the drug needs around the world. Although with some reservations concerning the possibility of undue self-medication, there has been a rise in online drug stores, which has made certain pharmaceuticals available. Desai (2016) reiterated some of the benefits of online drug stores, including increased access, relatively lower product costs, convenience and anonymity for consumers. It is further observed that accredited online pharmacies "have well-defined safety and quality benchmarks, uncomplicated privacy and security policies, a verifiable physical address and licensed pharmacist on roll" (Desai, 2016: p. 615).

A free flow of information, especially health-related information, has empowered individuals to make healthy choices. Advancements made in information and communication technologies are a significant driver of globalization and have helped in the spread of health information and knowledge. Internet access is a significant part of modern culture, which facilitates social connectivity and information sharing on a global scale. Although internet coverage is quite low in Africa (Labonté et al., 2011), it has been improving gradually since the beginning of the 21st century. The Global South is also benefitting from this free flow of information, which is an essential mechanism of how globalization impacts health.

Another important mechanism is the globalized flow of people. Labonté et al. (2011) observed that increased human mobility had accelerated the flow of pathogens. Both people and pathogens flow due to migration involving trade, tourism and military campaigns. There is increased movement of people looking for greener pastures around the world. The first aftermath of migration is increasing urbanization, which is a factor in the spread of infectious diseases. The high concentration of people in urban settings expedites frequent social contacts, which can increase susceptibility to some infectious diseases. The next section will focus on the actual manifestation of globalization and health. It will also describe the significant faces of globalization of health.

2.3   Faces of Globalization of Health

The critical question is about the impact of globalization on health, herein termed as faces of globalization of health. There are a number of these "faces" that can be explored to establish the link between globalization and health further (see Table 2.3). Therefore, this is an attempt to explore the numerous dimensions of how globalization impacts population health. As Woodward et al. (2001) argued, it is often hard to agree on the pathways and mechanisms through which globalization affects health, as there is no consensus. Perhaps, it is appropriate to argue that the mechanisms are complex. It is possible to check the literature on the general manifestations of the link between globalization and health. Such manifestations are realities as there have been a series of reports on the links and manifestations (see Cornia, 2001; Taylor, 2018; Youde, 2020). The next few subsections will examine, in concrete terms, some of the critical areas of globalization of health. Such areas are not new; they have been receiving attention for decades.

2.3.1   Globalization of Health Risks/Vulnerabilities

Health risks are factors or situations that increase the probability of contracting a disease; such factors can be ecological, economic, physiological or social. Beyond the risk of actual diseases, there is constant global vulnerability, the spread of conditions that expose individuals to diseases and the inability to cope with a disease condition or disasters in general. This subsection will focus more on the risks of infectious diseases, which are more prevalent in the Global South rather than the Global North. WHO (2009) reported that "traditional risks"—risks associated with poverty and inadequate social amenities (such as unsafe water and poor sanitation)—are common in low-income countries. Living conditions and access to basic amenities explain vulnerability to most communicable diseases. Malaria and cholera are two examples of diseases of poverty, highly prevalent only in low-income regions of the world, where they account for high morbidity and mortality rates.

The global community is confronted with global risks and vulnerabilities. Globalization compresses time and space; an infection in one region of the world can, in a matter of hours, spread to other regions. Lee (2004) observed that the Global North is often concerned about the perceived threat of certain infectious diseases, including human immunodeficiency virus (HIV) and tuberculosis, from the Global South. Wealthy regions are also bothered by the health condition of migrants from the developing world. This concern is always one-directional and discriminatory because it gives the impression that only developing nations pose threats to the other regions. Lee (2004) observed that, in fact, a complex equation of pluses and minuses exists for each society. For instance, population mobility benefits high-income countries more than low-income countries, but health risk is equally distributed.

Social proximity affects the spread of diseases. Infections can move around the world within hours due to improved modern transportation systems. The outbreak of severe acute respiratory syndrome (SARS) in 2002–2003 was of global concern, as it affected 37 countries with up to

10,000 reported cases and over 1,000 deaths between November 2002 and July 2003 (Smith, 2006). Beyond the region where the outbreak was initially reported, there was global apprehension about the outbreak, with every country taking measures to curtail a possible spread. With just one index case, the whole world could potentially be affected. The case of novel Coronavirus disease of 2019 [COVID-19] is a typical example (see Chapter 7).

Smith (2006) also observed that globalization not only increases the likelihood of a multi-country spread of disease but can also impact the global economy. The fear posed by the spread of a particular infection might reduce the global flow of people and trade within a few days, through travel bans or rigorous screening at border points. Sometimes, the perception of risk alone has an impact on human migration and economic activities. Such perception is often accentuated through the media (including social media), with a lot of lay permutations about the threats. The rise of social media speeds news spread about any form of (perceived or real) disease threats on a global scale.

In sum, despite global efforts to combat infectious diseases with vaccines and other public health measures, health risks from infectious disease still constitute a major global concern. HIV/AIDS, Ebola, tuberculosis and cholera still pose a tremendous threat in the global space. Infectious diseases tend to become global health emergencies. While the disease can spread quickly, the response can also be as quick. There can also be a quick global assessment and mobilization of resources to counter the spread when outbreaks occur. The capacity of the affected countries can be assessed and reinforced by other countries or global bodies. Such global cooperation and mobilization occurred during the SARS and Ebola outbreaks.

2.3.2 *Globalization of Lifestyle Diseases*

There is a growing burden of lifestyle diseases, which are also referred to as noncommunicable diseases (NCDs). Lifestyle diseases are related to the way people live. WHO (2009: v) revealed some leading global risks for mortality due to NCDs, including

> high blood pressure (responsible for 13% of deaths globally), tobacco use (9%), high blood glucose (6%), physical inactivity (6%), and overweight and obesity (5%). These risks are responsible for raising the risk of chronic diseases such as heart disease, diabetes and cancers. They affect countries across all income groups: high, middle and low.

The significant risk factors of lifestyle diseases seem to flow from the Global North to the Global South. There is a gradual risk of transition (like epidemiological transition), especially in the Global North, which explains the rise in the risk of lifestyle diseases. It is a transition from "traditional risks" to "modern risks". Bischoff (2008) averred that the complexities of globalization also lead to the changing pattern of risks in different regions of the world.

While infectious diseases of the Global South are uncommon in the Global North, the Global North does have a high burden of NCDs (including lifestyle and degenerative diseases), which are generally manageable but not curable. NCDs present a dangerous trend because of their attributes. The diseases are most not self-limiting; such diseases get worse with time (i.e., degenerating with time). Unless detected at a very early stage, most lifestyle diseases are not reversible. When such diseases reach an advanced stage, there is no cure. Lifestyle diseases often have protracted courses lasting up to several years or throughout the lifespan. In general, chronic diseases accrue a high economic burden because of the required prolonged care. Such diseases might push individuals in low-income countries into economic catastrophe due to the low capacity of the health system, care might not be sustainable and the mortality rate might be unusually high.

WHO (2009) also observed that the success recorded against infectious disease and the use of modern health technologies has led to an increase in life expectancy. Hence, in nearly all high-income countries, populations are aging with a life expectancy of more than 70 years of age. Modern development also leads to changes in the pattern of living. The developments in the food, alcohol and tobacco industries have drawn much attention regarding some health consequences. WHO (2009) further reiterated that low- and middle-income countries also face an increasing double burden of chronic and infectious conditions. Impliedly, individuals in the Global South face both traditional and modern risks. According to WHO (2009),

> eight risk factors, namely alcohol use, tobacco use, high blood pressure, high body mass index, high cholesterol, high blood glucose, low fruit and vegetable intake, and physical inactivity, account for 61% of cardiovascular deaths … Although these major risk factors are usually associated with high-income countries, over 84% of the total global burden of disease they cause occurs in low- and middle-income countries.

Expectedly, the adverse manifestations of the burden of lifestyle diseases are more pronounced in the Global South, largely because of the weak health systems.

The Global North has been implicated in the spread of lifestyle diseases through advertising and marketing of specific risk products such as tobacco and alcohol (WHO, 2007). For instance, the big tobacco industries are in the Global North, and there is rising tobacco-related morbidity and mortality in the Global South. Globalization has also transferred some western lifestyle and food to the Global South, leading to health consequences. There is constant media projection of the western way of life as the ideal, and hence, the Global South is highly westernizing.

Table 2.3 Faces of globalization of health

Globalization of health risks/ vulnerabilities	Social proximity facilitates widespread health because of the compression of space occasioned by globalization as infection could move around the world within hours due to improved modern transportation systems.
Globalization of lifestyle diseases	There is a risk transition from traditional (infectious diseases) to modern (non-communicable diseases) risks, prompted by the spread of western lifestyles.
Globalization of healthcare	Healthcare is like other services flowing across national boundaries.
Globalization of health technology	Globalization enhances the spread of health technology, including the possibility of telehealth, which enables the distribution of health-related services, through the use of information and communication technology.
Globalization of health indicators and targets	Standardized health indicators and targets meant to ensure effective monitoring of population health, decision-making and health policy.
Globalization of health policies and partnerships	Multiple partners, actors/stakeholders and organizations pool their resources (material and non-material) with set goals and frameworks to address global health concerns.
Globalization of medicalization	With the breakthrough in medical and information technology, all aspects of social life are increasingly medicalized, i.e., approached from medical purview.
Globalization of health rights	Global recognition of health rights as part of fundamental human rights which serve as inspiration for many global institutions (especially civil society) to call for improvement in health services around the world

2.3.3 Globalization of Healthcare

Just as health risks and vulnerabilities are globalized, so too is healthcare. Globalization is gradually compressing boundaries in terms of healthcare. Choices and preferences are improving not only within the community, but healthcare can now be accessed globally. Healthcare is like any other product flowing across boundaries. The same way food and tobacco flow from the North to the South, so do healthcare services, though with some barriers (mainly financial and travel barriers). In general, there is the possibility of patient transfer from one location to the other. Pharmaceuticals and other health-related institutions are becoming liberalized. Diagnosis and drugs can be accessed online. The health market is wide open for more possibilities in creating some access which, otherwise, without globalization and its drivers, might not be available.

Health insurance companies now operate on a global scale. There is a possibility of global health coverage, anywhere and anytime. Increasing access to healthcare can range from a routine check-up to a lengthy hospital stay in any country of the world (Jain, 2012). Insurance coverage can be made boundless, depending on the premium. There is a gradual movement toward global pooling of risk. In some socialized healthcare systems, there is more comprehensive health coverage without much discrimination. The principle of non-discrimination has been a global yardstick in terms of population healthcare. Global health insurance is a sure driver to achieve global health goals. Such insurance holds the potential to eliminate geographical and economic barriers to healthcare.

The new era witnesses increasing international travel and coverage of healthcare. From students traveling to the North to expatriates traveling to the South, and tourists to other categories of migrants, all can access healthcare with global health insurance coverage. The medical procedure not allowed or available in one country might be accessed in another country. This is the kind of freedom of choice that the globalists envisage; when prevailing laws constitute a barrier, a journey to another region might resolve the barrier. Globalized health services might be described as value to the end-users. Quality care is the focus of global health institutions, without any form of barrier in terms of boundary or distance. End-users are happier when health services are delivered at an affordable cost. Not only are services provided, but globalized health services also guarantee a standardized quality of healthcare, irrespective of the place or person (see Jain, 2012). Considering the quality of healthcare available in the Global North, it is most often the wealthy from the Global South who access healthcare in the Global North. Such medical tourism creates a kind of intra-country divide and inequality.

There is a strong global movement to eliminate all forms of discrimination in healthcare; to activate the altruistic principle to enable care for undocumented migrants and provide healthcare charity to the needy. In most instances, however, such services come at substantial financial costs, which might constitute a barrier. Globalized healthcare is not only related to clinical care, but also to improving population health through various forms of global aid or interventions that might increase personnel and equipment in underserved areas. It also includes global campaigns to fight against certain diseases (including malaria, HIV and poliomyelitis).

2.3.4 Globalization of Health Technology

The modern era has witnessed substantial development of medical technology and medicaments. The development of technology not only improves medical training. It is also a significant factor in the development of modern medicine in the modern era. In general, medical technology plays a crucial role in the state of health and healthcare. Medical technology is about innovations, whether tangible or not, that help in sustaining health. The technological breakthrough occasioned by the industrial revolution is ongoing and has improved beyond the vision of the early scientists during the industrial revolution. Diagnosis and treatment are getting easier with the use of various technologies. The substantial increase in medical devices and equipment has made significant contributions to human health. The broad areas of development include information technology, pharmaceuticals and biotechnology. The technology is not only about sophisticated techs such as robotic surgery and artificial organs but also the simple ones, including smart inhalers, adhesive bandages, ankle braces, crutches and corrective glasses, among others. For instance, despite the doomsters' prophesies of pestilence and famine due to geometric rise in the human population against the arithmetic growth of food production, the development of modern medical technology has been a significant counter-force against such prophecies. Improvements in contraceptive technology have allowed people to control the timing of childbirth and enhance family planning in general.

It is essential to acknowledge the incredible advances in transplantation medicine, cosmetic surgery, and emerging xenotransplantation, among others. The Healthcare Business and Technology (2016) acknowledged that medical practice is improving with the introduction of medical doctors to innovative technologies (both sophisticated and simple technologies). The use of technologies makes medical practice easier. Modern medical practice is, in fact, technologically driven. Medical technology has helped to connect doctors and clients thousands of miles apart through telecommunications. The client–physician connection is one area where globalization is enhancing health. The Healthcare Business and Technology (2016) further reiterated that patients could hold videoconferences with physicians in another city or continent for medical assistance. It is also possible to send health information and assistance instantaneously to any specialist or doctor in the world. Such a virtual connection saves time and money. The birth of telemedicine, involving remote diagnosis and treatment of clients, is one major area that connects technology with globalization and medicine. Telehealth enables the distribution of health-related services through the use of information and communication technology. Beyond client–physician (virtual) contact, there are other opportunities, including real-time health assessment and consultations, reminders, education, referrals and other forms of intervention.

The major development is that globalization is enhancing the spread of health technology. This is another primary face of globalization of health, which has drawn the South and North closer concerning the quality of healthcare. The apparent consequences include improved accessible, cost-effective and high-quality health care services (WHO, 2010), which otherwise might not be available. Globalization of health technology helps in overcoming distance as a barrier to healthcare. WHO (2010) noted that globalization of health tech favors improved health services to rural and underserved communities in the Global South and vulnerable groups that traditionally suffer from lack of access to healthcare. Globalization of health technology is not just about the use of information and communication technology (ICT), but the global spread of various forms of health technologies. The entire future of healthcare will be defined by digital technologies because of the immense potential such technologies have to revolutionize access to healthcare. For instance, there is gradual the applications of blockchain technology for electronic medical records, pharmaceutical supply chain and remote patient monitoring, including medical diagnostics (see Tando et al., 2020); and artificial intelligence (AI) including machine learning for diagnosis, risk assessment and disease surveillance to improve the inequities and access to quality healthcare in the Global South (see Schwalbe and Wahl, 2020).

2.3.5 Globalization of Health Indicators and Targets

One major area of globalization is the unified basis or indicators for assessing population health. When there is a discussion about global health, there is a need to discourse the health indicators and indices. The Canadian Institute of Health Information (CIHI) (2019) defined a health indicator as "a measure designed to summarize information about a given health priority in population health or health system performance". A global health indicator is, therefore, a measure designed to assess health priorities across the world. It is an attempt to provide a general picture of health needs assessment on a global scale. It serves as a comparative basis to understand population health and healthcare system performance in different regions. The CIHI (2019) averred that health indicators are essential because they provide comparable and actionable information across diverse geographic, organizational, or administrative boundaries and/or can track progress over time. The debate about health inequalities is all about differential health statistics in different geographical regions, which shows the performance of the regions in terms of disease burden and healthcare. It is possible to use such indicators to compare the Global North and the Global South. Table 2.4 shows some selected indicators. Some health indicators measure health directly, while others are demographic indicators. Development indicators (poverty, education and sanitation) can also be included because they are vital determinants of health (as distal indicators). Several global bodies, including WHO, UNICEF, Global Health Council, United Nations Development Program [UNDP], US Center for Disease Control and Prevention [CDC]) and national bodies (especially Ministries of Health) are responsible for tracking health indicators. Typically, the global bodies also provide support in monitoring the indicators, especially in the developing countries where there is limited infrastructure to do so. While some of these indicators are global in nature, country- or region-specific indicators are also available. For instance, Larson and Mercer (2004) indicated that the health situation in

Table 2.4 Some global population health indicators

Indicator	Meaning
Maternal Mortality Ratio (MMR)	The ratio of maternal deaths, defined as the death of a woman as a result of pregnancy or childbirth, during pregnancy or within 42 days after delivery.
Child Mortality Rate (CMR)	The probability of dying between the first and the fifth birthdays (the sum of the probabilities of dying in the second, third, fourth and fifth years of life).
Under-five mortality rate (U5MR)	Probability that a newborn child will die before reaching his or her fifth birthday (the sum of probabilities of dying in the first, second, third, fourth and fifth years of life).
Crude birth rate (CBR)	Number of births per 1,000 population over a specified period (usually in a year).
Crude death rate (CDR)	Number of deaths per 1,000 population over a specified period (usually a year).
Crude growth rate (CGR)	Also referred to as the natural population growth, it is determined by subtracting the CDR from the CBR for any given year and converting the result to a percentage.
Life expectancy	The number of years that a person born today (or at any other designated point in time) is expected to live, given the age-specific death rates for the country in which he or she lives at the time of birth.
Contraception prevalence rate (CPR)	Proportion of women of childbearing age (15–49 years) using some form of modern contraception (sometimes reported with traditional methods included).
Access to health services	Access is often determined by distance, time, cost and socio-cultural factors.
Children immunization coverage	Often represented as the percentage of children in a country who are fully immunized.

Source: WHO, 2021.

developed countries is better captured with health indicators reflecting lifestyles and individual behavior such as diet, smoking, physical exercise, or substance and alcohol abuse.

Larson and Mercer (2004) observed that population health is considerably improving in developing countries, especially within the last two decades. Such improvements have been observed in the maternal and child mortality rate, but more efforts still need to be invested in SSA and some parts of South Asia, where health indicator scores are poorest. Malaria incidence and mortality have also decreased over the last two decades, although current malaria death rates are still alarmingly high. Global efforts in the control of HIV are also yielding some positive results both regionally, specifically in SSA, and at the global level. Larson and Mercer (2004: p. 1199) inferred, "global monitoring of changes in the health of various populations requires the use of 'tried and true' global health indicators".

The primary importance of this globalization of health indicators is to ensure effective monitoring of population health, decision-making and health policy. The indicators are often checked against a set of global health targets, for example, "health for all" by the year 2000; health aspect of the Millennium Development Goals (MDGs) by 2015, and health aspects of Sustainable Development Goal (SDGs) by 2030. The global targets ensure some shared efforts and serve as a guiding measure for global efforts. For instance, Goal 3 of SDG aims to "ensure healthy lives and promote well-being for all at all ages". The targets include reducing maternal mortality to less than 70 per 100,000 live births and under-five mortality to less than 25 per 1,000 live births, ending the epidemics of AIDS, tuberculosis, malaria and achieving universal health coverage (among others) by 2030.

2.3.6 Globalization of Health Policies and Partnerships

Due to common identified priorities and targets, there is also a global movement toward universal health policies and partnerships. Youde (2014) observed that the increasing globalization of health also amounts to an expansion of the number and types of actors involved in addressing global health concerns. There is increasing attention on resolving some "global *bads*", including poor health indicators in some quarters. Hence, improving population health is a significant way of delivering global public goods. With the realization of the spread of global risk of disease, global action is more appropriate to tackle a global problem. The united front would help beyond domestic policy to tackle global health issues. Since most issues (including poverty, climate change, nuclear proliferation, human and national security, disease risks and economic crisis) are on a global scale and adversely affect global health, the sustainability of global action is paramount (Brown et al., 2004).

Brown et al. (2004: p. 1) further observed that "the traditional multilateral policy models are too strained to sufficiently tackle these global problems". Hence, there is an intensive call from all stakeholders to broaden the existing "structures of global governance, global public policy formation, and global policy implementation" (Brown et al. 2004: p. 1). The call is meant to address the issues mentioned earlier, including global health. Brown et al. (2004) further stressed that the media attention to H1N1 (swine flu), H7N9 (bird flu) and TDR-TB (drug-resistant tuberculosis) also necessitates the development of global policies to tackle health priorities. Lee (2004) noted that domestic policies could not adequately cater to the seemingly global health shifts. Therefore, global policies are necessary as far as they adapt to local contexts to address health issues. Such global health policies also need to respect the increased sharing of principles, ethical values and standards that underpin decision-making about health.

A global health partnership is a meaningful way for multiple partners, actors/stakeholders and organizations to pool resources, both material and non-material, to address global health concerns. The world has witnessed the birth of global health partnerships, such as the

Global Fund to Fight AIDS, Tuberculosis and Malaria, the Global Alliance for Vaccines and Immunization (GAVI) and The Vaccine Alliance, which address specific health issues on a global scale. The Global Fund is pooling resources to intensify the fight against malaria, tuberculosis (TB) and HIV. A minimum of $4 billion a year is earmarked to support programs championed by local experts in over 100 countries to improve the global efforts against AIDS, Tuberculosis and Malaria (The Global Fund, 2019). The Global Fund aims to specifically target the SDG goal of ending the epidemics of these diseases by 2030. The goal is to "fight harder, smarter and together".

With the realization that health problems span geographies, the drive toward global partnerships and policies or frameworks has intensified. There continue to be some gaps, but the movement is growing stronger. Although a number of the health targets of the MDGs were not met in many Third World countries, due partly to insufficient resources from the (global) partners, with the renewed efforts, the hope of meeting the SDG target is still bright. And although it is easier said than done, sustainability of the commitments and intensified local support from severally affected countries might change the story by 2030.

On the other side, globalization can also adversely affect the health system and thereby impede access to health services (Chapman, 2009). The adverse effects might result from the neoliberal stance, which promotes some reduction in public expenditure and supports the commodification of health. For instance, most global institutions (including the World Bank) often promote a market-oriented health sector, which is detrimental to the efforts to secure universal healthcare, especially in the Global South (Chapman, 2009).

2.3.7 Globalization of Medicalization

As the world becomes increasingly globalized, it is also evolving rapidly medicalized. Medicalization is a process where more and more ordinary issues are defined as medical issues and therefore require medical attention. Therefore, many aspects of human life, not previously considered pathological, are regarded as medical problems (Maturo, 2012). Medicalization is about the expansion of the medical gaze with the increasing roles of the medical doctors beyond the four walls of the hospital to all aspects of social life. There is an increasing medical gaze of food, sex, body, travel and other social events and problems. For instance, aging is a natural event that has been highly medicalized. Since aging begins at the moment of birth, the entire life course is medicalized. There is increasing research on aging, some to develop the medical means of reversing it. This idea of professional medical dominance of the medical gaze is also connected to globalization, and therefore, a significant manifestation of globalization of health.

Technologization is one of the engines of medicalization (Conrad, 2007), and thus serves as a driver of globalization. Technological development infiltrates all aspects of human life not only from birth to death but pre-birth until after death. The rise of genetic testing implies that more diseases are discoverable even long before such diseases are symptomatic. A typical example is prenatal genetic testing meant to discover the health status of the embryo, which could predict many life health situations. Another critical aspect of medicalization is pharmaceuticalization, which involves increasing the use of drugs, even in non-pathological conditions. For instance, there is the pharmaceuticalization of sex and beauty. There is increasing marketing and advertisement of lifestyle drugs. The body has become a medical project. The body is continuously under a medical gaze, especially with the rise of cosmetic surgery, which is not meant for "correction" but improvement or enhancement. There is a possibility of "extreme makeover" to touch-ups from time to time. "Beauty" can now be manufactured in the surgical room, and there are increasing demands from customers who have been convinced through advertising of medical possibilities. Conrad (2005) noted that medicalization is "driven more by commercial and market interests than by professional claims-makers". Medicalization is a "symptom" of capitalist expansion into the medical field, with a gradual shift from "patients" to "persons". There is also a gradual individualization of social problems, biological reductionism and changing the notion of what is normal or pathological (Maturo, 2012).

Through globalization, medicalization is spreading quickly, and is thus a significant aspect of globalization of health. With the flow of information and advances in medical technologies, the number of medical options is increasing, and therefore, medicalization is a major consequence. There is a flow of information and mass media projection of "utopia" conditions, which can be achieved through medical interventions. Globalized medicalization is a reality as the world is increasingly medicalized. One aspect of globalization is increasing "harmonization", the tendency for a common standard. Some individuals try to achieve common standards through medical interventions. The argument here does not criticize the globalization of medicalization or medicalization itself. It is an event or a process, which is context-specific: It is neither always good nor bad. There is no strict ethical rule on medicalization; it is a reality that needs to be evaluated from time to time to track its progress and consequences.

2.3.8 Globalization of Health Rights

The discussion around the right to healthcare is global. There is a strong movement to affirm the legal basis of the right to health everywhere in the world (Amzat and Razum, 2018). This global discussion is meant to fashion a way to universal coverage of healthcare, which confers responsibility or obligation on governments and other stakeholders to ensure the availability of healthcare; a kind of global duty to ensure quality health services. The global movement started with the enactment of the right to health in the WHO's constitution. The WHO (1948) affirmed the right to the enjoyment of the highest attainable standard of physical and mental health as one of the fundamental human rights. There have been other documents, which also document the right to health, including the Universal Declaration of Human Rights (Article 25) and International Covenant on Economic, Social and Cultural Rights (Article 12). The practical essence is to ensure that everyone, irrespective of any personal attributes, has access to healthcare.

The declaration of health for all by 2000 was a global declaration. The introduction of primary healthcare also followed the declaration as a practical and policy approach to ensuring health for all. Human rights have become the obligation of the government. With the discourse about human rights in the context of globalization, It is observed that human rights are not evenly guaranteed. So, also, the benefits of globalization are not equal across regions, which invariably affect the full implementation of human rights in the Global South. Health as a human right is also poorly exercised in the Global South. The realization of this inadequate access to health services also draws attention to some specific aspects of human rights not adequately attained. The persistence of health inequalities between the regions is a primary yardstick of measuring the extent of world inequalities. It can be argued that globalization has drawn attention to the health disparities around the world, and therefore, can serve as instrumental to the realization of the right to health.

On the other hand, Chapman (2009) observed that human rights norms form inspirations for some global institutions (especially civil societies) to call for improvements in health services. Chapman reiterated that the human rights paradigm is another basis for contesting the effects of globalization. The dimension of globalization of health (including the globalization of healthcare and technology) points to the complementary role that globalization can play in the realization of universal healthcare. Attaining this universal healthcare also hinges on human rights principles, including non-discrimination, the dignity of the human person and equality. There are emerging global institutions and civil societies that monitor various conditions around the world, propose interventions and ensure the attainment of human rights, including the right to health. Since human rights are interwoven, all global efforts to stop the violation of fundamental rights are connected to ensuring the attainment of a reasonable standard of health (see Amzat and Razum, 2018).

2.4 Summary

- Global health is defined as a way of understanding population health and healthcare within a global context. Global health serves as a bridge, linking the South and North but with unequal power and benefits. Global health could be global considering its basic scope (see Table 2.2) when compared with other domains, especially public and international health.
- The Global South experiences relatively poor health services., in many instances making the population (e.g., in SSA) highly susceptible to various adverse health conditions, mainly preventable diseases such as malaria, diarrhea and cholera. In many developing countries, the health system is not adequate to cater to the health needs of the population.
- It is often hard to agree on the pathways and mechanisms through which globalization affects health, as there is no consensus. The mechanisms are complex. However, the chapter demystifies the complexities by identifying some manifestations of the impacts of globalization on health.
- The global community is confronted with global risks and vulnerabilities. Globalization compresses time and space; an infection in one region of the world can, in a matter of hours, spread to other regions. HIV/AIDS, Ebola, tuberculosis and cholera still pose a tremendous threat in the global space. Infectious diseases tend to become global health emergencies.
- The significant risk factors of lifestyle diseases seem to flow from the Global North to the South. There is a gradual risk transition (like epidemiological transition), especially in the Global North, which explains the rise in the risk and burden of lifestyle diseases.
- Healthcare is like any other product flowing across boundaries. The same way food and tobacco flow from the North to the South, so do healthcare services, though with some barriers (mainly financial and travel barriers). The health market is wide open for more possibilities in creating some access which, otherwise, without globalization and its drivers, might not be available.
- Medical technology has helped to connect doctors and clients thousands of miles apart through telecommunications. Globalization of health technology helps in overcoming distance as a barrier to healthcare, which favors improved health services to rural and underserved communities in the Global South and vulnerable groups that traditionally suffer from inadequate access to healthcare.
- There is also the globalization of health indicators meant to ensure effective monitoring of population health, decision-making and health policy of different regions.
- With the realization that health problems span geographies, the drive toward global partnerships and policies or frameworks has intensified. The increasing globalization of health also amounts to an expansion of the number and types of actors involved in addressing identified priorities and targets (i.e., global health concerns).
- There is also global expansion of medicalization or medical gaze with the increasing roles of the health workers beyond the four walls of the hospital to all aspects of social life. Medicalization is a "symptom" of (global) capitalist expansion into the medical field, with a gradual shift from "patients" to "persons".

- Health rights discourse is also a global phenomenon. Human rights abuse adversely affects health globally and ensuring universal healthcare is a global target.

Critical Thinking Questions

- What is global health? Evaluate the scope of global health and suggest how to strengthen such scope to make it more global.
- Differentiate traditional from modern risks. To what extent can we apportion blame for the transmission of either modern or traditional risks between the global divide (North and South)?
- Within the context of unequal power relations, do you think that global health can be truly global? Why do you think inequality of power or concern should be downplayed in global health?
- The pathways and mechanisms through which globalization affects health is complex. Irrespective of such complexity, examine some specific areas of manifestation of the impact of globalization on health.
- To what extent is healthcare shifting from "patients" to "persons". Assess medicalization as a "symptom" of globalization and capitalist expansion into the medical field.
- In what specific ways is the growth of medical technology promoting globalization of health? Do you observe a balance between the North and South with respect to the growth of medical technology?
- To what extent do you agree that the right to health is a fundamental human right? Can the right to health be truly global?

Suggested Readings

- Chapman, A. R. (2009). Globalization, human rights, and the social determinants of health. *Bioethics*, *23*(2), 97–111. This article reviews the importance and challenges of human rights to achieving greater equity in shaping the social determinants of health on a global scale.
- Conrad, P. (2007). *The medicalization of society: On the transformation of human conditions into treatable disorders*. Maryland: Johns Hopkins University Press. This is an authoritative book that explains the meaning and dimensions of medicalization.
- Kawachi, I., and Wamala, S. (Eds.). (2006). Globalization and Health. Oxford: Oxford University Press. DOI:10.1093/acprof:oso/9780195172997.001.0001. The book presents health as a sensitive mirror of globalization. The various chapters examine how health is an important criterion for monitoring and evaluating the process of globalization.
- Woodward, D., Drager, N., Beaglehole, R., and Lipson, D. (2001). Globalization and health: A framework for analysis and action. *Bulletin of the World Health Organization*, *79*(9), 875–881. This article presents a conceptual framework for the linkages between economic globalization and health
- Youde, J. (2014). Global health partnerships: The emerging agenda. Brown, G. W., Yamey, G., and Wamala, S. (Eds.) *The Oxford handbook of global health policy* (pp 505-518). Oxford: Oxford University Press. The chapter is very good in understanding the politics of global health cooperation.
- Youde, J. (2020). *Globalization and Health*. London: Rowman and Littlefield Publishers. This book examines the various political dimensions of the intersections between globalization and health.

References

Amzat, J., & Razum, O. (2018). The right to health in Africa. In *Towards a Sociology of Health Discourse in Africa*. Cham, Switzerland: Springer International Publishing. doi: 10.1007/978-3-319-61672-8_2.

Bartelson, J. (2000). Three concepts of globalization. *International Sociology*, *15*(2), 180–196.

Beaglehole, R., & Bonita, R. (2010). What is global health? *Global Health Action, 3*, 5142. doi: 10.3402/gha.v3i0.5142.

Bischoff, H. (2008). Introduction. In Bischoff, H. (Ed.), *Risks in Modern Society* (pp. 1–16). Dordrecht: Springer.

Brown, G. W., Yamey, G., & Wamala, S. (2004). Introduction. In Brown, G. W., Yamey, G. & Wamala, S. (Eds.), *The Handbook of Global Health Policy* (pp. 505–518). Sussex: Wiley Blackwell.

Brown, T. M., Cueto, M. & Fee, E. (2006). The World Health Organization and the transition from "international" to "global" public health. *American Journal of Public Health*, *96*(1), 62–72. doi: 10.2105/AJPH.2004.050831.

Canadian Institute of Health Information (CIHI) (2019). Health indicators. www.cihi.ca/en/health-indicators. Accessed on July 29, 2019.

Chan, M. (2011). The increasing importance of global health. www.who.int/dg/speeches/2011/globalhealth_20110613/en/. Accessed on July 24, 2019.

Chapman, A. R. (2009). Globalization, human rights, and the social determinants of health. *Bioethics*, *23*(2), 97–111.

Conrad, P. (2005). The shifting engines of medicalization. *Journal of Health and Social Behavior*, *46*, 3–14.

Conrad, P. (2007). *The Medicalization of Society: On the Transformation of Human Conditions into Treatable Disorders*. Baltimore, MD: Johns Hopkins University Press.

Cornia, G. A. (2001). Globalization and health: Results and options. *Bulletin of the World Health Organization*, *79*(9), 834–841.

Desai, C. (2016). Online pharmacies: A boon or bane? *Indian Journal of Pharmacology*, *48*(6), 615–616. doi: 10.4103/0253-7613.194865.

Ferguson, M. (1992). The mythology about globalization. *European Journal of Communication*, *7*(1), 69–93.

Healthcare Business and Technology (2016). Health technology. www.healthcarebusinesstech.com/medical-technology/. Accessed on July 29, 2019.

Jain, S. H. (2012). What is strategy in global health care? www.healthaffairs.org/do/10.1377/hblog20120312.017575/full/. Accessed on July, 27, 2019.

Javed, N. (2014). Globalization or cultural colonialism. *International Journal of Development Research*, *4*(4), 825–827.

Kickbush, I. (2006). The need for a European strategy on global health. *Scandinavian Journal of Public Health*, *34*, 561–565.

Kickbusch, I., & Buse, K. (2001). Global influences and global responses: International health at the turn of the 21st century (pp. 701–738). In Merson, M. H., Black, R. E. & Mills, A. J. (Eds.), *International Public Health: Diseases, Programs, Systems, and Policies*. Gaithersburg, MD: Aspen Publishers.

Koplan, J. P., Bond, T. C., Merson, M. H., Reddy, K. S., Rodriguez, M. H., Sewankambo, N. K. & Wasserheit, J. N. (2009). Towards a common definition of global health. *Lancet*, *373*, 1993–1995.

Labonté, R., Mohindra, K. & Schrecker, T. (2011). The growing impact of globalization for health and public health practice. *Annual Review of Public Health*, *32*, 263–283.

Larson, C., & Mercer, A. (2004). Global health indicators: An overview. *Canadian Medical Association Journal*, *171*(10), 1199–1200.

Lee K. (2004). Globalisation: What is it and how does it affect health? *The Medical Journal of Australia*, *180*(4), 156–158.

Maturo, A. (2012). Medicalization: Current concept and future directions in a bionic society. *Mens Sana Monographs*, *10*(1), 122–133.

Schwalbe, N., & Wahl, B. (2020). Artificial intelligence and the future of global health. *Lancet*, *395*(10236), 1579–1586. doi: 10.1016/S0140-6736(20)30226-9.

Smith, R. D. (2006). Responding to global infectious disease outbreaks: Lessons from SARS on the role of risk perception, communication and management. *Social Science and Medicine*, *63*(12), 3113–3123.

Tandon, A., Dhir, A., Islam, A.K.M.N., Matti, M. & Kari, H. (2020). Blockchain in healthcare: A systematic literature review, synthesizing framework and future research agenda. *Computers in Industry, 122*, 103290. doi: 10.1016/j.compind.2020.103290.

Taylor, S. (2018). "Global health": Meaning what? *BMJ Global Health, 3*, e000843. doi: 10.1136/bmjgh-2018-000843.

The Global Fund (2019). Set up the fight. www.theglobalfund.org/en/stepupthefight/. Accessed on July 29, 2019.

World Health Organization (WHO) (1948). *Constitution of the WHO*. Geneva: WHO.

WHO (2007). *Obesity: Preventing and Managing the Global Epidemic*. Technical Report Series No. 894. Geneva: WHO.

WHO (2009). *Global Health Risks: Mortality and Burden of Disease Attributable to Selected Major Risks*. Geneva: WHO.

WHO (2010). *Telemedicine: Opportunities and Developments in Member States*. Report on the second global survey on eHealth (Vol. 2). Geneva: WHO.

WHO (2021). *Global Health Observatory Visualizations: Indicator Metadata Registry*. apps.who.int/gho/data/node.wrapper.imr?x-id=1. Accessed on January 29, 2019.

Woodward, D., Drager, N., Beaglehole, R., & Lipson, D. (2001). Globalization and health: A framework for analysis and action. *Bulletin of the World Health Organization, 79*(9), 875–881.

Youde, J. (2014). Global health partnerships: The emerging agenda. Brown, G. W., Yamey, G. & Wamala, S. (Eds.), *The Handbook of Global Health Policy* (pp. 505–518). Sussex: Wiley Blackwell.

Youde, J. (2020). *Globalization and Health*. Lanham, MD: Rowman and Littlefield Publishers.

3   Social and Global Determinants of Health

3.1 Introduction

Health is contextual in the sense that there are myriad factors that influence it. These factors are known as social determinants of health (SDH). Some of these factors even constitute the causes of diseases because they exact direct influence on the likelihood of developing a disease. It is in recognition of the SDH that the World Health Organization (WHO) instituted the WHO Commission of Social Determinants of Health (CSDH). It is essential to understand these contextual factors called SDH to understand population health in general. The SDH are the prime factors that, if improved, can possibly improve population health outcomes. Many countries of the Global South (especially sub-Saharan Africa [SSA]) are still confronted with traditional risks of infectious diseases, largely as a result of living conditions related to poverty and inadequate infrastructures, such as water and power supplies. In SSA, such inadequate infrastructure becomes a significant determinant of health. There are several communities without potable water, which explains the risk of guinea worm and other water-borne diseases. It is in this light that SDH is sometimes regarded as the fundamental causes of diseases.

Specifically, SDH refers to the social circumstances and conditions in which people are born, grow, live, work and play that invariably account for human health (CSDH, 2008). The social conditions even determine if a child will be born alive and for how long that child will likely live. Child mortality has been closely linked to social circumstances. It starts with maternal dietary behavior; whether or not the pregnant woman has access to adequate food required to sustain good health and development for both the fetus and herself. In some poor regions, famine and/or poor nutrition are common, impacting both the mother and unborn child. Inadequate access to healthcare also promotes home delivery in SSA, which also accounts for the high rate of maternal mortality and stillbirth. During delivery, many women do not have the opportunity to have skilled attendants. The issues of dietary behavior and access to a skilled attendant at birth constitute circumstances that can influence health outcomes. The focus on SDH in improving population health is receiving considerable attention across the world, both at a global level and within-country action (Donkin et al., 2017).

Beyond the preceding illustrations, globalization is another dominant social reality that has been implicated as a significant determinant of health. Globalization is a multifactorial concept with multiple mechanisms of influence on health. A closer look at globalization can help explain the relationship between SDH and globalization. This becomes the foundation of the notion of global determinants of health (GDH). The idea is to discuss some factors that operate at the global level, which affect population health (on a global scale). There will also be an attempt to situate several SDH within the global context. The chapter will proceed with the understanding of social determinants of population health and, finally, explains some specific global determinants of health.

DOI: 10.4324/9781003247975-3

3.2 Social Context of Population Health (Within the Global Context)

The primary constituent unit of the population is the individual. An understanding of population health starts with examining the individual. How are individuals faring in term of health status and access to healthcare? This is a fundamental question that every society would like to answer when considering the state of healthcare. At the individual level, the biology, ecology, social and political circumstances are critical. The first level is the biological or physiological well-being, which could provide immunity or vulnerability to specific health conditions. It is in this light that WHO stresses the importance of physiological well-being in its definition of health (see Section 1.2.2). Moreover, diseases can be detected through a competent diagnosis. Also important is the social aspect or condition, which is about income, living environment and lifestyles (dietary, smoking and sexual behavior, among others). There are fundamental determinants of health for the individual. Invariably, the aggregate of individuals constitutes a community or society, and by extension, what we call community health.

"Community" is used in this context to imply the neighborhood where individuals thrive, the immediate environment. Community is "a group of people with diverse characteristics who are linked by social ties, share common perspectives, and engage in joint action in geographical locations or settings" (MacQueen et al., 2001: p. 1929). Community implies residence or locality, workplace and other forms of dimensions, including work and spiritual dimensions. Community health is about a geographical space, i.e., environmental, social and economic resources to sustain emotional and physical well-being among people in ways that advance their aspirations and satisfy their needs in their unique environment (WHO, 1986). The community is a place of people-centered primary healthcare, and a major building block in the understanding of population health (see Goodman et al., 2014).

The summation of individual and community health accounts for national health or population health for a given country. This is why Georges et al. (2018) observed that illness and health should be understood in a multilevel context. The household production of health is applicable in the sense that individual health is produced and reproduced within the household. Georges et al. (2018) described the household production of health as the locus of health production toward the maintenance or restoration of health of household members. The daily process of health production involves many coordinated activities geared toward detection, protection and promotion of health within the household. Georges et al. noted that it is a dynamic process that internal resources (e.g., knowledge about health, health-related behaviors) are linked to external resources (e.g., information, resources, health services) (Figure 3.1).

The national level is a macro level, which involves the aggregate of individuals, communities, districts or counties. From the micro (individual) to the macro (national) level, health

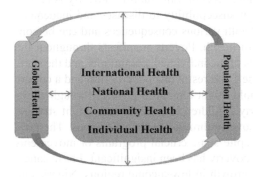

Figure 3.1 Population health within the global context

production is a complex process involving multilevel activities to maintain population health. Within the geographical space, therefore, the individual is the starting point, then the community, national and international levels, then a combination of all makes population health (see Figure 3.1). Global health is, however, a combination of all: The global level is the super-macro level (see Figure 3.1). Population health is influenced by several factors operating both at micro-macro and the super-macro levels. The discussion here is on the SDH and GDH, reflecting all the levels mentioned. The next section will describe some social determinants of health, focusing on significant factors at the micro-macro level (individual and community level) before examining the factors operating at the super-macro (global) level.

3.2.1 Social Determinants of Health

Understanding the social context or determinants of health is a prerequisite to understanding population health, whether in the Global South or the Global North. The SDH are responsible for health inequalities, especially within the country and between countries. The determinants are often used to explain the uneven distribution of diseases among individuals and between communities. The factors operate both at the individual and community levels. The SDH are factors undermining or promoting population health and such factors explain social inequality in general, and health inequalities in particular (Graham, 2004; Islam, 2019). A considerable improvement in the SDH, through policies and other forms of intervention, can considerably impact health inequalities (Solar and Irwin, 2010). The efforts to improve health must be multifactorial to consider both proximate, including lifestyle, behavior and personal characteristics and distal factors, such as the provision of social amenities and health facilities.

The availability (both quality and quantity) and distribution of social resources (including basic amenities) function to a large extent to determine citizens' health and prevalence of diseases (Islam, 2019). "Social determinants of health" has become a common term to understand population, public and global health. It is essential to briefly explain those factors in the context of the Global South.

3.2.1.1 Poverty in the Global South

Poverty is a global reality, but poverty is overrepresented in the Global South. Poverty is a very loaded concept with various meanings and dimensions. The primary yardstick of measuring poverty is a per capita income of less than US$1 or US$2 a day (Kacowicz, 2007). Concisely, poverty refers to a socio-economic condition concerning inadequate funds to secure the necessities of life, such as food, clothing and shelter. Poverty is a state of deprivation of material possessions or personal needs that account for a high level of vulnerability. Poverty is related to most social and health problems, including high susceptibility to diseases and inadequate access to healthcare. Poverty is multidimensional with various consequences and can be considered one of the notorious social determinants of health. Poverty manifests throughout the life course with obvious adverse effects at the levels of the individual, community and the state.

Poverty is a vicious cycle that can reproduce itself and result in a poverty trap and a culture of poverty. A child growing up in a poor household might remain in poverty through adulthood, subsequently raising their children in poverty. Children born in poverty might struggle with minimal or no state support and remain in poverty throughout their lifespans. The poverty trap is common in low-income countries. Despite some crucial programs or movements against poverty, the rate of improvement in world poverty has been insignificant. For instance, the incidence of poverty is rising with population growth in low-income regions. Nigeria and India have been repeatedly branded as the headquarters of poverty with the highest incidence of poverty. Other countries with high extreme poverty rates include DR Congo, Ethiopia, Tanzania, Mozambique, Bangladesh, Kenya and Indonesia.

The tragedy of poverty is the dehumanizing effects or consequences on all aspects of life. Grant (2005) documented the nexus between poverty and ill-health. Poverty impacts negatively on the physiological and psychological development of an individual. For Grant (2005), the indication of poverty starts with inadequate nutrition, which weakens human immunity to fight diseases. Many children in low-income countries die of hunger and malnutrition-related diseases (e.g., kwashiorkor and anemia). In the Arab regions (including Syria, Egypt, Lebanon, Tunisia, Jordan and Yemen), a study reported the prevalence of undernutrition, inadequate intake of nutrients and unhealthy dietary habits leading to growth retardation among young children and micronutrient deficiencies (Musaiger et al., 2011). Like in Africa, undernourishment is a significant problem in the Caribbean, with 18% of the people and 11% of under-five children classified as underweight (Sastre et al., 2014). In low-income regions, malnutrition, undernutrition or hunger among children is often a result of poverty, subsequently leading to intergenerational micronutrient deficiencies with adverse physiological pathologies.

Another significant indication of poverty is the inadequate capacity to meet healthcare costs. In low-income countries and even some high-income countries, such as the United States, healthcare expenditure is often financed through out-of-pocket payment due to a lack of or inadequate health insurance schemes. For most people, illness often results in financial catastrophe as funds meant for other needs might need to be diverted to healthcare. People may resort to self-medication or present late at the health facility, due to fear of hospital bills. The unfortunate paradox is that while the poor more often get sick, their access to healthcare is worse. Poor households bear the highest brunt of infectious diseases, primarily acute, thereby accounting for higher morbidity and mortality than other segments of the population. The health afflictions of poverty also significantly lead to the reproduction of poverty. The diminished capacity to function or work as a result of poverty-related hunger, morbidity or deficient mental development leads to inadequate resources or provisions to attain a good standard of living.

3.2.1.2 *Education and Health Literacy*

Level of educational attainment influences human well-being and is, therefore, considered a social determinant of health. Education exposes people to life skills and knowledge meant for personal and social development. Educational attainment is often calculated as the number of years of schooling, mostly in a formal setting. While informal education is also important, formal education is more standardized and follows an organized pattern in imparting knowledge. The most important aspect of basic education is the ability to read and write. The poorest literacy rates are found in countries of the Global South. While the last five decades have seen some improvement in the global literacy rate, some countries, including Afghanistan, Burkina Faso, Niger and South Sudan still have literacy rates below 50%. Deprivation of education is one of the worst forms of human deprivation; it is damaging to all human rights conventions. Education is also multifaceted with manifestation in all aspects of life. It is related to the rate of poverty since education is a significant means of fulfilling life aspirations. As education is a measure of knowledge, health literacy is also a related aspect.

Education helps to facilitate health literacy, which is the ability to understand basic health information to make health decisions. Education affects life choices, including health choices. Education holds direct and indirect implications for health. One indirect way is that education is one of the critical resources that could enormously facilitate an escape from the poverty trap. Low level of education and poverty are interrelated correlates of health measures and life expectancy. The number of years spent in school is related to social position and qualifications to secure white-collar jobs in many countries. An escape from the poverty trap translates to life opportunities, which can facilitate better health choices. In a general review, Telfair and Shelton (2012) observed that the health disparities between the educated and the less educated are highly significant. The authors observed that, from childhood, education instills certain lifelong beliefs and behaviors, which can enhance positive health outcomes. The health disparities are observable in both chronic and acute diseases, but the magnitude is greater for chronic conditions (such as cancer and diabetes). The educated are more likely to follow medical instructions and general therapeutic regimes. The educated are also expected to develop some health-protective behavior against certain risks.

Health promotion activities and behavior (such as personal hygiene and good nutrition) are strongly correlated with the level of education. The returns from education are higher in low-income countries with a high prevalence of diseases of poverty and ignorance (see Appleton, 2000). Low levels of education are related to vaccine hesitancy or resistance among children in many countries in the Global South. The main problem is that many people still hold to traditional superstitions, which prevent a clear understanding of certain health information. Low level of education is also correlated with human immunodeficiency virus (HIV) and tuberculosis (TB) prevalence in the Global South, especially in SSA; the burden of HIV and TB is greater among the uneducated (see Vandemoortele and Delamonica, 2002). Home delivery without a trained birth attendant is also related to lower education. Poor maternal education is related to maternal mortality and child mortality (UNESCO, 2010). It follows then that the major global health indicators are very poor in places with low literacy rates. In general, educational attainment influences the understanding of health information and behavior. Education is also an indicator of socio-economic status; education improves social positions and facilitates access to resources, which might improve health.

3.2.1.3 Employment and Working Condition

Work is a central aspect of human life and a social determinant of health. Employment and working conditions manifest in many ways. The first dimension is employment status: Whether someone is employed, under-employed or unemployed. Unemployment touches individuals worldwide. Many people are qualified, willing and able to work, but without any gainful employment. Unemployment is a major cause of urban poverty. The three factors: Occupation, income and education, are the significant measures of socio-economic status. The three factors are significantly related, and therefore, it is not surprising that all are determinants of health. The unemployed often have limited access to recourses that could sustain their health. The second dimension is under-employment, in which an individual's capacity is not fully utilized. Under-employment is also correlated with poverty. Those who are gainfully employed are better-placed in the social hierarchy and, therefore, prone to making better health decisions.

Another critical dimension relating to employment is working conditions. In low-income countries, a high percentage of people are employed in the unorganized and unregulated informal sector, including roadside trading. Such a work environment is not safe for human health because of the incessant possibility of accidents and other safety issues. A poor working condition also extends to the physical environment, such as working in places without appropriate safety gear (Mona et al., 2019). Many factories are stuffy and safety measures and regulations are not adequately observed, including a lack of gloves for cleaners, helmets for construction workers and fire extinguishers on the premises. Many workers around the world face safety hazards daily. Due to a high rate of poverty and unemployment, both workers and employers regularly participate in compromising safety measures, which account for a high percentage of work-related injuries in low-income countries (ILO, 2012, 2019). Globally, the

ILO reported that up to 2.78 million deaths and 374 million non-fatal work-related injuries are recorded annually. The ILO notes that Asia and the Pacific region account for almost four out of ten deaths from occupational accidents and work-related diseases affecting frequently the vulnerable groups (children, women, people living with disabilities, migrants and minority groups).

The primary occupation in a typical low-income country is agricultural work, which is often not mechanized. While it can be observed that there are usually safety issues in agricultural work, there is insufficient data on the number of deaths or injuries (Cole, 2006; Bhattarai et al., 2016; Prado et al., 2017). A study in rural Nepal reported that 69% of farmers had work-related injuries within a year preceding the survey. Farmers in low-income countries are at high risk of many diseases, including schistosomiasis, sleeping sickness, ascariasis and hookworm because of exposure to disease agents in soil, wastewater/sewage and dirty tools. Workers in the formal sector also face many rights and work condition issues. Working conditions are also about the legal rights and responsibilities of both employees and employers. In many instances, the rights of the workers are not protected. The ILO has often advocated that provision of safety measures for workers should not be merely based on economic considerations. For instance, the right to medical treatment in case of injury should not be negotiable. Migrants are a significant category of the vulnerable group who work in hazardous conditions. There is an increasing prevalence of unwholesome labor practices, including casualization of labor, in which there is no job security and limited obligations from the employer since there is no full legal employment contract with the workers. The majority of casual workers may even be outsourced from a third party. The main concern is about the various impacts of working conditions on human health. Employment and working conditions have been identified as a significant determinant of health. Therefore, there must be interventions to improve working conditions in order to enhance population health.

3.2.1.4 Environment and Living Conditions

The place of residence, neighborhood and living environment constitute another determinant of health. The primary aspect of the living condition is housing/shelter. Poor socio-economic status implies that the individual is likely to live in low-income areas, the majority of which are poorly planned. In a typical Third World country, poor areas are designated as slums or ghettos. A slum is simply an area that is deficient in one or more basic amenities, such as water, bathing and toilet facilities, power supply and necessary sanitation facilities. UN-HABITAT (2003) described a slum household as a group of individuals living under the same roof and lacking one or more of the following conditions: Access to clean water, access to sanitation, secure tenure, the durability of housing and sufficient living area. While six to seven out of ten urban dwellers in SSA live in slums (UN-HABITAT, 2003; Ramin, 2009; Zerbo et al., 2020), the housing situation is even poorer in typical rural areas. Many rural dwellers depend on open defecation and streams for their water supply for daily use. In the absence of potable water, other sources of water, mostly open sources, are utilized. Unfortunately, in such open sources, contamination is common, which makes water-borne diseases highly prevalent. Housing without a toilet or bathroom also makes the environment not conducive for healthy living. Open bathing and toileting are usually the norm, thereby contaminating the environment. For instance, waterlogs facilitate the breeding of mosquitoes, the vector of malaria. Such a favorable environment for mosquito breeding also partly explains the high prevalence of malaria in SSA.

Neighborhoods infested with cockroaches and bugs, visible mold and dampness are not favorable for healthy living (Oudin et al., 2016). Poor housing conditions are associated with respiratory infections, asthma, difficulty in falling asleep and mental health in children (Krieger and Higgins, 2002). In the Global South, sub-standard housing is still obvious in urban slums and rural areas in general. The markers of sub-standard housing are inadequate safe drinking water and water for cleaning, washing and bathing, ineffective waste disposal and the incursion of disease vectors (e.g., insects and rats) (Krieger and Higgins, 2002). Crowding and inadequate ventilation, associated with TB and respiratory infection, are also features of poor housing or neighborhoods (Krieger and Higgins, 2002). A poor neighborhood is also unplanned, and therefore might not be freely accessible in times of emergencies (e.g., flooding and fire). Most urban centers in the Global South are experiencing an influx of people without a commensurate increase in supporting infrastructure. Sastre et al. (2014) noted the problem in the Caribbean Island nations when they observed that most urban cities are overcrowded, which aggravates health problems as a result of worsening living conditions and sanitation.

Another critical dimension of poor living condition is homelessness. Millions of people who are homeless live on the street or under bridges. While those who are living in sub-standard housing lack some basic amenities, those on the street have nothing; they live in deplorable conditions. There are street households with all family members living on one street corner. The children on the street are in the most challenging circumstances and constitute a large category of the street population. The homeless, in particular street children, are frequently at a higher risk of disease. Cumber and Tsoka-Gwegweni (2015) documented the critical health challenges facing street children in Africa. They observed that street kids beg for food and other means of livelihood on the street and sometimes engage in all sorts of menial jobs for survival. They sleep in uncompleted or abandoned structures or open places. Street children (and all the homeless people) are highly vulnerable to risky sexual behavior and abuse, substance abuse, growth and nutritional disorders, physical injuries, violence, water-borne diseases, malaria, respiratory diseases, neglected tropical diseases, mental health issues, reproductive health disorders, and sexually transmitted infections, including HIV/AIDS (Cumber and Tsoka-Gwegweni, 2015). The disease burden among the homeless is more significant than in the general population. Overall poor living conditions produce all sorts of adverse health events.

3.2.1.5 Access to Healthcare and Social Protection

The ease with which people can access healthcare is another major social determinant of health. Inadequate access to healthcare is a big concern around the world. Health is instrumental to daily life and well-being, but still, its availability is very scarce in many regions. A high disease burden and consequent short life expectancy can partially be explained by inadequate access to healthcare. Universality has been a core principle in terms of healthcare; that healthcare should be available to everybody everywhere he/she may be. No one should travel more than 30 minutes or 5 kilometers to access healthcare. As much as possible, all barriers to accessing healthcare should be subjugated by the local authorities. Removing such barriers has been a significant battle for all concerned agencies, but there are still many communities underserved with healthcare. In some communities, modern health facilities are not available at all (Amzat and Razum, 2014b).

Many studies have focused on dimensions of access to healthcare (Obrist et al., 2007; Levesque et al., 2013). The first dimension is whether a health facility is physically available. The reality in developing countries is that there are many communities, especially rural communities, without any kind of health facility. Community members must trek a very long distance or for several hours to access a primary healthcare center. The question of geographical distance between the users and services is paramount. Another dimension is about affordability, which involves both direct and indirect costs involved in accessing healthcare. In many countries in the Global South, healthcare is still accessed through direct expenditure (i.e., out-of-pocket payment). Healthcare is, like any other commodity, accessed on a "cash and carry" basis. The implication of out-of-pocket payment is the lack of or inadequate health insurance coverage. With a high rate of poverty in the developing world, the inability to pay for healthcare costs prevents many households from accessing healthcare. The question of acceptability is paramount in access to healthcare. When healthcare is available, do people accept the services as a means of preventive and curative care? Are there cultural impediments to accessing healthcare? Are there issues relating to cultural beliefs, notions or norms preventing access to healthcare? There continue to be cultural barriers stymieing the utilization of modern healthcare in Africa (Amzat and Razum, 2018a). For instance, in Muslim-dominated areas, many people hold religious beliefs that prevent them from practicing modern family planning.

Although the notion of universal healthcare is gaining momentum, there are still critical gaps in access to healthcare. In South Asia, for example, there are large gaps in essential services, such as skilled birth attendance, routine childhood immunizations and family planning (Zaidi et al., 2017). Uneven coverage of health services translates to lower life expectancy, higher morbidity and undernutrition among those with limited access to healthcare. Like in SSA and the Caribbean, rural areas have fewer functional health services, forcing most people to travel a long distance to access healthcare, coupled with the problem of inadequate transport services, gender norms and low health literacy (Amzat and Grandi, 2011; Zaidi et al., 2017). Out-of-pocket expenditure accounts make up 56% of total health expenditure in Pakistan, 62% in India, 64% in Afghanistan and 67% in Bangladesh (Zaidi et al., 2017). Because of inadequate government health services, there is a heavy reliance on the private health sector. Unfortunately, health insurance in South Asia ranges from 0% of total health expenditure in Afghanistan to 7.7% in India.

An additional major factor relating to access to healthcare in the Global South is inadequate social safety nets. Social protection schemes are meant to provide coverage against risks of poverty, vulnerability, unemployment, sickness, disability and old age, but many social protection schemes are grossly inadequate and ineffectual. The ILO observed that about 73% of the global population is not, or is only partly, covered by social protection. With the exception of Botswana, Swaziland and Bangladesh, social protection schemes are very poor in the Global South, (ILO, 2014; Schmitt, 2019). A major social protection scheme is health insurance. Many countries of the Global South are still debating how to improve health insurance schemes. Inadequate social protection is not just a public health tragedy but also a global health tragedy. Unless there are intensified efforts to improve social protection schemes, access to healthcare and healthy living, in general, will continue to suffer.

3.2.1.6 Lifestyle Factors

Individual behaviors regarding lifestyle are part of micro level social determinants of health. Individual factors are those issues which individuals, through human agency, have some control, although influences at the macro level cannot be discounted. Lifestyle factors include alcohol and drug use, health and illness behavior, dietary, sexual and smoking behavior and physical activities (Amzat and Razum, 2014a). Alcohol and drug use are pervasive problems worldwide. Drug misuse or abuse involving alcohol, tobacco, marijuana and even prescription drugs is prevalent among all age groups and genders (Schulte and Hser, 2014). There is always the possibility of overdose, accidents and mental problems (e.g., antisocial personality disorder, bipolar disorder and anxiety disorders), among other health effects (Schulte and Hser, 2014).

Drug misuse and abuse often start during adolescence, with the effects accruing throughout the lifespan. Significant health effects manifest after repeated or long-term use, often in the later years. Dependence and addiction are usually the immediate effects that adversely affect the social well-being of the users. Uchtenhagen (2004) concisely reported that in Asia, Africa and Latin America, the urban population is increasingly vulnerable to substance abuse problems. The high rates of poverty, as a result of unemployment, social deprivation and low education, contribute to a higher prevalence of substance abuse, including heavy drinking or alcoholism. In most countries of the South, 7 out of 10 street children drink heavily, and alcohol consumption is causally linked to over 60 types of disease and injury (Uchtenhagen, 2004). Another addictive behavior is tobacco smoking, which WHO describes as one of the most dangerous public [global] health threats of the 21st century, killing up to half of its users. Annually, direct smoking kills over 8 million people, while indirectly, through second-hand smoke, 1.2 million non-smokers die (WHO, 2020b). Sadly, around 8 out of 10 smokers live in the Global South, where the burden of tobacco-related morbidity and mortality is heaviest (WHO, 2020b).

Sexual behavior is also a significant component of lifestyle and can make individuals vulnerable to certain diseases, including HIV, which is a global health problem. Wellings et al. (2006) stressed some differences in sexual behavior between the Global South and North: A general trend of late marriage, high prevalence of premarital sex and monogamy are more dominant in the Global North. While condom use has increased globally, it remains relatively low in many countries of the Global South (Wellings et al., 2006). Over the years, condom use has increased in SSA and Latin America, but not enough to significantly impact HIV incidence (Hindin and Fatusi, 2009). The low practice of safe sex, i.e., condom use, can partly explain the higher prevalence of HIV in the Global South, especially in SSA.

The prevalence of obesity, accumulation of excessive body fat that presents risk to health usually defined as a body mass index (BMI) greater than or equal to 30 in adults (WHO, 2020a), is linked to several health problems (including diabetes mellitus, hypertension, respiratory problems and cardiovascular disease), is connected to dietary behavior and physical activities. Bhurosy and Jeewon (2014) noted that obesity is not confined to the Global North but has become a significant health challenge in the Global South, affecting over 100 million people. The authors also observed that lower Body Mass Index (BMI) trends (since the 1980s) are more predominant in African and Southeast Asian countries, but there is an imminent increasing trend. In general, the prevalence of lifestyle diseases is related to health and illness behavior; what people do to retain their perceived health condition and to recuperate when they feel ill. For instance, to maintain good health, physical activities, medical check-ups, a balanced diet and other measures are recommended, but inadequate economic capacity, low education, and limited access to healthcare constrain health and illness behavior.

3.3 Global Determinants of Health (GDH)

Like population health, the determinants of health operate at different levels: Micro (individual), meso (community or society), macro (national) and the super-macro (global). This section will highlight some determinants of health at the global level. Globalization has emerged as a powerful force shaping population health. Chapman (2009) reiterated that globalization as a process affects health systems and the social determinants of health in ways that are sometimes detrimental to health equity between nations. The impacts of globalization can be seen in areas of power, resources, policies and trade, all of which reshape SDH (Chapman, 2009). Irrespective of the direction of the impacts, there are specific determinants known as Global Determinants of Health (GDH). While most of the social determinants described earlier operate at the local or community level, some global processes are consequential for local health conditions. The next few subsections elaborate on some global determinants.

3.3.1 Economic Regulations and Health Markets

A previous section (Section 3.2.1.1) examined poverty as an SDH. Unfortunately, the poverty in the Global South is not unconnected to specific processes at the global level. The idea is not to shift the direct blame of poverty of individuals to another group. The apprehension is about how global economic regulation impacts national economies. In many instances, such impacts are negative, thereby generating poverty and limited access to healthcare for the weak and vulnerable. Global economic regulations come with concerns and opportunities, but more concerns for the weak and vulnerable. For instance, while there is increasing global trade for health services through the globalization of healthcare (see Section 2.3.3), vulnerable populations are mere onlookers, i.e., without active participation that would improve overall population health. Medical tourism is for the affluent, because it comes with exorbitant costs beyond the reach of ordinary citizens of the Global South. The globalization of healthcare is not based on charity or aid; it is typically for-profit and foreign exchange.

There have been pressures on a global scale for the provision of healthcare as a right to all individuals through the provision of adequate health infrastructures. Sometimes, the move is contradictory to some economic policies, such as deregulation, structural adjustment programs (SAP) and other liberalization policies. Deregulation policies, whereby limiting government regulations allows market competition among key players, have been popularized over the years. Government regulations are sometimes stiff and coercive. The argument for deregulation has always been that the government should create opportunities and fertile environments in which players can operate. Another view is that opening the market will attract means that more investment opportunities, subsequently enhancing economic growth. The critical question is: Can deregulation also work in the health sector, especially in the Global South? In countries with a high poverty rate, can deregulation help the vulnerable in improving healthcare access? To be clear, the move toward deregulation has been highly controversial and might not be a core solution to the health crisis in low-income countries.

Most states have embraced structural adjustment programs in the Global South. The core aspect of SAPs is the reduction in subsidy and public expenditure. The global capitalist system, through the World Bank (WB) and International Monetary Fund (IMF), dictates the terms of SAPs, which include the drive to make the developing economies more market-oriented, i.e., promoting deregulation and reducing governments' profligacy (expressed in terms of excessive charity spending) (Amzat and Olutayo, 2009; Forster et al., 2020). Many scholars have implicated SAPs in decline in the African economy and thereby responsible for the suffering facing the rural and urban poor, women, children and other vulnerable groups (Onimode, 1992). Thomson et al. (2017) explained the problem of global economic regulations focusing on the impact of SAPs on healthcare. The study submitted that SAPs have adverse effects on health spending and, consequently, on health systems (Forster et al., 2020). Reductions in government spending affect health infrastructure and, invariably, also the quantity and quality of care available to vulnerable populations in the Global South. The first apparent consequential manifestation is the reduction in the fiscal space in which healthcare systems operate. The glaring effects reflect in weak responses to epidemics, such as to HIV in SSA (Thomson et al., 2017).

In addition, Thomson et al. (2017) highlight that global deregulation and SAPs undermine access to affordable healthcare and the worst consequences are felt among the social determinants of health, such as income, education and social protection schemes, especially in the Global South. Since there have been heavy criticisms of SAPs, the WB and IMF replaced its enhanced structural adjustment facilities with a new one called Poverty Reduction Strategy and Growth Facilities (PRGF) (Bretton Woods Project, 2003). Low-income Global South still swims against the same tide as the policies, and interest rate and repayment conditions are the same. The unfavorable conditionalities are still attached to loans (Bretton Woods Project, 2003; Forster et al., 2020). Unfortunately, low-income countries are perpetual borrowers. The conditionalities cannot be the same and the partners would expect a different result.

Imbalanced trade and trade regulations are problematic, but it is certain economic schemes, imposed with hypothetically "good" intentions, which in the short and long run are detrimental to general well-being and healthcare. The reason for the failure of the imposed schemes is that social goals are often relegated for fiscal targets (Kentikelenis et al., 2015). Another cause is that population health is not usually a significant consideration of such economic regulations. While in the beginning, the consequences were regarded as "teething problems", unfortunately, the problems, now assuming a magnitude of a global problem, have persisted for several decades. The poor state of health infrastructure in the Global South is not just a function of social determinants of health at the macro level but also at the super-macro level, herein referred to as GDH.

3.3.2 Global Flow of People and Information

A major consequence of globalization is the increased flow of humans, facilitated by developments in transportation and information systems. The compression of time and space are core aspects of globalization, and they imply that messages are transmittable to a far distance within the twinkle of an eye and people (through modern transportation) can cover a vast distance within a few hours. Via the flow of people across international borders (for resettlement, study, trade, tourism), global mobility is increasing. Global mobility is also about global trade involving the movement of goods, services and capital. Global trade patterns will inevitably impact many of the known determinants of health, including employment, social capital and education (Smith and Henefeld, 2018).

Global mobility negatively impacts global health through communicable diseases. Globalization has been implicated in the outbreaks of infectious diseases, including severe acute respiratory syndrome (SARS), HIV, Ebola and COVID-19. The 2014–2016 Ebola outbreak affected several countries beyond Africa, leading to over 28,000 cases and 11,310 deaths (WHO, 2016b). Ebola reached Nigeria during this pandemic when a traveler entered the country on a flight from Liberia, putting the entire country in national panic (Amzat and Razum, 2018b). It took some drastic national efforts and international partnerships to stop the Ebola outbreaks (2014–2016).

Human-to-human transmission is significant in the spread of infectious diseases. Without the global flow of people, most infectious diseases would remain confined to the area of origin. Global mobility has also been implicated in the spread of HIV/AIDS concerning the risky sexual behavior of migrants. HIV/AIDS has also been globalized. Therefore, globalization facilitates the rapid dissemination of HIV infection across national borders (Coovadia and Hadingham, 2005). For instance, Docquier et al. (2014) discussed the role of international migration in the spread of HIV in SSA. Historically, migration to, and consequent return from, some high-prevalence areas accounted for an increase in HIV prevalence in many SSA countries. Docquier et al. (2014) observed that in many African countries, emigration to high prevalence countries increases infection rates at origin throughout the 1990s. However, globalization also ensured global partnerships in the fight against HIV/AIDS, giving the developing world more access to funding and the technologies required to fight the disease.

Thus, the impacts of globalization, in terms of the flow of people and information, are not always negative. While globalization can facilitate the spread of infectious diseases, it can also facilitate quick response to outbreaks, as resources can be more quickly mobilized and channeled to curtail the spread. Through information technology and communication (ICT), people can be informed within minutes to prepare for any outbreak. Responding to an outbreak requires global cooperation for adequate geographical coverage, resource mobilization and surveillance (Huynen et al., 2005). In this light, global health bodies, including the WHO, are gaining more relevance by providing leadership in the mitigation of outbreaks. For instance, during the SARS and Ebola outbreaks, the WHO provided global alerts, geographically specific travel advisories and monitoring (Huynen et al., 2005). Jani et al. (2019) observed that there has been a gradual decline in the prevalence of infectious diseases in the Third World due to global partnerships and technology transfer, occasioned by the globalization process. In short, the global flow of people and information is a major global determinant of health.

3.3.3 *Global Culture and Health*

There is an emerging global culture. The concept of a global culture might sound, to some sociologists and anthropologists, like an over-ambitious grand narrative. Such an impression is because of postmodern ideology, which dwells more on mini-narratives and activation of differences. Also, globalization is not about homogenization; at least in its real sense of uniformity. What is true, however, is the drive toward harmonization, not homogenization, and differences are recognized and respected even in harmony. There are diversities in harmony, a kind of gradual acculturation and cultural exchange across the world. The idea of global culture is not about one heavenly way of life; it is about harmonization of standard values and best practices. Therefore, global culture signifies certain cultural denominators that are generally valued and respected, cutting across all borders and territories. There are global cultural precepts of peace, success, respect, virtues, rights, partnerships/cooperation and love, among others. Global culture also goes beyond virtues—it can be observed in technology, education and policies, among others.

Cultural globalization is the formation and transmission of ideas, values and meanings, which intensify interconnectedness among different cultures and populations (see Manfred, 2005; Sarthak, 2006; Soborski, 2012). Global culture marks the gradual formation of shared values, norms, knowledge and practices around the globe. The gradual emergence of global culture is historically traced to colonialism, international or global trade, media, global mobility and development of ICT. All of these historical antecedents have led to cultural diffusion or gradual cultural exchange. Particularly noteworthy are developments in the media, especially the visual media, which have led to the propagation of cultural values and materials across the globe. Mobility is also a significant factor responsible for cultural globalization. People learn and unlearn through social contacts and migration, leading to some form of cultural refinement, modification and sophistication. The circulation of cultures (including languages) has broadened human social relations and, consequently, holds implications for human health.

The reality of global culture does not nullify the local but often places it within a global landscape (Airhihenbuwa, 2010). The co-existence of local and global culture is not entirely in terms of comparison but complementarity, or what Airhihenbuwa (2010: p. 52) called the "examination of the location of the local and its global vantage point". Understanding the local health condition is always in comparison with the global standard; therefore, global culture is not about the imposition of certain predetermined precepts. Importantly, respecting the local narrative does not preclude sifting norms that favor the risks of various diseases. For instance, certain gender norms in SSA and the Middle East adversely affect maternal health, risk of HIV and mental health. Some cultural norms, through the understanding of their impacts, have also been designated as harmful (Amzat and Razum, 2018a). There is a global movement to sift such cultural norms. Globalization is transformation; therefore, the formation of global culture is (sometimes) corrective, instrumental and interventional. There are many global principles and precepts developed through thorough scientific thinking, which often form the basis of implementation or interventional research or policy.

On the other side, global culture is (sometimes) perceived as coercive and disruptive, hence, there is the possibility of resistance to change. There is always the thinking that every individual should be co-opted into the global culture. Some critical areas have always been food habits, technological dependence and lifestyle in particular; all of which have health consequences. The presumption is that global standards exact pressure on local communities, thereby disrupting lifestyle and community arrangements. Irrespective of the presumption, there is an emerging global culture, which, without controversy, influences population health. Global culture is thus a global determinant of health. As previously argued, globalization is a contextual factor of health.

3.3.4 Environmental Change and Challenges

A previous section (Section 3.2.1.4) examined living conditions as a social determinant of health. SDHs are related to the environment, i.e., where people are born, grow up, play and work. The focus on living conditions, addressed at the micro level, is also a component of environmental issues. The argument here will focus more on issues on a global scale and how global ecological conditions affect overall human health. Environmental issues, both natural and built, have always been a major concern in global health. The area of environmental health addresses all sorts of issues of physical, biological and chemical factors external to an individual but impacting human existence and behavior. The topic of environmental health is vast, including many issues, such as sanitation and waste management, toxic and vector control, air quality, biosafety, climate change, pollution (air, noise, water), food safety, disaster preparedness and housing, among others. A close look points to the fact that some issues tend to take a global dimension and are better addressed at the global level.

The WHO (2016a) estimates that approximately 12.6 million deaths can be attributed annually to unhealthy environments (Africa: 2.2 million; Southeast Asia: 3.8 million; Western Pacific: 3.5 million; and Europe: 1.4 million). WHO (2016a) identified common environmental risks, such as air, water and soil pollution, chemical exposures, climate change and ultraviolet radiation, that account for more than 100 types of diseases (including cancer and asthma), injuries and disasters (such as droughts and famines). The environment is inextricably linked to human health. One significant global dimension is about greenhouse gasses emissions responsible for the depletion of the ozone layer, which is globally consequential for human health. The Global South has a lower emissions rate but shares the consequence. It is because of this burden that The Global Health Council (2013) observed that the "world around us" has severe implications for human health. The Global Health Council (2013) and Ritchie and Rosser (2019) stressed the global concerns about the environment with specific points, including:

1. The Global South (primarily low-income populations) is disproportionately exposed to environmental perils like pollution from local [and sometimes, international] power plants or waste treatment sites. The environmental situation translates to and explains health inequalities within the global divide. The Global South also serves as a dumping site for outdated and environmentally dangerous materials, with adverse implications for health.
2. There are still over 1.1 billion people without access to clean water. Water is central to human livelihood; therefore, lack or inadequate access (to clean water) signifies deplorable livelihood. Regions with high estimates without access to clean water include East Asia and the Pacific (133 million), SSA (326 million), and South Asia (133 million).

3. As of 2015, more than 2.5 billion people in developing countries had very minimal access to improved/modern sanitation facilities: (East and the Pacific (519 million), Latin America and the Caribbean (106 million), South Asia (963 million) and SSA (705 million). A significant manifestation of lack of improved sanitation is open defecation, which is hazardous for human existence.

4. Environmental factors (including unsafe water and air pollution) are responsible for 1/3 of the burden of childhood diseases. This partly accounts for high childhood morbidity and mortality in the Global South.

5. The world is much concerned about climate change primarily as a result of ozone layer depletion as a result of greenhouse gasses emission. The highly industrial world (including the United States, China, Germany, the United Kingdom and India) is culpable of global environmental crisis.

6. During the last century, population growth has mirrored the growth of greenhouse gasses responsible for climate change. If current trends do not change, the global population will hit 9.2 billion in 2050. The growth is with enormous consequences on the environment and, consequently, human health.

3.3.5 *Health Technology Transfer and Exchange*

A previous section (Section 2.3.4) described globalization of health technology as a major face of globalization of health. Globalization ensures collaboration and partnership in terms of exchange of technical know-how. The inadequate health technology has been a significant impediment to access to quality healthcare in the Global South. The extent of globalization of health technology, primarily focusing on underserved areas, might improve health indicators. It has been observed that global health heavily relies on humans (biomedical scientists and public health workers) and materials (equipment) to solve health problems, both at the local and global levels (Harris and Tanner, 2000). Harris and Tanner (2000) noted that many countries in the Global South face several obstacles to healthcare, including limited financial, material and human resources, scientific isolation, insufficient technical training and research tools and inadequate scientific information. There is a need for partnerships for the transfer of up-to-date and sustainable technologies and other materials necessary to facilitate quality healthcare.

Transfer of sustainable and compatible technology can improve health in underserved areas. It is not always about sophisticated technology, especially in rural areas. Equipment can only be useful if it is modified and simplified to suit the local condition (Harris and Tanner, 2000). The fact remains that technology-transfer gaps do exist, ranging from a complete lack of equipment to grossly inadequate equipment. The implication is that investment and capacity-building are urgently required to promote the production of health products to fill the existing gaps in the Global South. The best form of support to fill the gap is also to encourage local production of such health products. Local production is a sure way of promoting accessibility and affordability of health products. The move might involve the transfer of license agreements and technical materials. One crucial area of technology transfer involves research and development. There are many international or global research centers across the Global South, mostly supported by the organizations in the North. This is a way of building local capacity to address health challenges, which will invariably lessen the global burden.

Historically, modern healthcare has been a product of the Global North that has been transferred to the Global South. Over the years, modern healthcare has often proven superior to traditional medicine in addressing global health challenges. In SSA, colonialism marked the introduction of modern healthcare systems and the relegation of traditional healthcare. Since the independence of most African countries in the 1950s and 1960s, modern healthcare has been the mainstay in the prevention and control of health problems. The region has also struggled vehemently to update its technology in line with modern health challenges. Health indicators generally reflect the level of technical know-how, political will and financial investment in national healthcare. The health indicators in the Global South also partially mirror the inadequate technology transfer and exchange from the Global North.

3.3.6 Global Politics and Policies of Healthcare

The politics and policies of healthcare at the global level are additional global determinants of health. A previous section examined the globalization of healthcare policies and efforts in the control of diseases. The focus in this section is on how such policies and politics are major global determinants of health. Politics is, simply put, about who gets what, where, when and how. It concerns regions of the South and North, different component units (countries), inequalities (the global divide), prioritization (what diseases should be prioritized and why) and quantities and types of resources available. In the same way, individuals prioritize at the household level, and nations make decisions about the allocation of health resources nationally, global decisions are made at the global level. As resources, material and non-material, are finite, priorities must be set. The starting point is agenda setting, defining what constitutes a health condition of global significance and what resources are available to tackle such conditions. The global health governance bodies, including the WHO and other numerous affiliates, administer the main politics and policies. The primary concern is about the representation of interests: What is the power relation of the component units (Member States)? Is it balanced or not? Are certain stakeholders powerful enough to direct the course of action against the will of others?

Globalization has significantly shaped the politics of healthcare. For instance, in terms of priority setting, the focus on HIV, malaria and TB is a result of global politics. The diseases (HIV, Malaria and TB) with a low burden in the North have the propensity to become a global pandemic. The fear of epidemics is a significant concern, which leads to the securitization agenda of the North. Sparke (2020) corroborated the preceding assertion about global health politics that the epidemiological situation of possible globalized outbreaks is a significant factor shaping the global health policies. For instance, the malaria problem appears as one of the MDGs with a specific target to reduce the burden of the disease among the affected population to halt a possible re-emergence in the North. It is in the same vein that 2001–2010 was declared as the United Nations' (UN) decade to roll back malaria. Sparke (2020) further observed that, beyond the global health security concern, politics is also about how to extend drug access and health services to the world's poor (especially in low-income countries). Sparke (2020) further noted that the political gesture is often "tied to ideational globalisation through a humanitarian concern with globalising human health rights".

While acknowledging the political gesture of support, there is also a problematic politics of neoliberalization implicated in the crisis of the health system in the Global South. It is like the gesture of giving with the right hand and retrieving with the left hand. Neoliberalization is a double-edged sword: Sharp and soft at the same time. It is sharp enough to create global health vulnerabilities/problems through structural violence and soft enough to steer the delivery of global health responses (see Sparke, 2020). The sword is soft enough to declare a global health plan with lofty health goals, and sharp enough to expand the global pharmaceuticals, often draining the meager resources of the poor back to the North. Unfortunately, despite the neoliberal tragedy, there are shortages and gradual cuts in global health funding (evident in the former president Trump's 2017 budget) (see Sparke, 2020), which would affect meeting the global health goals.

3.4 Summary

- Health is contextual in the sense that there are myriad factors, regarded as social determinants of health (SDH) influencing it. Some of those factors even constitute the causes of diseases because they exact direct influence on the likelihood of ill-health.
- Globalization is another dominant social reality, which has been implicated as a significant determinant of health. The un-equalizing process of globalization manifests in the poor social determinants and the exploitative global determinants of health in the Global South.
- Understanding the social context or determinants of health is a prerequisite to understanding population health, whether in the Global South or North. The SDH are responsible for health inequalities, especially within the country and between countries.
- Many countries of the Global South are still confronted with traditional risks of infectious diseases, largely as a result of living conditions related to poverty and inadequate infrastructures (such as water and power supplies) compounded by limited access to healthcare and social protection.
- The determinants of health operate at different levels: Micro (individual), meso (community or society), macro (national) and the super-macro (global). Globalization has emerged as a powerful force shaping population health. Globalization as a process also affects health systems and other social determinants of health in ways that are sometimes detrimental to health equity between nations.
- The global determinants of health examined include economic regulation and health markets, the global flow of people and information, global culture and health, environmental change and challenges, health technology transfer and exchange, and global politics and policies of healthcare, among others.
- In general, social and global determinants of health must be mitigated to improve population health on a global scale.

Critical Thinking Questions

- How are individuals faring in terms of health status and access to healthcare in your community?
- What four factors do you consider the most significant of social determinants of health in your locality?
- How does globalization influence any four social determinants of health in your locality?
- Liberalization and deregulation policies are major features of capitalism, which is a global socio-political system. How do such capitalist policies influence healthcare policies and strategies on a global scale?
- People and information are unstoppable in this globalized era. Discuss how this flow (of people and information) portends some positive and negative consequences for global health. How is the global flow of people and information a major global determinant of health?
- Why does the "world around us" in terms of environmental concerns constitute a global determinant of health? Why is the Global South carrying the heaviest burden of such environmental concerns?
- To what extent can you argue that the health indicators in the Global South mirror the inadequate technology transfer and exchange from the Global North? Does the Global South have to wait for such technology?

Suggested Readings

- Amzat, J., and Razum, O. (2014). Social determinants/context of health. In: *Medical sociology in Africa.* Cham, Switzerland: Springer International Publishing. DOI 10.1007/978-3-319-03986-2_4. The chapter discusses in details the social determinants of health in Africa.
- CSDH. (2008). Closing the gap in a generation: Health equity through action on the social determinants of health. Final Report of the Commission on Social Determinants of Health. World Health Organization. A World Health Organization's document detailing the social determinants of health.
- Cockerham, G., and Cockerham, W. (2010). *Health and globalization.* Cambridge: Polity. The book examines the impact of global processes (such as pollution, modernization and technological change) on health.
- Collin, J., and Lee, K. (2005). *Global change and health.* New York: McGraw Hill. The books argues that determinants of health circumvent, undermine or are oblivious to the territorial boundaries of states and discusses how global changes affect human health on a global scale.
- Labonté, R., and Arne Ruckert, A. (2019). Globalization as a "determinant of the determinants of health". In: *Health equity in a globalizing era: Past challenges, future prospects.*Oxford: Oxford University Press. DOI:10.1093/oso/9780198835356.003.0002. The chapter relies on two different frameworks to unpack globalization processes as meta-determinants of health inequities within and between nations.
- Lee, K. (2003). *Health impacts of globalization: Towards global governance.* London: Palgrave Macmillan. The book relies on specific case studies to discuss the impact of globalization on health.
- Forster, T., Kentikelenis, A. E., Stubbs, T. H., and King, L. P. (2020) Globalization and health equity: The impact of structural adjustment programs on developing countries. *Soc Sci Med.,* 267:112496. doi: 10.1016/j.socscimed.2019.112496. The chapter provides a deeper understanding of international-level health determinants: Economic globalization and the organizations that spread market-oriented policies to the developing world.

References

Airhihenbuwa, C. O. (2010). Culture matters in global health. *The European Health Psychologist, 12,* 52–55.

Amzat, J., & Grandi, G. (2011). Gender context of personalism in bioethics. *Developing World Bioethics, 11*(3), 136–145.

Amzat, J., & Olutayo, O. A. (2009). Nigeria, capitalism and the question of equity. *The Anthropologist, 11*(4), 239–246.

Amzat, J., & Razum, O. (2014a). Health and illness behaviour. In *Medical Sociology in Africa.* Cham, Switzerland: Springer International Publishing. doi: 10.1007/978-3-319-03986-2_3.

Amzat, J., & Razum, O. (2014b). Social determinants/context of health. In *Medical Sociology in Africa.* Cham, Switzerland: Springer International Publishing. doi: 10.1007/978-3-319-03986-2_4.

Amzat, J., & Razum, O. (2018a). African culture and health. *Towards a Sociology of Health Discourse in Africa.* Cham, Switzerland: Springer International Publishing. doi: 10.1007/978-3-319-61672-8_5.

Amzat, J., & Razum, O. (2018b). Healthcare emergencies in Africa: The case of Ebola in Nigeria. In *Towards a Sociology of Health Discourse in Africa.* Cham, Switzerland: Springer International Publishing. doi: 10.1007/978-3-319-61672-8_10.

Appleton, S. (2000). Education and health at the household level in sub-Saharan Africa. In CID Working Paper no. 33, Explaining African Economic Growth Performance Conference Series, Cambridge, UK: Center for International Development at Harvard University.

Bhattarai, D., Singh, S.B., Baral, D., Sah, R. B., Budhathoki, S. S., & Pokharel, P. K. (2016). Work-related injuries among farmers: A cross-sectional study from rural Nepal. *Journal of Occupational Medicine and Toxicology*, *11*, 48. doi: 10.1186/s12995-016-0137-2.

Bhurosy, T., & Jeewon, R. (2014). Overweight and obesity epidemic in developing countries: A problem with diet, physical activity, or socioeconomic status? *The Scientific World Journal*, 964236. doi: 10.1155/2014/964236.

Bretton Woods Project (2003). *Poverty Reduction Strategy Papers (PRSPs): A Rough Guide*. London: Bretton Woods Project.

Chapman, A. R. (2009). Globalization, human rights, and the social determinants of health. *Bioethics*, *23*(2), 97–111.

Cole, D. (2006). Understanding the links between agriculture and health: Occupational health hazards of agriculture. In *International Food Policy Research Institute, Focus 13, Brief 8 of 16*. Washington, DC: International Food Policy Research Institute.

Coovadia, H. M., & Hadingham, J. (2005). HIV/AIDS: Global trends, global funds and delivery bottlenecks. *Globalization and Health*, *1*, 13. doi: 10.1186/1744-8603-1-13.

Commission on Social Determinants of Health [CSDH] (2008). *Closing the Gap in a Generation: Health Equity through Action on the Social Determinants of Health. Final Report of the Commission on Social Determinants of Health*. Geneva: World Health Organization.

Cumber, S., & Tsoka-Gwegweni, J. (2015). The health profile of street children in Africa: A literature review. *Journal of Public Health in Africa*, *6*(2). doi: 10.4081/jphia.2015.566.

Docquier, F., Vasilakis, C. & Munsi, D. T. (2014). International migration and the propagation of HIV in sub-Saharan Africa. *Journal of Health Economics*, *35*, 20–33. doi: 10.1016/j.jhealeco.2014.01.004.

Donkin, A., Goldblatt, P., Allen, J., Nathanson, V. & Marmot, M. (2017). Global action on the social determinants of health. *BMJ Global Health*, *3*, e000603. doi: 10.1136/bmjgh-2017-000603.

Forster, T., Kentikelenis, A. E., Stubbs, T. H. & King, L. P. (2020) Globalization and health equity: The impact of structural adjustment programs on developing countries. *Social Science and Medicine*, *267*, 112496. doi: 10.1016/j.socscimed.2019.112496.

Georges, D., Kreft, D. & Doblhammer, G. (2018). The contextual and household contribution to individual health status in Germany: What is the role of gender and migration background? In Doblhammer G. & Gumà J. (Eds.), *A Demographic Perspective on Gender, Family and Health in Europe* (pp. 193–232). Cham: Springer.

Goodman, R. A., Bunnell, R. & Posner, S. F. (2014). What is "community health"? Examining the meaning of an evolving field in public health. *Preventive Medicine*, *67*(Suppl 1), S58–61.

Graham, H. (2004). Social determinants and their unequal distribution: Clarifying policy understandings. *Milbank Quarterly*, *82*, 101–24. doi: 10.1111/j.0887-378X.2004.00303.x.

Grant, U. (2005). *Health and Poverty Linkages*. Chronic Poverty Research Centre.

Harris, E., & Tanner, M. (2000). Health technology transfer. *BMJ*, *321*(7264), 817–820. doi: 10.1136/bmj.321.7264.817

Hindin, M., & Fatusi, A. O. (2009). Adolescent sexual and reproductive health in developing countries: An overview of trends and interventions. *International Perspectives on Sexual and Reproductive Health*, *35*(2), 58–62.

Huynen, M. M., Martens, P. & Hilderink, H. B. (2005). The health impacts of globalization: A conceptual framework. *Globalization and Health*, *1*, 14. doi: 10.1186/1744-8603-1-14

International Labour Organization (ILO) (2012). *Estimating the Economic Costs of Occupational Injuries and Illnesses in Developing Countries: Essential Information for Decision-Makers*. Geneva: International Labour Office.

ILO (2014). *World Social Protection Report. Building Economic Recovery, Inclusive Development and Social Justice*. Geneva: ILO.

ILO (2019). *Safety and Health at Work*. Geneva: International Labour Office. www.ilo.org/global/topics/safety-and-health-at-work/lang--en/index.htm. Accessed on August 5, 2019.

Islam, M. M. (2019) Social determinants of health and related inequalities: Confusion and implications. *Frontiers Public Health*, *7*, 11. doi: 10.3389/fpubh.2019.00011.

Jani, V. J., Joshi, N. A. & Mehta, D. J. (2019). Globalization and health: An empirical investigation. *Global Social Policy*, 1–18.

Kacowicz, A. M. (2007). Globalization, poverty, and the North-South divide. *International Studies Review*, *9*(4), 565–580.

Kentikelenis, A. E., Stubbs, T. H. & King, L. P. (2015). Structural adjustment and public spending on health: Evidence from IMF programs in low-income countries. *Social Science and Medicine*, *126*, 169–176. doi: 10.1016/j.socscimed.2014.12.027.

Krieger, J., & Higgins, D. L. (2002). Housing and health: Time again for public health action. *American Journal of Public Health*, *92*, 758–768. doi: 10.2105/AJPH.92.5.758.

Levesque, J., Harris, M. F. & Russell, G. (2013). Patient-centered access to health care: Conceptualising access at the interface of health systems and populations. *International Journal for Equity in Health*, *11*,12–18.

MacQueen, K. M., McClellan, E., Metzger, D. S., Kegeles, S., Strauss, R. P., Scotti, R., Blanchard, L. & Trotter II, R. T. (2001). What is community? An evidence-based definition for participatory public health. *American Journal of Public Health*, *91*, 1929–1938.

Manfred, B. S. (2005). Ideologies of globalization. *Journal of Political Ideologies*, *10*(1), 11–30. doi: 10.1080/1356931052000310263.

Mona, G. G., Chimbari, M. J. & Hongoro, C. (2019). A systematic review on occupational hazards, injuries and diseases among police officers worldwide: Policy implications for the South African Police Service. *Journal of Occupational Medicine and Toxicology*, *14*, 2. doi: 10.1186/s12995-018-0221-x.

Musaiger, A. O., Hassan, A. S. & Obeid, O. (2011). The paradox of nutrition-related diseases in the Arab Countries: The need for action. *International Journal of Environmental Research and Public Health*, *8*, 3637–3671. doi:10.3390/ijerph8093637.

Obrist, B., Iteba, N., Lengeler, C., Makemba, A., Mshana, C., Nathan, R., Alba, S., Dillip, A., Hetzel, M. W., Mayumana, I., Schulze, A. & Mshinda, H. (2007). Access to health care in contexts of livelihood insecurity: A framework for analysis and action *PLoS Medicine*, *4*(10), e308. doi: 10.1371/journal.pmed.0040308.

Onimode, B. (1992). *A Future for Africa: Beyond the Politics of Adjustment*. London: Earthscan.

Oudin, A., Richter, J. C., Taj, T., Al-Nahar, L. & Jakobsson, K. (2016). Poor housing conditions in association with child health in a disadvantaged immigrant population: A cross-sectional study in Rosengård, Malmö, Sweden. *BMJ Open*, *6*(1), e007979. doi: 10.1136/bmjopen-2015-007979.

Prado, J. B., Mulay, P. R., Kasner, E. J., Bojes, H. K. & Calvert, G. M. (2017). Acute pesticide-related illness among farmworkers: Barriers to reporting to public health authorities. *Journal of Agromedicine*, *22*(4), 395–405. doi: 10.1080/1059924X.2017.1353936.

Ramin, B. (2009). Slums, climate change and human health in sub-Saharan Africa. *Bulletin of the World Health Organization*, *87*, 886–886. doi: 10.2471/BLT.09.073445.

Ritchie, H., & Roser, M. (2019). Water Use and Sanitation. Published online at *OurWorldInData.org*. https://ourworldindata.org/water-use-sanitation [Online Resource]. Accessed on August 9, 2019.

Sarthak, A. (2006). *Transport, Geography, Tribalism*. London: Aditua Publications.

Sastre, F., Rojas, P., Cyrus, E., De La Rosa, M. & Khoury, A. H. (2014). Improving the health status of Caribbean people: Recommendations from the triangulating on health equity summit. *Global Health Promotion*, *21*(3), 19–28. doi: 10.1177/1757975914523455.

Schmitt, C. (2019). The coverage of social protection in the Global South. *International Journal of Social Welfare*, 1–14. doi: 10.1111/ijsw.12374.

Schulte, M. T., & Hser, Y. I. (2014). Substance use and associated health conditions throughout the lifespan. *Public Health Reviews*, *35*(2). https://web-beta.archive.org/web/20150206061220/http://www.publichealthreviews.eu/upload/pdf_files/14/00_Schulte_Hser.pdf.

Smith, R., & Henefeld, J. (2018). Globalization, trade and health economics. *Health Economics*. doi: 10.1093/acrefore/9780190625979.013.35.

Soborski, R. (2012). Globalization and ideology: A critical review of the debate. *Journal of Political Ideologies*, *17*(3), 323–346. doi: 10.1080/13569317.2012.716632.

Solar, O., & Irwin, A. (2010). A conceptual framework for action on the social determinants of health. In *Social Determinants of Health Discussion Paper 2 (Policy and Practice)*. Geneva: World Health Organization.

Sparke, M. (2020). Globalization and the politics of global health. McInnes, C., Lee, K. & Youde, J. (Eds.), *The Oxford Handbook of Global Health Policy*. New York: Oxford University Press.

Telfair, J., & Shelton, T. L. (2012). Educational attainment as a social determinant of health. *North Carolina Medical Journal, 73*(5), 358–365.

The Global Health Council (2013). Linking global health with the globe: Environmental health. https://globalhealth.org/linking-global-health-with-the-globe-environmental-health/. Accessed on August 30, 2019.

Thomson, M., Kentikelenis, A., & Stubbs, T. (2017). Structural adjustment programmes adversely affect vulnerable populations: A systematic-narrative review of their effect on child and maternal health. *Public Health Reviews, 38*, 13. doi: 10.1186/s40985-017-0059-2.

Uchtenhagen, A. (2004). Substance use problems in developing countries. *Bulletin of the World Health Organization, 82*(9), 639–718.

UNESCO (2010). *EFA Global Monitoring Report: Reaching the Marginalized*. Paris: UNESCO and Oxford University Press.

United Nations Human Settlements Programme (UN-HABITAT) (2003). *The Challenge of Slums: Global Report on Human Settlements*. London: Earthscan Publications Ltd.

Vandemoortele, J., & Delamonica, E. (2002). Education vaccine against HIV/AIDS. *Current Issues in Comparative Education, 3*(1), 6–13.

Wellings, K., Collumbien, M., Slaymaker, E., Singh, S., Hodges, Z., Patel, D. & Bajos, N. (2006). Sexual behaviour in context: A global perspective. *Lancet,* 11, *368*(9548), 1706–28.

World Health Organization (WHO) (1986). A discussion document on the concept and principles of health promotion. *Health Promotion, 1*(1), 73–76.

WHO (2016a). An estimated 12.6 million deaths each year are attributable to unhealthy environments. www.who.int/news-room/detail/15-03-2016-an-estimated-12-6-million-deaths-each-year-are-attributable-to-unhealthy-environments. Accessed on August 12, 2019.

WHO (2016b). Situation report: Ebola virus disease. http://apps.who.int/iris/bitstream/10665/208883/1/ebolasitrep_10Jun2016_eng.pdf?ua=1. Accessed on August 12, 2019.

WHO (2020a). Obesity and overweight: Key facts. www.who.int/news-room/fact-sheets/detail/obesity-and-overweight. Accessed on August 12, 2020.

WHO (2020b). Tobacco: Key facts. www.who.int/news-room/fact-sheets/detail/tobacco. Accessed on August 11, 2020.

Zaidi, S., Saligram, P., Syed, A., Egbert, S. & Kabir, S. (2017). Expanding access to healthcare in South Asia. *BMJ, 357*, j1645.

Zerbo, A., Delgado, R. C., & Gonzál, P. A. (2020). Vulnerability and everyday health risks of urban informal settlements in Sub-Saharan Africa. *Global Health Journal*. doi: 10.1016/j.glohj.2020.04.003.

4 Globalization and Health

A Theoretical Lens

4.1 Introduction

It is important to situate the discussion of globalization and health within certain theoretical precepts. This will provide a guide to further understanding the mechanisms or correlation between globalization and health, impacts of globalization on health and health on globalization, especially in the Global South. The understanding of globalization is often premised on the notion of global inequalities. Global regions are divided into high-, middle- and low-income countries. All three blocs are active players, but with differential levels of participation occasioned by differential capacities (Wallerstein, 2004). The rich countries are generally in the Global North while the others, middle- and low-income countries, are in the Global South. The relationships between the different blocs have been that of cooperation, conflict and consensus. Cooperation refers to partnerships in tackling issues of common concern around the world. This is why there are global health goals or targets set to be achieved within a set period. There were Millennium Development Goals (MDGs) between 2000 and 2015, and then there are Sustainable Development Goals (SDGs) between 2015 and 2030, which every nation set to achieve with some form of global cooperation. There is a fundamental consensus on the need to improve population health in terms of health goals and rights. The degree of actualization of the set health goals differs from one region to another.

Conflict is common in the global health arena. Tension and suspicion sometimes exist around health goals and the methodologies required to improve population health. Accusations might be exchanged in the face of health tragedies because of unfavorable policies and practices. Instead of being viewed as providing benefits, partnerships are sometimes perceived as disadvantaging the weak. There are conspiracy theories of western ulterior motives to worsen the health condition in the Global South further. For example, there is no consensus among the highly industrialized countries to minimize greenhouse gas emissions and commit commensurate funds to tackle the problem. While the problem affects all nations, the Global South suffers a greater burden from industrial emissions and waste (Ritchie and Rosser, 2019). Another argument is that health crises may generate differential interest and benefits for some players, for example, global pharmaceutical companies potentially profiting from disease outbreaks in low-income countries. Another point of contention is whether the Global South carries its equal share of responsibility in population health. Most low-income nations have not been able to provide the appropriate health governance necessary, especially at the national level, to achieve the desired health goals.

The preceding highlights some of the prevailing arguments from the different theoretical approaches to globalization and health. In contrast, a typical materialist approach focuses more on the prevailing conflicts and profiteering in the globalization process, and how that impacts significantly the health of populations in disadvantaged nations in terms of the indicators of

DOI: 10.4324/9781003247975-4

population healthcare. The primary materialist assumption is that global inequalities lead to global health inequalities. The works of Immanuel Wallerstein can be adapted to reflect a typical materialist approach to explaining global health. The Wallerstein approach examines the historical antecedents, such as colonialism, in the build-up to the current global disparities. A structuralist approach examines levels of responsibility and how structural arrangement influences population health. Having highlighted some critical issues, it is necessary to examine some of the theories in detail, to put the discussion within some perspectives.

4.2 Structuration Theory and Globalization of Health

Structuralists have always focused on how social structures act to determine human actions. They view social structures as social facts that are coercive of human behavior. Unlike most structuralists, Anthony Giddens (1984) links human agency with structures. Giddens' perspective is important because of the close linkages and importance attributed to both agency and structures in the understanding of social life. It is applicable in this sense because health issues operate at multiple levels, and cannot be described, therefore, as merely structural problems developed only through globalization. The tradition in interpretive sociology is to underestimate the power of structures; hence, there is less discussion around structural constraints (Giddens, 1984). In structural-functionalism, however, structures have primacy over actions, and their constraining attribute is emphasized. This macro–micro debate is as old as social science itself. In health social sciences and public health, the critical question is whether individual health conditions are determined by societal arrangements or by individual behavior. Questions around individual lifestyles, such as smoking and sexual behavior, remain open for debate: Are such behaviors self-determined by the actors, or determined by their social circumstances?

In his seminal work, *The Constitution of Society*, Giddens examined what makes societies in terms of the process of action and various influences. To Giddens, the social structure is the playground of human actors: A platform for the creation and re-creation of actions. In this theory, the individual actors create the playground; realities that enable or constrain human actions are the handiwork of the actors. Human action creates structures and structures guide actions. In and through their activities, agents reproduce the conditions that make these human actions possible (Giddens, 1984: p. 2). The conditions are the so-called structures that involve the creation of some set of rules to guide subsequent actions. Giddens defines structure as a sum of "rules and resources, organized as properties of social systems" that exist only as structural properties (Giddens, 1984: p. 23). The rules and resources are implicated in the production and reproduction of the social system. The structure is but a framework that enables the enactment of action, which is judged according to the prevailing rules and resources. The resources are vast, including the knowledge that people hold in a particular context about rules and consequences. Specifically, according to Giddens, structure exists as knowledge about how things are to be done, said or written.

The first characteristic of the structure is that it is dominating. This is why it is agreed that it is coercive of human behavior. The knowledge of "how things are done" might not necessarily be coercive in the real sense but provide the basis and justification which most people do not want to change instantaneously. Social structures also attach significance to action. Individuals would do "things" as far as those things are "important" for self and the system in the context of the actors' judgment. The structure is also a process of legitimation in the form of norms and values attached to action. The structure is defined in terms of the power of domination. The macro-level of society is about how the structures are deterministic of human action. Sometimes, it is often about the mechanical model of man, as if the individual has less choice to make. Giddens (1984) embraced the duality of the purpose of structures; it is about a dependent choice. While the structure exacts power, the human agency is also significant.

Agency is not the attribute of individuals but the outcomes of an action, i.e., the consequences of their activities or interventions. It is a process that reflects in the capacity of an individual to enact actions. Social life is about a series of interactions, actions and inactions and of doing and undoing. Agency is about the power to produce action, i.e., what individuals are doing and the capability of doing those things. The recognition of human agency and structure signifies a macro–micro orientation: Recognizing the macro and micro at the same time. Human agency is not static; it is a process or a flow (Giddens, 1984). While agency is about breaking free or independent choices, it is still bounded in structure in the sense that it is about limitations and opportunities within which the actions take place.

The structure influencing human action is very broad; the macro aspect of social life is expanded to wide coverage in the era of globalization. This is why a previous section described globalization as a super-macro level, a form of superstructure dominating an individual in the process of their agency. Globalization as a structure, the super-macro is a process of rules and resources enabling and constraining at the same time. Giddens also asserts that globalization emerged from complex processes. Globalization is a product of modernization that Giddens (2002) also defined in terms of intensification of social relations, social connectivity, dissipation of distance and grand influence originating from everywhere.

In short, structuration explores the question of how both individuals and social forces shape social reality. The importance of macro and microstructure is accentuated—the impacts of globalization manifest in most aspects of life, including health. For example, there are lifestyle factors (including sexual and smoking behavior) that determine health. People are not entirely free to act on self-will because of the coercive tendency of social forces and limited knowledge. Irrespective of the situation, humans are partially responsible for their condition. Individuals need to absorb global influences to experience its impacts. The critical question to ask is "what" is changing "what".

Both individuals and social forces shape globalization, and globalization influences human action. Hence, Giddens notes, the line of causality runs in both directions. Globalization is not a natural event but a social product. People make society and globalization, and realistically, both constrain or encourage individuals. The process of reflexivity of structure and agency is what Giddens (1984) referred to as "duality of structures". The duality of structures implies that structures are created, maintained and changed through actions, while actions are given meanings only through the embedded rules within the structure. Duality is about the simultaneous existence or interplay of micro–macro, which mutually constitute each other. To Giddens (1984: p. 25), "the notion of the duality of structure, the structural properties of social systems are both medium and outcome of the practices they recursively organize". Giddens further noted that the duality of structure is the basis for the "continuities in social reproduction across time-space". He stressed that the world is muddled up, in the sense that large-scale social encounters also produce unintended consequences. It could be part of the unintended consequences that some regions are exploited and, thereby, disadvantaged.

Within the context of the duality of structure, the process leading to health outcomes is circular (Figure 4.1). There are recursive relationships among the availability of health facilities, health practices and health outcomes. The health profile of a community is a function of health practices and levels of access to quality health services through health facilities (Oppong, 2014). The three factors become inseparable: When there are inadequate health facilities, individual health practices (e.g., health and illness behavior) will be poor, which will account for a poor community health profile. The health profile might also determine the investment of health resources (e.g., provision of a health facility) in a particular community. In this sense,

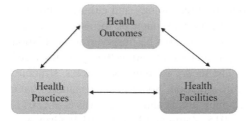

Figure 4.1 Giddens' Structuration Theory applied to health (Source: Oppong, S., 2014:114)

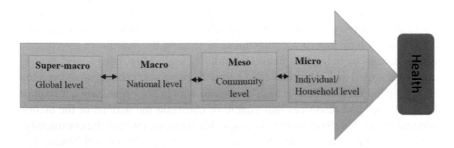

Figure 4.2 Levels of health determinants

globalization becomes a context of the duality of structure, thereby influencing health practices, organization of healthcare and invariably health outcomes.

The concept of agency also involves the process of risk accumulation. For lifestyle diseases, a human agency can be partially responsible. The essence of human agency is to condone or repel the influence from the global level or macro issues promoting access to risk factors (e.g., tobacco or alcohol). Does a "global process" involve human agency or their products? Agency is about choices and decisions dependent on specific forces. For example, in some predominantly Muslim regions of the Global South, access to alcohol is constrained. Such a proscriptive rule could lead to compliance with such Islamic provisions, but, in some cases, it leads to the smuggling of such restricted products. Thus, a proscriptive rule may help to curtail certain behaviors, thereby enabling others or promoting inevitable unintended consequences such as human and drug trafficking. The choice is also a function of knowledge, although in healthcare there is a difference between theoretical knowledge and practical action. Self-efficacy is the ability to implement action after some theoretical knowledge. Therefore, there are both micro and macro linkages in risk accumulation.

Figure 4.2 shows the complexity of the micro–macro process. Within the discourse of globalization and health, a two-level analysis includes globalization as a macro process, and individual nations as a micro process. However, a multilevel process is probably more apt than the micro–macro process. While Giddens did not introduce either the meso or the super-macro level, it is important not to reduce the process to just two levels, micro and macro. Giddens (2002) extensively examined globalization as an emerging force reshaping the social context often subsumed as part of the macro process. It is just for emphasis in the context of globalization and health that the former is recognized as a super-macro structure. The bi-directional arrows in Figure 4.2 signify a cycle of influence of super-macro–macro–meso–micro. The cycle of influence has now been expanded as four-fold or in quadrants. With globalization, the cycle of influence is getting broader or multilevel, and thus should always be so recognized in the process of determining social outcomes or conditions.

Giddens, among others, also recognized the diffusion of technology and cultures, and their implications for globalization. The diffusion has significant consequences for aspects of day-to-day life and material development. The consequences can also be observed in population health and organization of healthcare. It is in this light that structuration theory is described as meta-theory to describe globalization and health. The theory is about the process, structure and agency, and their interaction to produce a definite situation. Some previous studies have used structuration theory to examine some aspect of population health (see Groves et al., 2011; Sharma et al., 2012; Oppong, 2014; Bodolica et al., 2015; Zanin and Piercy, 2019). Groves et al. (2011) studied safety culture through the lens of structuration theory, observing that safety conditions involve both individual actions and organizational structures. People create rules and are constrained by the rules. Rules are shared through communication, thereby (re)producing a corporate safety culture system in terms of patient safety. For Bodolica et al. (2015), the concern was also about micro–macro connectedness in shaping the healthcare governance structure and health outcomes of individual patients. Bodolica argues that macro level healthcare infrastructures are changed and reproduced over time through micro encounters between patients and physicians (Bodolica et al., 2015). The overall healthcare organization becomes the structure with some rules and resources that enable or constrain the actions of the actors. Furthermore, Zanin and Piercy (2019) examined how specific structures within the community-based model of mental health care enable and constrain people living with mental illness. The study noted the existence of structural barriers, but people try to re-create structures to meet their mental health needs.

This is a grand approach to situate the structuration theory beyond some internal processes. The focus is more on the impact of the external on some macro, meso and micro processes. The interplay of these levels produces consequences, both intended and unintended. The global actors enact actions while operating within the context of some influences, which invariably account for population health. The main concern of the structuration perspective is not about the nature of such action, whether positive or negative; it is about the process of creating and reproduction of "contents", which account for a definite situation.

4.3 Risk Society Theory

The risk society theory is often traced to the works of Ulrich Beck (1992: *Risk Society* and 1999: *World Risk Society*) and Anthony Giddens (1990: *The Consequences of Modernity* and 2002: *Runaway world*). In *Runaway World: How Globalization is Shaping the World*, Giddens (2002) made some important observations about the succession of alterations as a result of globalization. The initial presumption of the theory is that the human capacity to take charge of the world is the most crucial product of scientific revolution. The world started as what is now termed primitive but, with innovations and inventions, the world has recorded massive development that those in the primitive era could not have imagined. Development is a continuous process; the next 1,000 years cannot be imagined in terms of technological breakthroughs. In sociology, the central causal polemic is that social problems are modern, i.e., byproducts of the industrial revolution and modernization. Industrialism is continuous; the world is becoming more industrialized, urbanized and globalized. It is a runway world, a world departing swiftly from its original form. Development is evolutionary, usually gradual, but modern industrial development is seen as drastic. As humans have to live with the joys of the breakthrough, individuals also have to live with pains. Such "pains" are basically unintended or latent consequences of inventions and development. Both intended and unintended consequences become highly "generalized conditions of system reproduction", which is of global importance for control (Giddens, 2002: p. 68).

The foregoing discussion relates that the globalized world offers both opportunities and catastrophes, which are not limited in geographical coverage. Opportunities and risks are two sides of a coin. It is almost impossible to discuss one without the other. It is a matter of high proportion of undeniable risks, whether consciously manufactured or not. In many instances, the risk is unpredictable, which puts people in the dilemma of the unknown to a large extent until the manifestation of the risks bit by bit. It is often problematic or challenging to draw on past historical experience to measure future risks. The past is unlike the present; invention or development only has historical antecedents but has not existed in the past. It is all about the new risk brought by new development. For example, the emergence of the mobile phone reshaped the patterns and intensity of communication. Apart from health hazards and the disappearance of traditional patterns of communication, criminal activities are easily facilitated using the same technology. Due to the development of information and communication technology (ICT), there is a growing field of cybercriminology. Unlike before, crime can be committed without physical contact with the victim. Information is now available electronically and can be hacked or accessed the same way. The world loses billions of dollars to cybercrime or internet fraud annually, up to $2.7 billion and $3.5 billion in 2018 and 2019, respectively, in the US alone (see Norris et al., 2019; FBI, 2019).

Giddens (2002) extensively discussed the concept of manufactured risks, which are products of modernization or globalization. Science and technology are driving the world, giving room for more possibilities and opportunities which were unavailable in the premodern era. Through human activities and advancement in technology (including ICT) risks are manufactured, and such risks are ubiquitous in the globalized era. Therefore, the production and reproduction of risks eventually lead to the making of a risk society. A risk society is "a systematic way of dealing with hazards and insecurities induced and introduced by modernization itself" (Beck, 1992:21). For Beck, "risk" is used in the contexts of hazard and vulnerability. There is epidemiology of risk; it is not evenly distributed, and both internal and external factors positively influence its distribution. Another central argument is that risks are manufactured continuously. The primary manifestation of risk is on the quality of life and social order. How to mitigate risks becomes a significant global challenge. There is also increasing concern about the accumulation of risk in different regions of the world. The capacity to manage threats also differs across the regions.

Giddens (2002: p. 80) clarified that "risk is not the same as hazard or danger. Risk refers to hazards that are actively assessed concerning future possibilities". Risk is not a problem of traditional societies, which are less exposed to the risks of modern societies. The only danger is that traditional societies are driving toward modernity, or are assessed as traditional or primitive in comparison to the modern ones. Risk accumulates as society tries to break away from its past form. It is often argued that change is a reality that every society must contend with. Social change, in general, follows the strain of movement from primitive or traditional to modern. Breaking away from the past is, therefore, inevitable as a sign of social progress. Societies develop from simple to complex, and primitive or traditional to modern. All societies are future-oriented and, therefore, must be concerned about risk. Modern civilization is pervasive and a product highly subscribed to in assessing the state of development and human welfare. Giddens observed that the fate of society is left to science, not religion or traditional authority. Humans perpetuate activities that modify the world with the use of human intelligence. There is materialist epidemiology of risk as the accumulation of risk is dependent on the level of socio-economic development or the socio-economic system. For instance, capitalism is partial and irregular; the system generates vulnerability because of some of its inbuilt contradictions, including capital accumulation, alienation and pauperization. According to Giddens (2002: p. 83), "modern capitalism embeds itself into the future by calculating future profit and loss, and therefore risk, as a continuous process".

To further explain risk society, Giddens (2002: p. 86) differentiated between two types of risk: external and manufactured risk. He defined external risk as risk experience coming from outside, i.e., from the fixities of tradition or nature. Although in traditional societies, people get sick, to some extent, some sickness can be attributed to external risk, calculable and insurable. The social epidemiology has buttressed that many diseases are not as a direct result of industrialization but could also be attributed to human activities. Some external risks are also manufactured. For example, malaria is as a result of human activities, especially agricultural activities and geographical expansion of residence to new areas. For instance, Wellcome (2002: p. 30) summarized Day Karen's research report about the origin of malaria. The human invasion of the rainforest, during the dawn of agriculture in Africa about 3,200–7,000 years ago, coincided with the emergence of the *falciparum* parasite. The massive ecological change, communal living and the cutting down of the rainforest for slash-and-burn agriculture coincided with "major change in the mosquito vector at that time when it began biting humans instead of animals" (Wellcome, 2002: p. 30). The *falciparum* then traveled around the world through human migration. The narration about malaria shows the importance of human activities and migration in the spread of disease. Coincidentally, migration is a crucial aspect of globalization.

Of central concern to Giddens (2002:86) were the manufactured risks "created by the very impact of our developing knowledge upon the world. Manufactured risk refers to risk situations that humans have very little historical experience of confronting. Most environmental risks, such as those connected with global warming, fall into this category. The intensifying globalization directly influences them. The "nature" has been in the purview of technological development, with every aspect amenable to technological intervention. Invariably, all aspects of human life and the human body have been affected by technological development. The world is growing out of the "natural" to the artificial creation of processes and events. This process of change or massive alteration of nature and tradition is termed as denaturalization and detraditionalization, respectively. The world is losing its traditions, paving the way for modernity. He observed that there is virtually no aspect of the human environment (physical, material and non-physical) that has escaped human intervention. There is nothing completely natural anymore, from the air that individuals breathe to the food that humans eat. Giddens observed that the intensification of many natural disasters, including flooding and volcanos, is not wholly natural.

Beck (1992) proposed some more in-depth reflection on the notion and characters of risk society, as summarized by Etkin (2016: pp. 77–78) as follows:

1. Accumulation of wealth is fundamentally different from that of risk. Wealth accumulates more at the top of society; risk settles at the bottom. In a world divided into high-, middle- and low-income countries, the reality is that risk tends to settle more at the lower quantile of the society where there is an inadequate capacity to deal with it.
2. The manufacturing of risk and its accumulation is beyond controllability. These risks are, in Beck's words, "systematic and often cause irreversible harm". Modernization, and by extension, globalization comes with unintended uncertainties, which have become a reality the world has to contend with.
3. Risk inequality is a global reality. As globalization is an unequal process, so the risk escalation is unequal across various divides. "There are both losers and winners, and the winners are mainly big business" and high-income countries. "There is a systematic attraction between extreme poverty and extreme risk".
4. "Dealing with risks is fundamentally a political process and can only be meaningfully discussed within an ethical framework". This explains the globalization of health policies

and polities with the view of mobilizing government, agencies and other stakeholders to mitigate disease burden on a global scale.

5. "Risks display a 'social boomerang effect'; even the rich and powerful are not safe from them, although wealth can buy various degrees of safety from some hazards". For example, infectious diseases (such as severe acute respiratory syndrome [SARS] and Ebola) know no boundary. There is only a fundamental difference in terms of the degree of exposure and vulnerability and response to risks.

6. "Through the unrestrained production of modernization risks, a policy of making the earth uninhabitable is being conducted in continuing leaps and bounds". There are continuous production and reproduction of health hazards, beyond individuals but jeopardizing human living conditions.

Scientific traditions, through their dominance, also generate risk in some ways. The world is dominated by scientific traditions, with many scientific or expert opinions on daily life and activities. As scientific knowledge overcomes tradition, it pushes people to respect scientific suggestions about how to live, eat, play and sleep. The culture of science also influences the process of risk reproduction. Most aspects of social life are now scientifically regulated; science has hijacked human life and existence. It is part of what is termed as medicalization (see Section 2.3.7). There is a reification of scientific tradition as an antecedent to globalization—science exacts significant control on human life. Giddens (2002) submitted that science and technology intrude into human lives on a global level. The less exciting aspects, but those that are still of great concern, are the conflicting messages, which support the incalculable manufactured risk. Giddens observed some contradictory evidence about the benefits of red wine, and the worst, future evidence might contradict what is known today. Other examples abound: Homosexualism was previously abnormal and, therefore, medicalized. It has since been de-medicalized and normalized. There is no absolute assurance that eating an egg a day is beneficial or not—or that it is only helpful for a particular age group. Even if there is some evidence, future evidence might show otherwise. The scientific world comes with immense uncertainties, with falsifiable or provisional knowledge.

Figure 4.3 presents a simple model of risk society and global health. The Figure identifies the drivers of globalization as science, technology and modernization. The Figure depicts that

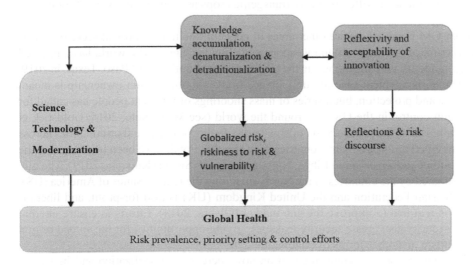

Figure 4.3 Risk society and global health

the accumulation of knowledge is related to denaturalization and detraditionalization processes or human intervention in all spheres of life. The first dilemma is the reflexivity and acceptability of innovations. The reflexive situation is when little or nothing is known about any adverse consequences of innovation concerning denaturalization. With time, concern emerged, leading to some reflections or risk discourse. The critical issue is about globalized risk, riskiness to risk and vulnerability, which affects global health.

Giddens (1999) noted that science and technology create as many uncertainties that cannot merely be "solved" by yet further scientific advances. He observed that the creation of risk is a continuous and perpetual process: There is always new riskiness to risk.

> In a social order in which new technologies are chronically affecting our lives, and an almost endless revision of taken-for-granted ways of doing things ensues, the future becomes ever more absorbing, but at the same time opaque. There are few direct lines to it, only a plurality of future scenarios (Giddens, 1999: p. 4).

For example, the world is in the era of genetically modified (GM) food: Most agricultural products are no more natural. Agricultural innovation comes with improved seedlings and breeds to increase production and profits. There have been numerous concerns about the safety of genetically modified organisms (GMOs). Despite the concerns, both the North and South must embrace new technologies to be competitive and adopt the best practices to ensure improved food production to avert famine.

Food is produced from animals or plants whose deoxyribonucleic acid (DNA) has been genetically altered with the aid of genetic engineering. GM foods have been globalized, with several countries now growing it, and it is consumed all over the world. The promise is about meeting the food needs of the world. Bawa and Anilakumar (2013) reported that there are many transgenic crops that have been modified, including fruit and nut trees that mature years earlier. Despite the promises of GM foods, the scientific breakthrough comes with some observable concerns regarding safety, environmental and ecological risks and health hazards. There is still ongoing research on the long-term effects of GM foods on the human body—of future consequences, yet to unfold, but expected and incalculable. GM food is a typical example of breaking from the "natural". Bawa and Anilakumar (2013) observed that many community members often perceive transgenic crops as an unnatural way of producing foods.

Apart from GM Foods, there are other areas of concern, including national security threatened by terrorism, proliferation of gun/weapons and climate change. The world has witnessed gun violence incidents, with the highest in the US. The mass shooting in El Paso, Texas, in 2019, killing 22 people, is a typical case of gun violence (mass shooting). Gun ownership is meant for self-defense and protection, but a series of mass shootings of innocent people has called for a rethink of gun control in the US and around the world (see Wintemute, 2015; Goldstick et al., 2019). There is also the proliferation of small arms fueling conflict and criminalities across the globe. Smuggled arms into many countries of the Global South have been implicated in the continuous conflict and terrorism in Libya, Nigeria and South Sudan (Kuwonu, 2019). The gun industry, dominated by the countries of the North, including the United States of America (US), France, the Russian Federation and the United Kingdom (UK) is also for-profit, and liberalization policy is required to improve the gun market (Olvera, 2014). Efforts to ensure internal and personal security also create security leakages, giving opportunities for the spread of gun violence, terrorism and other forms of criminalities.

The risk society theory is mainly focused on how increasing globalization and its significant drivers, technology and science, are generating risks. Due to globalized proximity of various world regions, risk-sharing is highly pervasive. Although the distribution of those risks is uneven, as evident in the South–North divide, risk is ubiquitous and overwhelming. As Beck (1992) and Giddens (1999) observed, the next step is to take global responsibility by limiting risks (e.g., ecological, economic or health risks) or adopting the precautionary principle.

4.4 Political Economy of Globalized Health

Political economy has emerged as a distinct theoretical perspective in the understanding of various socio-economic and political events. The economic aspect of globalization has been a major yardstick of measuring globalization over the years. The political economy is often traced to the Frankfurt School theorists who have been heavily influenced by the philosophies of Kant, Hegel and especially Marx (Hayden and el-Ojeili, 2006). Karl Marx developed a variant of political-economic perspective, described as historical materialism or conflict perspective, which has been applied to the understanding of "everything and anything", especially macro processes (Amzat and Omololu, 2012). The Marxian perspective is relevant in the analysis of inequality and inequity from a structural perspective. The view builds some strictures about capitalism, observing that it has some inbuilt contradictions, including capital accumulation, exploitation and alienation (see Lovell, 2004; Schweickart, 2014). The idea of political economy is that the state of the nation, individual and, by extension, the global world is based on the economic stage of development. Therefore, the economic substructure is the base which gives rise to the superstructures, including law, politics, religion, family, media and education. The emergence of class structure is a significant consequence, with some individuals (bourgeoisie) at the top, while others (proletariats) are at the bottom of society. The inequality does not only operate at the individual level but also between nations concerning income, education and health (see Wallenstein, 2004; Roser, 2019).

Political economy is often about economic and political systems as determinants of the character and structure of the society. The heaviest hammer of the Marxists falls on capitalism. Hayden and el-Ojeili (2006) observed that capitalism is an "economic system based on the generalized production and circulation of commodities"—a privately driven market of goods and services—for profit motive. Capital accumulation is a result of surplus value derived from profit maximization. The existence of capital also implies the existence of wage laborers who work to earn a living. The foremost criticism of capitalism describes it as having an overriding logic of self-interest and profit at the expense of the well-being of human society (Hayden and el-Ojeili, 2006). The capitalist system is chaotic, thereby responsible for several social problems of the modern world, and socially divisive as the basis for socioeconomic inequality and inequity in human society. According to Axford (2013: p. 11) "Marxist globalists treat the making of a global, market-driven economy as the latest twist in the development of capitalism as an exploitative system of wealth creation and uneven development". To the Marxists, globalization is yet another effort toward the furtherance of the capitalist agenda of expansion, inequality and unequal progress.

Marxist globalists also use the dependency theory, which emerged in the 1950s to examine socio-economic underdevelopment in the Global South. The perspective emphasized the putative bottlenecks, designed by the global political and economic powers of the North, on the way to the development of the South (Amin, 1976; Frank, 1978; Olutayo and Omobowale, 2007; Amadi, 2012; Jalata, 2013). The dependency theorists noted the major adverse manifestations of the socio-economic bottlenecks, including the relapse in agricultural and small-scale enterprises, monoculturalism and unequal international specialization in terms of productive activities, i.e., the specialization on cash crops and structural imbalances in the political and social relationships. Cardoso and Faletto (1979) also observed the extent of technological penetration of the South, imbalance terms of economic exchanges which limit self-sustained growth in the periphery, i.e., the low-income countries. One of the major consequences is aid and loan dependency, which further strangulate economic development in the South (Abdullahi and Amzat, 2011). Therefore, dependency promotes underdevelopment. The propagation of the dominant neoliberal reforms of open markets, foreign direct investment and deregulation promote further incorporation into the capitalist system with its cyclical fluctuations and persisting contradictions in the South (Tausch, 2019). Globalization is, therefore, a mere extension of the capitalist system with its adverse neoliberal reforms, which are detrimental to the development of low-income countries.

For Marxist globalists, the question of whether globalization is good or bad is settled. The whole process started with the incorporation of other parts of the world into the capitalist system with the powerful nations exploiting the weak countries, and promoting an agenda that would make them more vulnerable. The agenda aims to create a network of capitalist units but with unequal stake and benefits within the network. Globalization is about the capitalist ideological sentiments, and it is thus a potent development in watering the seed of world capitalist expansion and sustainability. To Axford (2013: p. 9), globalization is inimical to progressive and humanitarian goals for regional gains at the expense of other regions. The glaring results will be subjugation and further oppression of the weak nations. Global capitalism generates poverty and other emerging problems, such as human trafficking or child labor and inequalities, which reflect in all aspects of social life, including population health.

In addition, globalization should signify a single transnational political economy, but global polarization is evident along the line of economic and political power (Adams and Gupta, 1997). Unfortunately, the gaps in major development indicators between high- and low-income countries, far from narrowing, has more than tripled during the last 30 years (Adams and Gupta, 1997). While there has been a steady improvement in the Global North, the progress is at a snail's pace in the Global South. The significant problems have remained the same: Poverty, inequality and poor health indicators. The persistence of the problems necessitates the movement from unmet goals of MDGs to SDGs, and most serious attention should be diverted to many countries in the Global South if SDGs would be achieved by 2030.

The idea of political economy of globalized health is meant to understand the role of the socio-economic system's condition on population health. It is a macro analysis exploring the impact of resource allocation and economic power on population health (Janzen, 1978). Global inequalities in economic power and condition of living manifest in health inequalities on a global scale. Global health can be examined within the context of class and imperialist relations inherent in the capitalist world system (Baer, 1982). Globalization further promotes this world system. In general, a political economy of health is a "historical perspective for analyzing disease distribution and health services under a variety of economic systems, with particular emphasis on the effects of stratified social, political, and economic relations within the world economic system" (Morgan, 1987:132).

The first significant aspect is about the unequal distribution and incidence of diseases in the regions. Baer (1982) noted the two aspects of the political economy of health: the political economy of illness and healthcare. The political economy of illness is historical materialist epidemiology, concerned with the structural factors responsible for the distribution, prevalence and incidence of diseases in various human societies (Amzat and Razum, 2014:109). Disease burden is not even across the populations, within and between countries. Materialist epidemiology is an attempt to provide the "holistic understanding of fundamental causes of diseases and the distribution of risk behaviors as well as the incidence of morbidity and mortality in human society". Class and power relations have been implicated in the distribution of diseases with the lower class bearing higher disease burden. The second aspect is the political economy of healthcare, how the structural factors determine the distribution and consumption of health services. The political economy of healthcare examines "the impact of (capitalist) modes of production on the production, distribution, and consumption of health services and the influence of class relations within which medical institutions are organized" (Amzat and Razum, 2014:109). Therefore, the political economy of health within the context of globalization is simply about how globalization and its drivers impact both epidemiology of diseases and access to healthcare. The core themes include the commodification of health, unequal economic powers, unequal disease burden, and unequal access to healthcare. One of the variants of the political-economic perspective is the world systems theory or analysis examined in the next subsection.

4.4.1 World System Analysis of Global Health Inequalities

Immanuel Wallerstein (1974, 2004) developed the World System Analysis (WSA) also known as World Systems Theory (WST) or the World Systems Perspective to analyze global inequality. It is a macro perspective and a variant of critical or Marxian theory in the social sciences in general and sociology in particular. The historical perspective is about how countries, especially of the South, were incorporated into the world capitalist system, which invariably determined the nature and pattern of their economic development. The global expansion of capitalism "established" sub-division or branches across the world through colonialism and other imperialist strategies to sustain the capitalist system and exercise control on the branches. A system is defined as a structure with component units. Therefore, the idea of world systems is a multiple cultural system of division of labor (including medical division of labor). The main argument is also that countries do not have economies but are part of the world economy through a global division of labor (Wallerstein, 2004). It is further argued that the world economy is in tripartite of the core (mostly the Global North), semi-peripheral and peripheral zones (Global South). Inequalities arise as a result of the division of labor because the core zone monopolizes the immensely profitable activities, and the other zones specialized in less profitable activities.

According to Wallerstein (1974, 2004), the world economic system is hierarchical, apportioned into a tripartite, i.e., three types of countries: core, semi-peripheral and peripheral. Most countries in the Global South constitute the semi-peripheral and peripheral zones and are like feeder nations for the advanced capitalist world. What sets the Global North and South apart include technology, level of industrialization, bureaucratic culture, the legal system, human rights and infrastructures, among other features. Also, more importantly, the core region exercises some political and economic control of the other regions. Most countries of the Global South are the peripheral, e.g., African countries and low-income countries in South America, characteristically agrarian, less industrialized and produce more raw materials to feed the Northern industries (Wallerstein, 1974, 2004). The other category is the semi-peripheral countries (e.g., South Korea, Taiwan, Mexico, Brazil, India, China and South Africa) with better development indicators than the peripheral but less than the core region. Apart from raw materials, the peripheral and semi-peripheral serve as the sources of cheap labor, and profit from direct investment and export markets (Chirot, 1986).

Medical imperialism also follows the same pattern of the world system. Healthcare is a major market product of capitalist expansion and domination, which has been extended on a global scale. The incorporation into the world capitalist system also comes with the adoption of a modern healthcare system. The adoption of a modern healthcare system is also a means of domination, and capitalist expansion encouraged the development and investment in western medicine as the best form of care. The previous traditional medicine was subjugated for the new medical system and had to give way for proper acceptability into the modern capitalist regime. The raw materials provided by other zones also include pharmaceutical raw materials, since the big pharmaceutical companies are in the core regions. Then the other zones serve as the export markets for the major drugs from the core regions. The big markets for pharmaceuticals and research sites for the development of new drugs are mostly in the Global South. Due to high wages in the core zone, there is a continuous brain drain in the form of movement of health workers from other zones to the core areas (Mohyuddin et al., 2014). The health workers are in short supply in other zones; hence, the health workforce situation is further jeopardized by the exodus.

One strategic goal of the core zone is to further the "modernization" of the other zones to facilitate demands for modern goods, including modern healthcare. By implication, there is continuous manufacturing of modern risks (see Section 4.3). The development strategies explain the risk transition in the Global South. Mohyuddin et al. (2014) supported the assertion that most health interventions end up creating more markets for pharmaceutical products and medical assistance in the other zones. The global stakeholders' agenda, policies and politics are geared toward that of the capitalist systems. Collins (2013) confirmed the world system analysis of health that the system has perpetuated a decline in the "margin of safety" for people in the periphery. Unequal relations have reinforced differential living conditions, which has deteriorated health conditions in the South. The first significant observation is that the social determinants of health are deficient in the peripheral and semi-peripheral countries. The zones are characterized by a high incidence of poverty, low literacy and insufficient infrastructures, which incidentally are significant determinants of health.

Wallerstein (1996) also made some critical submissions about global health. He observed the "manufacturing" of diseases due to environmental changes as a result of industrial technologies. He observed the emergence of new disease patterns. The world "may thus be at the threshold of new dramatic plagues of a different kind" (Wallerstein, 1996: p. 76). He observed the improvement in life expectancy in the North due to advances in medical technology. Unfortunately, most countries in the South still have lower life expectancies despite the advancement in medical technology. In the case of many countries in sub-Saharan Africa (SSA), the envisaged plague observed by Wallerstein (1996) is brutally ravaging many communities. Differential longevity, a scourge of human immunodeficiency virus (HIV), infant and maternal mortality are typical illustrations of an uneven record of struggle against diseases (Wallerstein, 1996). Wallerstein (1996: p. 63) specifically observed that capitalism has led to "a massive increase in the margin of human safety … endemic dangers … and … erratic violence". Collins (2013) examined Wallerstein's assertion by assessing mortality data for countries in different zones using a set of health-related proxies. The bulk of Collins' data supported Wallerstein's assertion, especially in terms of mortality for chronic disease and sporadic violence but not for infectious diseases.

Another significant observation is about the commodification of everything. The primary justification of capitalist expansion is profit motive, not charitable welfare. The motive accounts for the objectification and commodification of health like any other product in the market space. Commodification accounts for the promotion of structural adjustment programs (SAP) and deregulation (see Section 3.3.1) reforms in the provision of infrastructure, despite the universal principle in healthcare. Within the capitalist motive, it is assumed that the private hands are more efficient and effective and would, therefore, ensure better delivery of quality healthcare. In the capitalist system, the essence of deregulation is to shift some of the burden from the government, and create space for investors; healthcare is a business, and the government should have less business in business. In the Global South, deregulation policies have been received with mixed feelings: More negative than positive (see Onimode, 1992; Amzat and Olutayo, 2009).

Figure 4.4 shows a simple model representation of the world system analysis of health. It is a simple adaptation of the perspective to explain global health inequalities. The peripheral

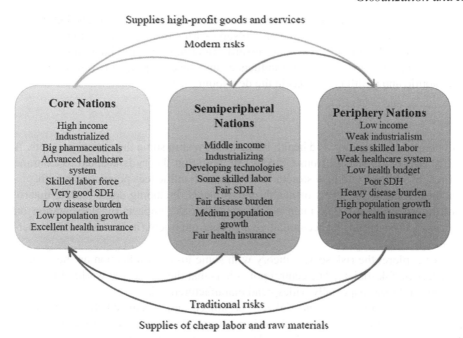

Supplies high-profit goods and services

Modern risks

Core Nations

High income
Industrialized
Big pharmaceuticals
Advanced healthcare
system
Skilled labor force
Very good SDH
Low disease burden
Low population growth
Excellent health insurance

Semiperipheral Nations

Middle income
Industrializing
Developing technologies
Some skilled labor
Fair SDH
Fair disease burden
Medium population growth
Fair health insurance

Periphery Nations

Low income
Weak industrialism
Less skilled labor
Weak healthcare system
Low health budget
Poor SDH
Heavy disease burden
High population growth
Poor health insurance

Traditional risks

Supplies of cheap labor and raw materials

Figure 4.4 World health-systems theory

nations are usually at the bottom, with a glaring manifestation of features of weak nations in terms of healthcare. A majority of the countries in the peripheral zone are fraught with weak industrialization, low income or per capita, less skilled labor (shortage of health workers), overall weak healthcare system and insufficient healthcare budget. The poor social determinants of health (see Section 3.2.1) explain the considerable burden of infectious diseases responsible for high morbidity and mortality and the spread of traditional risks. There is also high population growth with no commensurate increase in supportive infrastructure (such as health and education facilities, water and power supply). One of the worst characters of the healthcare system is out-of-pocket finance due to poor health insurance schemes. The semi-peripheral nations are faring better than the peripheral. There are gradual improvements and better socioeconomic and health indicators. Some of the semi-peripheral countries are transitioning gradually to become highly industrialized. The core nations are the advanced capitalist states with advanced health systems and low population growth. The core nations manufacture substantial modern risks, and produce the bulk of the pharmaceuticals and technologies required to support modern healthcare.

The hierarchical tripartite (of the world systems) reflects and reinforces health inequalities on a global scale. Like the dependency theory, the WST provides a macro explanation of the socioeconomic condition and healthcare in developing countries. As a solution, the critical Marxist theorists often suggest an "emancipatory socialist alternative and the establishment of de-commodified economic structures" (el-Ojeili, 2014: p. 7) not only in healthcare but a detotalization of the capitalist system. Health inequalities between countries and within a country are presented as a significant tribulation of the capitalist system. The unequal structural arrangements of the society put many people at a disadvantaged position, which negatively affect their health.

To be critical of the WST, the Marxian perspective in general and beyond the macro explanations, numerous micro processes also influence health. It is often tough to underrate the influence of super-macro or macro structures as determinants of life circumstances, but it does not mean that the total blame can be shifted on the super-structures; the meso and micro levels are also critical (see Figure 4.2). Looking inward might unfold some internal conditions responsible for the assimilation of external influences and specific problems responsible for poor socio-economic and health conditions in the developing world.

4.5 Summary

- The discourse of globalization and health is examined within some theoretical precepts. A structuralist approach, derived from Giddens' structuration theory is adapted to examine levels of responsibilities and how structural arrangement influences population health.
- The structural focus is on levels of health determinants, including super-macro, macro, meso and micro processes. The main argument is that the impacts of globalization on health occur as a sequential and accumulative process from micro (individual) to the super-macro (global) level.
- This chapter explores the risk society theory with some in-depth reflection on the notions and characters of risk society. The central polemic is that the globalized world offers both opportunities and risks, especially widespread manufactured risk.
- The world is becoming more industrialized, urbanized and globalized. It is a runaway world, a world departing swiftly from its original form. As humans have to live with the joys of the breakthroughs, individuals also have to live with pains. Such "pains" are most times unintended or latent consequences of inventions and development.
- A risk society is "a systematic way of dealing with hazards and insecurities induced and introduced by modernization itself". The primary manifestation of risk is on the quality of life and social order. There is also increasing concern about the accumulation of risk in different regions of the world. The capacity to manage threats also differs across the regions.
- Giddens (2002) differentiated between two types of risk: External and manufactured risk. External risk is a risk experience coming from outside, i.e., from the fixities of tradition or nature. Manufactured risk results from the process of change or massive alteration of nature and tradition termed as denaturalization and detraditionalization, respectively.
- The major thesis is that, due to globalized proximity of various world regions, risk-sharing is highly inescapable. Then, the distribution of the risks is uneven between the world regions. The mitigation efforts should be to take global responsibility by limiting risks (e.g., ecological, economic or health risks) or adopting the precautionary principle.
- The last perspective is the political economy of globalization and health. The chapter examines the notion that development inequalities lead to global health inequalities. The main focus is on Wallerstein's theory as a typical materialist approach to explaining global health, herein described as global health-systems perspective.
- The idea of political economy of globalized health or world health-systems theory is meant to understand the role of socio-economic system and condition on population health. Global inequalities in economic power and condition of living manifest in health inequalities on a global scale. Therefore, global health can be examined within the context of class and imperialist relations inherent in the capitalist world system.
- Medical imperialism also follows the same pattern of the world system. Healthcare is a major market product of capitalist expansion and domination, which has been extended on a global scale. The hierarchical tripartite (of the world systems) reflects and reinforces health inequalities on a global scale.
- Both risk society and political economy perspectives reiterate that due to global relations, profound adverse health consequences are more prevalent in the less developed regions.

Critical Thinking Questions

- The impact of globalization on health is accumulative from the micro to the super-macro level. To what extent does structuration perspective explain the consequential and accumulative impact of globalization on health.

- With reference to the risk society theory, how risky to global health is the world we live in? Make reference to the unintended consequences of globalization on health.

- By reflecting on any locality, evaluate and differentiate between external and manufactured risks. What are the implications of the two types of risk for global health in both the North and South?

- Discuss the thesis that the hierarchical tripartite (of the world systems) reflects and reinforces health inequalities on a global scale. Debate some specific mechanisms reinforcing such health inequalities.

- To what extent do you agree with the following notion: The world health system is an emerging theoretical disposition, which could help in the analysis and understanding of global health inequalities.

- Can the "emancipatory" socialist alternative in the health system be a panacea to global health crisis? How realistic is it in the Global South? Explain some pros and cons of such alternative.

Suggested Readings

- Amzat, J., and Razum, O. (2014). Social production of health. In: *Medical sociology in Africa*. Cham, Switzerland: Springer International Publishing. DOI 10.1007/978-3-319-03986-2_6. The chapter examines social production of health as a theoretical perspective in understanding human health.

- Beck, U. (1999). *World risk society*. Malden, MA: Polity Press. The book analyses the structural dynamics of the modern world, the global nature of risk and the future of global politics.

- Giddens, A. (1984). *The constitution of society: Outline of the theory of structuration*. Oxford: Polity Press. It is a theory book about the creation and reproduction of social systems based on the analysis of both structure and agents.

- Giddens, A. (2002). *Runaway world: How globalization is shaping the world*. London: Profile Books. The book evaluates the ever-increasing impact of globalization, showing how interdependence directly affects everyday lives.

- Hayden, P., and el-Ojeili, C. (2006). *Critical theories of globalization*. NY: Palgrave Macmillan. This book provides a comprehensive overview of globalization and its consequences from the perspective of social and political critical theory.

- Wallerstein, I. (1974). *The Modern World-System*. New York: Academic Press. The book presents a grand narrative of world historical development as a global geographical division of labor between the North and South.

References

Abdullahi, A. A., & Amzat, J. (2011). The problems and challenges of foreign aid in developing countries. *Bayero Journal of Social and Management Studies (BAJOSAMS)*, *14*(1), 108–119.

Adams, F., & Gupta, S. D. (1997). The political economy of globalization: An introduction. In Gupta, S. D. (Ed.), *The Political Economy of Globalization*. Boston, MA: Kluwer Academic Publishers.

Amadi, L. (2012). Africa, beyond the new dependency: A political economy. *African Journal of Political Science and International Relations*, *6*(8), 191–203.

Amin, S. (1976). *Unequal Development: An Essay on the Social Formations of Peripheral Capitalism*. New York: Monthly Review Press.

Amzat, J., & Olutayo, O. A. (2009). Nigeria, capitalism and the question of equity. *The Anthropologist*, *11*(4), 239–246.

Amzat, J., & Omololu, F. (2012). The basics of sociological paradigms. In Ogundiya, I. S. & Amzat, J. (Eds.), *The Basics of Social Sciences* (pp. 115–134). Lagos: Malthouse Press.

Amzat, J., & Razum, O. (2014). Social production of health. In: *Medical Sociology in Africa*. Cham, Switzerland: Springer International Publishing. doi: 10.1007/978-3-319-03986-2_6.

Axford, B. (2013). *Theories of Globalization*. Cambridge: Polity Press.

Baer, H. A. (1982). On the political economy of health. *Medical Anthropology Newsletter*, *14*(1), 1–17.

Bawa, A. S., & Anilakumar, K. R. (2013). Genetically modified foods: Safety, risks and public concerns-a review. *Journal of Food Science and Technology*, *50*(6), 1035–1046. doi: 10.1007/s13197-012-0899-1.

Beck, U. (1992). *Risk Society: Towards a New Modernity*. New Delhi: Sage.

Beck, U. (1999). *World Risk Society*. Malden, MA: Polity Press.

Bodolica, V., Spraggon, M. & Tofan, G. (2015). A structuration framework for bridging the macro–micro divide in health-care governance. *Health Expectations*, *19*, 790–804.

Cardoso, F. H., & Faletto, E. (1979). *Dependency and Development in Latin América*. Berkeley, CA: University of California Press.

Chirot, D. (1986). *Social Change in the Modern Era*. New York: Harcourt Brace Jovanovich.

Collins, A. N. (2013). Inequalities in global health: A world-system analysis, 1945-present. An Unpublished Doctoral Thesis submitted to Department of Sociology, Anthropology, and Social Work, Kansas State University, USA.

el-Ojeili, C. (2014). Reflections on Wallerstein: The modern world-system, four decades on. *Critical Sociology*, *41*(4–5), 679–700. doi:10.1177/0896920513497377.

Etkin, D. (2016). *Disaster Theory: An Interdisciplinary Approach to Concepts and Causes* (pp. 53–101). Oxford: Butterworth-Heinemann.

Federal Bureau of Investigation (2019). *Internet Crime Report 2019*. Washington, DC: Internet Crime Complaint Center. https://pdf.ic3.gov/2019_IC3Report.pdf. Accessed on August 12, 2020.

Frank, A. G. (1978). *Dependent Accumulation and Underdevelopment*. New York: Monthly Review Press.

Giddens, A. (1984). *The Constitution of Society: Outline of the Theory of Structuration*. Oxford: Polity Press.

Giddens, A. (1990). *The Consequences of Modernity*. Stanford, CA: Stanford University Press.

Giddens, A. (1999). Risk and responsibility. *The Modern Law Review*, *62*(1), 1–10.

Giddens, A. (2002). *Runaway World: How Globalization is Shaping the World*. London: Profile Books.

Goldstick, J. E., Zeoli, A., Mair, C. & Cunningham, R. M. (2019). US firearm-related mortality: National, state, and population trends, 1999–2017. *Health Affairs*, *38*(10), 1646–1652.

Groves, P. S., Meisenbach, R. J. & Scott-Cawiezell, J. (2011). Keeping patients safe in healthcare organizations: A structuration theory of safety culture. *Journal of Advanced Nursing*, *67*(8), 1846–1855. doi: 10.1111/j.1365-2648.2011.05619.x.

Hayden, P., & el-Ojeili, C. (2006). *Critical Theories of Globalization*. New York: Palgrave Macmillan.

Jalata, A. (2013). Colonial terrorism, global capitalism and African underdevelopment: 500 Years of crimes against African peoples. *The Journal of Pan-African Studies*, *5*(9), 1–43.

Janzen, J. M. (1978). The comparative study of medical systems as changing social systems. *Social Science & Medicine*, *12*, 121–129.

Kuwonu, F. (2019). Small arms fueling deadly communal violence: Local communities in search of lasting peace. https://reliefweb.int/report/world/small-arms-fueling-deadly-communal-violence. Accessed on August 12, 2020.

Lovell, D. (2004). Marx's Utopian legacy. *The European legacy 9*(5), 629–640. doi: 10.1080/1084877042000306398.

Morgan, L. M. (1987). Dependency theory in the political economy of health: An anthropological critique. *Medical Anthropology Quarterly*, *1*(2), 131–154.

Mohyuddin, A., Ambreen, M., Juhi Naveed, J. & Ahmad, D. (2014). World system analysis of biomedical hegemony. *Advances in Anthropology*, *4*, 59–67.

Norris, G., Brookes, A. & Dowell, D. (2019). The psychology of internet fraud victimisation: A systematic review. *Journal of Police and Criminal Psychology*, *34*, 231–245. doi: 10.1007/s11896-019-09334-5.

Olutayo, A. O., & Omobowale, A. O. (2007). Capitalism, globalisation and the underdevelopment process in Africa: History in perpetuity. *Africa Development*, *32*(2), 97–112. doi: 10.4314/ad.v32i2.57179.

Olvera, G. M. B. (2014). The security council and the illegal transfer of small arms and light weapons to non-state actors. *Mexican Law Review*, *6*(2), 225–250.

Onimode, B. (1992). *A Future for Africa: Beyond the Politics of Adjustment*. London: Earthscan.

Oppong, S. (2014). Between Bandura and Giddens: Structuration theory in social psychological research? *Psychological Thought*, *7*(2), 111–123. doi:10.5964/psyct.v7i2.104.

Ritchie, H., & Roser, M. (2019). Water use and sanitation. Published online at *OurWorldInData.org*. https://ourworldindata.org/water-use-sanitation [Online Resource]. Accessed on August 9, 2019.

Roser, M. (2019). Global inequality of opportunity. https://ourworldindata.org/global-inequality-of -opportunity. Accessed on August 12, 2020.

Schweickart, C. D. (2014). Marx's democratic critique of capitalism and its implications for a viable socialism. *Owl of Minerva*, *46*(1), 67–77.

Sharma U., Barnett, J. & Clarke, M. (2012). Using concepts from structuration theory and consequence of modernity to understand IS deployment in health-care setting. In Dwivedi Y., Wade M., & Schneberger, S. (Eds.), *Information Systems Theory*. Integrated Series in Information Systems, vol. 29. New York: Springer.

Tausch, A. (2019). Globalization and development: The relevance of classical "dependency" theory for the world today. *International Social Science Journal*, *68*(227–228), 79–99. doi: 10.1111/issj.12190.

Wallerstein, I. (1974a). *The Modern World-System*. New York: Academic Press.

Wallerstein, I. (1974b). *The Modern World-System I: Capitalist Agriculture and the Origins of the European World-Economy in the Sixteenth Century*. New York: Academic Press.

Wallerstein, I. (1996). *Historical Capitalism with Capitalist Civilization*. New York: Verso.

Wallerstein, I. (2004). World-systems Analysis. In George Modelski (Ed.), *World System History*. Encyclopedia of Life Support Systems (EOLSS). Oxford: Eolss Publishers.

Wellcome News (2002). *Research Directions in Malaria*. Supplement 6. London: Wellcome News.

Wintemute, G. J. (2015). The epidemiology of firearm violence in the twenty-first century United States. *Annual Review of Public Health*, *36*, 5–19.

Zanin, A. C., & Piercy, C. W. (2019). The structuration of community-based mental health care: A duality analysis of a volunteer group's local agency. *Qualitative Health Research*, *29*(2), 184–197.

5 Globalization and NCDs in the Global South

5.1 Introduction

Many antecedents and emerging factors of development are fueling the rise of noncommunicable diseases (NCDs). The increasing NCDs in the Global South are associated with increasing modernization and globalization (Fedacko et al., 2019; Labonté and Ruckert, 2019). Communicable diseases have been and continue to be a significant health challenge in the South; the health situation is compounded by the huge additional burden of noncommunicable diseases, generally chronic diseases. Such diseases degenerate, get worse with time. The disease onset is prolonged gradually and develops with time. The onset is not usually sudden; that is why early diagnosis is often the critical control strategy. Without early diagnosis, the disease might be out of control, thereby becoming irreversible and leading to mortality. Chronic diseases have a long-span and long-duration, primarily when appropriately managed. An individual can live with it for several years or throughout their lifespan. The diseases affect the quality of life with time. Chronic illnesses often lead to biographic disruption, incapacitation of individuals or a situation whereby the structures of everyday life are disorganized (Amzat and Razum, 2014). It leads to the inability of an individual to follow a regular pattern of usual behavior, routine or activity. For instance, cancer may disrupt one's existential being, life course and identity. Most chronic diseases are not curable but treatable or manageable. The management of chronic diseases requires enormous resources, especially in the context of the Global South, with limited health insurance coverage. Many poor households might experience financial catastrophe due to the financial burden of managing a chronic disease. For example, the costs of cancer treatment or kidney dialysis might be outrageous for a typical poor household. Another characteristic of a chronic disease is its noncommunicability—deriving its name from this characteristic. Most of the diseases cannot be contracted through contact with a sufferer. However, some of them (such as some types of cancer, autism and Huntington disease) can be genetically inherited. Despite this noncommunicability, the disease burden is very high. The lack of a (permanent) cure for many of them is a major problem.

Chronic diseases are often regarded as lifestyle diseases. Globalization plays a significant role in the prevalence of chronic diseases because of lifestyle and behavioral factors (see Sections 2.3.2 and 3.2.1.6). As previously regarded, globalization is a super-macro process that influences personal biography or, specifically, lifestyle. Some chronic diseases are a result of human lifestyle, a prominent social determinant of health often conceived at the micro level, but emerging evidence has shown that lifestyle has a lot to do with macro and super-macro factors, which are coercive of micro behavior. The continuous process of industrialization, urbanization, global markets and media technologies has altered realities of social existence beyond measure. Globalization is a factor of change, development and economic progress, but it affects all aspects of life, including nutrition, communication and human well-being. The Global South is

DOI: 10.4324/9781003247975-5

experiencing some socio-economic transitions or transformations in line with the moderniza-tion agenda. The premise is that the assimilation of modernization (or globalization) recipes hold several health implications. As previously discussed in Chapter 1, globalization comes with opportunities and uncertainties, including some unintended consequences. Within global health, the "unintended" consequences are now overwhelming and dictating human health conditions. One such overwhelming consequence is the high prevalence of lifestyle diseases. Such lifestyle diseases were previously termed as the diseases of the rich, but now typically have no class boundary, as the Global South also bears a heavy burden of such diseases. The next few sections will examine the burden of NCDs in the Global South, behavioral factors in NCDs and some theoretical explanations.

5.2 Burden of Noncommunicable Diseases (NCDs) in the Global South

WHO (2018a) reported that NCDs are responsible for 7 out of 10 deaths globally, specifically, 71% representing about 41 million deaths annually. Figure 5.1 supports the assertion that NCDs constitute a significant health threat of this era and will continue to influence the direction of the health discourse around the world. As previously pointed out, NCDs tend to be protracted, thereby constituting a financial burden for households and possibly leading to premature deaths. Since globalization has been implicated in the prevalence of NCDs, globalization becomes a major determinant of health. It is a single factor that unites the world and dictates the prevailing trend in terms of population health. The only reason why NCDs do not constitute health emer-gencies is because they are typically manageable.

While the diseases can be managed in the Global North, the story in the Global South is dif-ferent. The healthcare systems in the Global South are relatively weak, and most management of chronic diseases requires high-tech healthcare. In places where such advanced services are not available, people die prematurely. In other words, NCDs take on a more severe dimen-sion in the Third World, leading to premature deaths of people between 30 and 69. The WHO reported that about 15 million global deaths in 2018 were premature, with over 85% occurring in the Global South. Globally, NCDs cardiovascular diseases, cancers, respiratory diseases and diabetes are the four leading causes of death. Cardiovascular diseases and cancers account for up to 40% and 22% of the deaths, respectively (WHO, 2018b). There have been some declines in infectious diseases, but fatalities from NCDs have increased over the years. The possibility of a further increase is also indisputable.

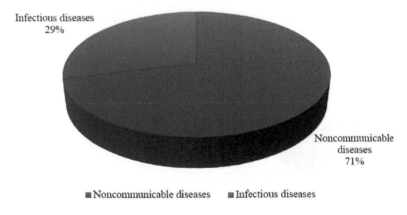

Figure 5.1 Global deaths (Source: WHO [World Health Organization], 2018a)

The diseases of globalization present the most significant global health challenge, but with unequal burden across the major divide: South and North. The South carries the heaviest burden of almost 78% (about 32 million of 41 million) of the deaths (see Figure 5.2) (WHO, 2018). This is in line with the assertion of the risk society theory which states that, while risk is ubiquitous, it settles more at the bottom of the society (see Section 4.3). The uncertainties and risks produced by the process of globalization are evident in the low-income regions of the world. The actual prevalence of NCDs might not be as high as in the North, but, due to weak health systems, the Global South suffers more mortalities from NCDs. The burden of mortality from NCDs is too heavy to bear for the Global South, considering the per capita income and the weak health system in general.

In Southeast Asia, the WHO (2002) observed that the ten-member countries in the region (Bangladesh, Bhutan, DPR Korea, India, Indonesia, Maldives, Myanmar, Nepal, Sri Lanka and Thailand) are experiencing a wave of globalization with the health consequences that come with it. The ten countries have recorded some success in the control of infectious diseases but are experiencing a rapid increase in the burden of NCDs. As of 1998, the burden of NCDs was relatively low, ranging from from7% in Nepal to 48% in Sri Lanka (WHO, 2002). The trend has since changed, however, with NCDs accounting for up to 62% of all deaths in the region, killing over 8.2 million people, the majority of whom die prematurely. Since 1998, the WHO has predicted NCD-related deaths will reach as high as 70% for the region by 2020.

In South Asia, the threat of NCDs is increasing (Narain et al., 2011; Siegel et al., 2014). Narain et al. (2011) claimed that NCDs constitute global health and developmental tragedies, which further draw South Asia backward in its development efforts. Narain et al. reported that the NCDs were the highest killer in the region, with almost 7.9 million deaths, and with cardiovascular diseases (CVDs) topping the list at 25% of the deaths. Siegel et al. (2014) also noted that the burden of NCDs in South Asia is rising above the global average. The researchers note the success regarded in the fight against infectious diseases, but NCDs pose serious threats as a result of increasing urbanization and socio-economic development occasioned by globalization. With the continuous globalization trends, the possibility of an increase in the burden of NCDs is expected. The death burden from NCDs is generally more than 50%. Siegel et al. (2014) noted that poverty and poor health systems constitute a significant barrier in the management of chronic diseases in South Asia. Low et al. (2015) observed that CVDs, cancer and diabetes are the three major NCDs in the Asia Pacific region, and that the poor are the ones who suffer more due to less healthcare coverage and related policies, legislations and regulations regarding NCDs.

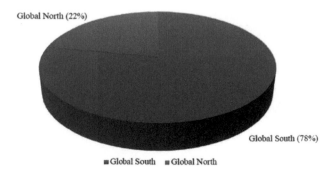

Global North (22%)

Global South (78%)

■Global South   ■Global North

Figure 5.2 Differential death burden from NCDs (Source: WHO [World Health Organization], 2018a)

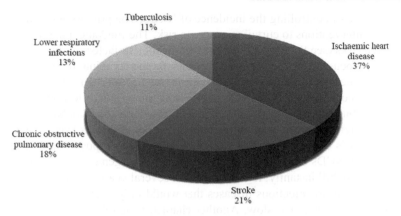

Figure 5.3 Top 5 causes of death in Southeast Asia (Source: WHO. (2018b). Global health observatory data)

The WHO (2018a) Global Health Observatory data for 2018 showed some patterns in Southeast Asia, the East Mediterranean Region and Western Pacific Regions. Figure 5.3 shows that, of the top 5 causes of death, 3 NCDs are responsible, accounting for 76% of all deaths. The two infectious diseases constitute only 24% of deaths. In the top 10 causes of death, an additional 3 NCDs appear, including diabetes, cirrhosis of the liver and kidney diseases. The data from Southeast Asia are similar to those of the East Mediterranean Region, where the top 2 causes of death are ischemic heart disease and stroke, together constituting 67% of the leading 5 causes of death in 2016. In the Western Pacific Region (including Cambodia and China), NCDs make up 100% of the leading 5 causes of death in the region. Of the top 5 NCDs, stroke and ischemic heart disease, each constituted 33%, totaling 66% of the causes of death.

Low- and middle-income countries (LMICs) of Africa are also struggling to manage the simultaneous challenge of NCDs and a high infectious disease burden. In some African countries, such as Algeria, Cabo Verde, South Africa, Sao Tome and Principe, Seychelles, Mauritius, Namibia and Seychelles, NCDs cause over 50% of all reported adult deaths (WHO, 2018c). There has been a reduction in the burden of infectious diseases in Algeria, but a heavy burden of NCDs (up to 76% of deaths) (WHO, 2018c). Seychelles has one of the heaviest burdens of NCDs in Africa, accounting for up to 81% of all deaths. In general, in addition to infectious diseases, the burden of NCDs is rising very fast in LMICs, devastating already weak economies (Juma et al., 2019). As highlighted in Figure 5.2, the Global South, of which Africa is a part, carries 78% of the global burden of NCDs. As of 2016, of the top ten causes of death in the African region, two NCDs, stroke and ischemic heart disease, appear as fourth and seventh, respectively. The remaining eight top causes of death were infectious diseases. The North Africa region has the highest burden of NCDs in Africa. The data for the region is usually combined with those of the Middle East, described as MENA (Middle East and North Africa). In MENA, NCDs account for 74% of the deaths in the region. Having examined the burden of NCDs, it is essential to discuss the major behavioral risk factors within the globalizing context.

5.3 Behavioral Factors in Noncommunicable Diseases

Lifestyle factors as social determinants of health were briefly discussed previously (see Section 3.2.1.6). The following section will further unpack the lifestyle factors to explain some that are connected with NCDs. From a sociological purview, behavioral factors are important causal factors in the risk of NCDs. Global and public health researchers also focus attention on behavioral factors as a measure of controlling the incidence of NCDs. The primary method of control has been behavioral interventions to curtail exposure to risk. The fundamental assumption is that the manufactured risks (see Section 4.3) are the significant risk factors in the spread of NCDs. Most interventions focus on the individual, rather than on the combination of macro and micro factors espoused in the structuration theory of Giddens (see Section 4.2). Discussions in global health must always consider the conceived levels (from super-macro to micro) for a successful fight against the burden of NCDs in all regions of the world. The Global South, however, requires particular attention, since it accounts for over 70% of all deaths from NCDs.

One characteristic of NCDs is the relatively long time-period between exposure and incidence. This is one reason that NCDs are problematic in terms of management and control. Smoking as a risk factor does not kill instantly; it generally takes several years or even decades before mortality occurs. Unlike most infectious diseases that would only take a few days to manifest, the onset of NCDs is gradual and slow. Another characteristic of NCDs conforms to the aphorism that "the road to hell is paved with good intentions". First, it is a long journey (accumulation of risk over time); second, several individuals engage in risk with some perceived leisure motives. The "good intentions" is that risk accumulates from perceived "sweet" adventures. People have advanced various subjective reasons for smoking. They justify their actions, unfortunately, without immediate consequence that would prove the perils of tobacco. The aphorism can also be considered in light of unhealthy nutrition. The third point is that most of the risk factors are very addictive. Once the risk journey starts, the damage begins, and it is highly challenging to stop. The fourth point is that everybody is entangled in the web of risk. It is not only the smokers at risk from smoking, the non-smokers who also inhale from the polluted air, thereby accumulating some risk. Almost everyone enjoys the "sweet risk journey" of alcoholic and non-alcoholic drinks, and processed foods, among others. All age groups are at risk of NCDs, although the risk increases with age.

Figure 5.4 shows the context of the risks of NCDs. The main box in Figure 5.4 presents the "risk factors". However, the risk factors exist within a global context and are highly a function of globalization. Globalization has been implicated in the high prevalence of the risk factors, which are consequential for the incidence of NCDs. Globalization also affects other contextual issues, including social determinants of health, policy/regulatory environment and health systems. There have been some policies to mitigate the effect of globalization of the risk factors, the extent of domestication and implementation of such policies are

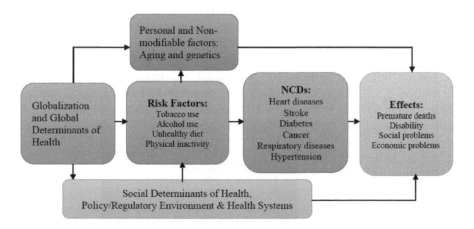

Figure 5.4 Context of risk of noncommunicable diseases

an essential determinant in the burden of NCDs in specific countries. The health policies and systems also significantly affect health outcomes of NCDs, since the diseases are typically manageable. There are also personal (e.g., gender and income) and non-modifying factors (aging and genetics), which affect disease outcome. The high mortality in the Global South is primarily due to the high burden in the context of weak health systems. Beyond morbidity and mortality, adverse health conditions lead to social and economic problems, which further affect development efforts. Simply put, the success of any intervention against NCDs depends on the consideration of the behavioral risk factors, which will be examined in subsequent subsections.

5.3.1 Smoking and Tobacco Use

The use of tobacco, in various ways, is a major risk factor, explaining susceptibility to many NCDs. Al-Ibrahim and Gross (1990: p. 214) defined tobacco use as "any habitual use of the tobacco plant leaf and its products. The predominant use of tobacco is by smoke inhalation of cigarettes, pipes, and cigars". Smokeless tobacco includes products that can be sniffed, sucked or chewed. Tobacco is the most common substance smoked, followed by marijuana and others. There are also several other substances, non-tobacco inhaled or smoked, including heroin and cocaine, among others. Smoking affects the entire human body, and exposes individuals to many adverse health conditions; smoking affects the circulatory, respiratory, reproductive and immune systems, and the skin, eyes, mouth and hair (Dresden, 2019). Smoking and tobacco use have also been linked to the global top-five chronic diseases: (lung) Cancer, (ischemia) stroke, heart diseases, diabetes and Alzheimer's diseases. The quantification of smoking is about the number of cigarettes smoked per day and for how many years. The other usage, chewed or sniffed, might be difficult to quantify (Al-Ibrahim and Gross, 1990).

The tobacco industry represents one of the biggest industrial manufacturing of risk. The products are usually explicitly marked as unsafe for human consumption—such inscriptions include "smokers are liable to die young" and "smoking is dangerous to health", among others. Despite the warning inscription, millions of individuals continue to smoke, consume risk and eventually die as a result of smoking. The tobacco use kills over 8 million people every year; 15% of whom are secondhand smokers; 80% of smokers live in the Global South, where tobacco-related morbidity and mortality are highest (WHO, 2019b). Between 1990 and 2015, smoking increased by more than 25%; by 2015, smoking was one of the top-five contributors to global DALYs (Disability-Adjusted Life Years) in 109 countries (GBDS 2015). In 2015, among men, smoking was the second-leading risk factor for cardiovascular and circulatory diseases, cancers and chronic respiratory conditions (GBDS 2015 Risk Factors Collaborators, 2016). Especially in the Global South, smoking is a part of male culture. Beyond the health risks of smoking, there are other socio-economic risks: Due to its habituating and addictive nature, smoking gulps household resources. In an addictive situation, individuals are no longer in control of the habit—it affects social relationships and pauperizes households.

Yach and Bettcher (2000) noted that the globalization of "tobacco marketing, trade, research, and industry constitute a gruesome threat to global health". China, Brazil, the USA and India are the top producers of tobacco products in the world. Tobacco products were aggressively marketed between the 1960s and the 1980s, and its usages have been globalized, spreading the risks and increasing related morbidity and mortality. The tobacco industry operates as a global force, buying influence and power, penetrating markets across the world (Yach and Bettcher, 2000). The previous loose regulation and global governance have facilitated the penetration of the tobacco market. The global stakeholders only intensified efforts after the damage has been done: Tobacco has become a global addictive brand with over one billion smokers, killing millions of people annually. The global tobacco markets make billions of US dollars in profits at the expense of global population health.

The world is witnessing tobacco industry globalization, which accounts for the global burden of related morbidity and mortality. The industry is perpetually seeking natural resources and product markets across the globe. Tobacco use penetrates as a lifestyle recipe, first starting as a class product—i.e., for the affluent, projected through the media. Smoking behavior penetrates through hegemonic domination, with many people imbibing the tradition both consciously and unconsciously. Lee et al. (2016) reported increasing targeting of LMICs for markets in the 1960s, marked by "the expansion of transnational tobacco companies (TTCs) into Latin America" and "newly industrializing economies of Asia in the 1980s, and Eastern Europe, the Middle East and Africa" from the 1990s. These periods marked the most aggressive expansion of global tobacco markets, with the use of "unethical" tactics and strategies, and a subsequent increase in related morbidity and mortality.

Smoking is a leading global health tragedy that requires some global efforts to stop it. There have been some global control efforts, including the adoption of the Framework Convention on Tobacco Control (FCTC), focusing on behavioral change rather than just personal responsibility (Lee et al., 2016). Tobacco control is within the domain of global governance led by many stakeholders, including the governments of various countries (who signed onto the treaty) and the WHO, among others. The primary demand of the treaty is the reduction in tobacco use. The major global strategy is called **MPOWER** (launched February, 2008): **M**onitor tobacco use and prevention policies; **P**rotect people from tobacco smoke; **O**ffer help to quit tobacco use; **W**arn about the dangers of tobacco; **E**nforce bans on tobacco advertising, promotion and sponsorship; and **R**aise taxes on tobacco. Lee et al. (2016) reported that at least 180 states' parties signed onto the treaty. As of the tenth year of the initiative, there have been some achievements, including a 14.8 million reduction in the number of smokers, averting over 7.3 million deaths (Chan, 2015). The current rate of mortality, however, shows a considerable gap that needs to be covered through intensification of global efforts.

5.3.2 *Harmful Use of Alcohol*

Harmful use of alcohol is about intoxication, dependence and addiction that increases health risks. Harmful use of alcohol is a global health tragedy accounting for up to 2.5 million deaths (about 3.7% of global deaths) per year (WHO, 2019d). Harmful alcoholic use is measured by the volume, extent and frequency of alcohol consumption. One significant way of manifestation is frequent intoxication or alcoholism (often called alcohol use disorder [AUD]). Alcoholism is a condition of perpetual desire to consume alcohol, despite negative impacts, or it can be defined as problem drinking, a condition of continuous drinking beyond body tolerance. The WHO reported that alcohol could damage every organ or system in the body and contribute to more than 60 diseases and conditions, including cancer, heart diseases, liver damage and memory loss, among others. Alcoholism also contributes to many social problems and consequences, such as impaired family relationships, traffic and work accidents, absenteeism, financial burden (poverty), unemployment, domestic abuse, risky sexual behavior and some mental health issues.

Despite the health problems associated with alcohol use, its yearly consumption is expected to increase over the next decade in more than half of WHO regions: From 8.0 to 8.4 liters in the Americas; 7.3 liters to 8.1 liters in the Western Pacific Region; and 4.5 to 6.2 liters in the Southeast Asia Region (WHO, 2018b). "Globally, an increase of 0.4 liters is expected in total alcohol per capita consumption in low-income countries by 2025" (WHO, 2018b: p. 58), portending an increase in alcohol-related problems. Globalization has also been implicated in the world alcohol problem; beer has been the most consumed alcoholic drink, and its consumption has increased significantly in the last five decades across countries (Cohen and Swinnen, 2015). There has been a significant increase in beer consumption in emerging economies, where the burden of alcohol abuse is most massive (Jernigan et al., 2000; Cohen and Swinnen, 2015).

Jernigan et al. (2000) reported that globalization significantly influenced the drinking culture at the local level. The open market for alcohol and the drive for profit have also promoted aggressive marketing, with some hidden and open strategies. For instance, popular alcohol brands sponsor various sport events to get the attention of young people who regularly engage in or follow sport events. In short, seeking new markets ensures expansion to the emerging economies, where the policy environment may be too weak to curtail the pressures from multinational companies (Jernigan et al., 2000). While alcohol has always been a traditional drink in most developing nations, globalization is modifying the new drinking culture to improve patronage with fewer cultural restrictions. Traditional drinking behavior occurs with some form of social control with drinking on a special occasion, open space and habitually by adults (Jernigan et al., 2000). Wilson (2004) submitted that alcohol is a global commodity and a significant symbol of the forces of globalization. It has become a major ceremonial commodity of all kinds of occasions. Alcohol consumption portrays foreign influence on local culture; sometimes, a brand (of alcohol) is a status symbol. Wilson (2004) noted that drinking (alcohol) had not received deserving attention in the southern socio-cultural context, especially with the consideration of its globalized positive representation of some branded liquor. While alcohol has some cultural meanings which promote its consumption, understanding its global health context is vital in efforts to curtail its adverse consequences. For instance, in addition to the 2.7 million deaths annually, alcohol use contributed to 9.7% of the Disability-Adjusted Life Years in Latin America, and 1.6–2.8% in Asia and Africa in the year 2000 (Jernigan et al., 2000). The tendency to consider alcohol as just an economic commodity needs to be aligned with public health considerations.

Pang and Guindon (2004) also confirmed that globalization has resulted in higher alcohol use in the Global South, especially among younger individuals. Therefore, global efforts to reverse the trend in terms of the adverse health consequences must be intensified. The global efforts to confront the harmful effects of alcohol started in 1983 when the World Health Assembly (WHA) recognized alcohol-related problems as one of the world's major health concerns (WHO, 2019d). On Friday, 21 May 2010, the WHA adopted by consensus resolution WHA 63.13, which endorses the global strategy focusing on some critical areas of policy options and interventions at the national level, including community action; drink-driving policies and countermeasures; control of availability and marketing of alcohol (WHO, 2019d). The resolution aims to reduce the adverse consequences of drinking and alcohol intoxication; improve health services' response; reduce the public health impact of illicit alcohol and informally produced alcohol (WHO, 2019d). The Global South needs to domesticate and reinforce the implementation of the global strategy against the adverse effects of alcohol use.

5.3.3 *Inadequate Physical Activity*

Adequate body movement to dispense some energy is required to service the skeletal system. This movement is simply referred to as physical activity. Inadequate physical activity (sometimes called a sedentary lifestyle) has been implicated as the fourth-leading risk factor for global mortality (6% of deaths globally) (WHO, 2019a). The WHO estimated that physical inactivity contributes, as a leading cause, to approximately 30% of ischemic heart disease, 27% of diabetes and 21–25% of colon and breast cancers. In other words, adequate physical activities would reduce the risk of these diseases, in addition to hypertension, stroke and depression.

The WHO identified other main benefits of sufficient physical activities to include improvement in bone and functional health, which is fundamental to energy expenditure (balance) and weight control. In general, the benefits of physical activity are immeasurable for functional health. Physical activities do not necessarily mean exercise, which is only one structured type of physical activity (WHO, 2019a). It is possible to have adequate physical activity without doing it in a structured or organized manner. Beyond exercise, physical activities also include walking, labor (formal and domestic) and playing (recreation or leisure) (WHO, 2019a). The general recommendation is that an adult should engage in moderate or vigorous physical activity of at least 150 or 75 minutes per week, respectively (or a combination of both moderate and rigorous activity) (Guthold et al., 2018). Physical inactivity in the context of increasing age leads to deterioration of human physiology (not only the joints but all organs of the body), which will later reduce physical capacity and function (see Figure 5.5). Physical inactivity is highly correlated with many NCDs, often irreversible and exhibiting a protracted course.

Guthold et al. (2018) analyzed data from 168 countries involving 1.9 million participants and observed differential patterns of physical activity based on sex and region. The study reported the lowest physical activity in men from Oceania, East and South Asia and sub-Saharan Africa (SSA). Within each region, women had less physical activity (compared to men) except in East and Southeast Asia; with a relatively wide gap between the sexes in central Asia, MENA and South Asia. There is some cultural context to insufficient activity. In MENA, for example, there is a general restriction on women engaging in activities outside the home because of some Islamic beliefs. Women are more active in the private than the public sphere; in most quarters, there is even restriction of movement as a cultural measure of "protecting" women from sexual harassment. Sharara et al. (2018) and Donnelly et al. (2018) also confirmed the high prevalence of inactivity, but higher among women in Arab countries. Sharara et al. (2018) reported reasons that keep Arab women from getting sufficient physical activity, including gender norms and conservative dress not suitable for some physical activities. Gender inequality also reflects in physical inactivity, which pushes women "towards a lifestyle centered on hospitality, excessive food consumption and sedentariness" (Sharara et al., 2018). The average prevalence (of physical inactivity) was more than 40% in all Arab countries, except for Comoros (21%), Egypt (32%) Jordan (5%); and up to 68% in Saudi Arabia and 87% in Sudan (Sharara et al., 2018). Social variables, such as age, gender and low income, are correlated with the high prevalence,

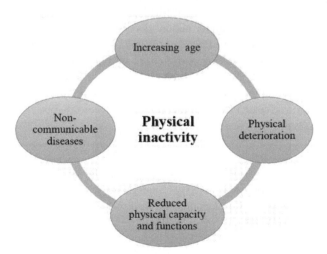

Figure 5.5 Vicious circle of physical inactivity and noncommunicable diseases

and it was noted that specific aspects of the cultural context discouraged physical activity (Sharara et al., 2018).

In general, the prevalence of insufficient physical activity in high-income countries was more than double the prevalence in low-income countries in 2016. The prevalence of insufficient physical activity has also increased in high-income countries, from 31.6% (27.1–37.2) in 2001 to 36.8% (35.0–38.0) in 2016, whereas it has been stable in low-income countries (Guthold et al., 2018). Guthold's report further highlighted that the prevalence of insufficient inactivity was more than 50% in Iraq, Kuwait, American Samoa and Saudi Arabia, and lower than 10% in Uganda, Mozambique, Lesotho, Tanzania, Niue, Vanuatu and Togo). Insufficient physical activity has been reported in more than one-third of the population in 55 (32.7%) of 168 countries. Between 2001 and 2016, although there were improvements in some countries (including Brazil, Bulgaria, Germany, Philippines and Singapore), a decline was recorded in others (including Cook Islands, Jordan, Tokelau, Samoa, Myanmar, Solomon Islands and Tonga).

The data from African countries also indicate a high prevalence of physical inactivity. The emerging development processes, including urbanization and globalization, are major factors in the prevalence of physical inactivity. Many of the African countries (notably, SSA) are just in the early stages of an emerging NCD epidemic (Barr et al., 2018). Africa is undergoing various forms of transition: Economic, demographic and even political transition, occasioned by some forces of globalization.

Globalization and its major drivers also affect the prevalence of physical inactivity across the globe. Improvement in technology has led to a drastic reduction in physical activities; labor is technologically driven with less use of physical human strength. Work, walking and playing processes are highly automated. The globalization era is that of digitalization, urbanization and automation (see Barr et al., 2018). There is increasing acceptability of electronic scooters instead of bicycles, computer games instead of physical games, preference for the elevator instead of climbing the stairs and automation of house chores (i.e., dishwashing and laundry). The penetration of technologies in daily human activities has reduced physical activities to a great extent. The use of technology has promoted ease of doing tasks but with some adverse consequences, including insufficient physical activity. Logically, countries with less industrialization should have higher physical activity, but the reverse is the case. The highly industrialized countries are also experiencing a gradual reduction in physical activity.

Insufficient physical activity is another global health tragedy that should be addressed on a global scale. The world needs to be engaged to be physically active daily. The first major step is that more information is required on the benefits of physical activities. Increased perceived benefits might likely improve physical activities around the world. Working, walking (transportation) and playing (recreation) need to be refined to ensure some active engagement. There has been a gradual development of a global response to the global pandemic of physical inactivity; Varela et al. (2017) observed that surveillance and monitoring of country-level progress would facilitate the development and implementation of programs that would foster physical activity. For instance, Oyeyemi et al. (2018) suggested the integration of physical activity surveillance into the existing national demographic and health survey in Nigeria and elsewhere in Africa. WHO is also leading the global partnership to promote active living and reduce the burden of NDCs related to physical inactivity.

5.3.4 Unhealthy Diet

An unhealthy diet is also a major risk factor for NCDs. Unhealthy diet includes overeating of fatty, greasy, raw and sweet foods (including beverages), highly flavored and pungent food, and with reduced intake of fiber fish and omega-3-fatty acids (Alisi et al., 2019). Unhealthy diet has also been linked to several NCDs, including obesity, CVDs, hypertension and cancer. Westernization, urbanization and globalization have been major drivers of the shift in dietary patterns all over the globe. The previous factor, physical inactivity or sedentary lifestyle, plays a significant role as an intermediate factor in the link between an unhealthy diet and the emergence of NCDs. The incidence of obesity is linked to unhealthy diet and physical inactivity. The shift in dietary patterns comes with health consequences, including rising obesity, worsening levels of metabolic risks and decreased physical activity (GBDS 2015 Risk Factors Collaborators, 2016). Obesity is a significant indicator of an unhealthy diet, linked to many health conditions, and it is increasing all over the world. The worldwide prevalence of obesity nearly tripled between 1975 and 2016, and it is no longer a problem confined to high-income countries; it is on the rise in low- and middle-income countries as well (see Ng et al., 2014, Haggblade et al., 2016; Misra et al., 2019). The WHO reported an increasing prevalence of overweight (usually defined as a BMI greater than or equal to 25 in adults), and obesity (usually represented as a BMI greater than or equal to 30) (among adults >15 years old) in the MENA region. The data show the highest rates of overweight people in Kuwait, Egypt, the United Arab Emirates, Jordan, Bahrain and Saudi Arabia, with the prevalence of overweight/obesity ranging from 74% to 86% among women and 69% to 77% among men.

Sub-Saharan Africa faces malnutrition issues, including both food insecurity and an emerging obesity crisis. With a high prevalence of hunger, malnutrition and obesity (typically as a result of overeating), the African continent is overweight and hungry at the same time, making the problem extremely complex. Haggblade et al. (2016) observed that SSA is undergoing a nutrition transition as a result of urbanization and globalization. Haggblade et al. focused on three countries, including South Africa—advanced, Ghana—intermediate, and Uganda—early, at different stages of the nutrition transformation. The experience of structural change in Africa's food systems is evident; Haggblade et al. observed an increase in urban food markets, mostly processed food, some sourced from the global chain of the food market. Therefore, more foods are stored, preserved, processed and packaged. Packaged food, a mark of global extension of the global food market, linked to urban space, has increased demand for prepared convenience foods. The African share of the overweight population has increased swiftly, from 17% in 1980 to 30% in 2008. Regional and sex differences have been reported with overweight and obesity levels, highest in Southern and Northern Africa and greater among women than men (Haggblade et al., 2016). The case of Africa (and MENA) is that of the emerging feminization of obesity. The health implications are also glaring; there is an increasing incidence of unhealthy diet-related conditions such as diabetes, hypertension and cardiovascular disease. Unfortunately, the problem of unhealthy diet has a double face in SSA—the simultaneous burden of undernutrition and overnutrition—both above 30% in Swaziland, Lesotho and South Africa (Haggblade et al., 2016).

The situation of the double burden of overnutrition and undernutrition is similar in South Asia (Misra et al., 2019). Obesity is higher among women than men. As in Africa, most people in South Asia also consider obesity or being overweight as a sign of good living or wealth. The prevalence of obesity ranges from 4.6% in Bangladesh to 43.5% in the Maldives and is higher in urban than in rural areas (Misra et al., 2019). The main explanation for the lower rate in rural areas is the insufficient access to globalized food (or so-called western foods), lower purchasing power and a more physically active lifestyle. In short, Misra et al. also implicated urbanization and globalization in the prevalence of an unhealthy diet in South Asia. Being overweight in South Asia is mainly due to the increasing consumption of globalized, western foods (including sweetened beverages, fried snacks and other high-calorie-dense western foods) coupled with physical inactivity (or sedentary behavior) (Misra et al., 2017).

Latin America and the Caribbean are not exempted from the problem of unhealthy diet. Using obesity and being overweight as major manifestations of an unhealthy diet, Latin America has an overweight prevalence rate of 57% in the adult population (54% and 70% in men and women, respectively) while obesity is 19% (14.6% in men and 24% in women) (Ng et al. 2014). The highest obesity prevalence in the region is in El Salvador (33%) and Paraguay (30.1%) for women, and Uruguay (23.3%) and Chile (22.0%) for men. The Caribbean nations also have high rates of overweight and obesity—with Barbados, Trinidad and Tobago, Antigua and Barbuda, all above 30% (Ng et al., 2014).

In summary, an unhealthy diet is a global problem requiring global actions. The changing food patterns, occasioned by globalization, have been implicated in all regions of the globe. As previously mentioned, increasing urbanization, modernization and the growth of global fast-food spell a common fate for the world in terms of a nutrition transition. One of the results is the hyper-increasing rate of obesity, which comes with related NCDs. The implication of globalization and global fast-foods further necessitates the examination of the McDonaldization theory, not only related to unhealthy diet but also other risk behaviors, including harmful use of alcohol and tobacco.

5.4 McDonaldization Theory

Since the inception of the fast-food giant in 1937, from which George Ritzer derived the concept, *McDonaldization* has penetrated over 100 countries of the world as a brand name, a culture of capitalist expansion or liberalization of trade, a prominent indicator of globalization or global village, an example of the globalization of manufactured risk and the power of global force on nutrition transition. Ritzer's theoretical concept goes beyond a particular brand; it concentrates more of the principles of fast-food and the proliferation of fast-food itself. The implication of the preceding is that there is almost no country free from McDonaldization. Ritzer conceived his McDonaldization thesis is 1983, before widespread Internet facilities. He observed a significant globalization trend, which now has a prominent perplexity in the world. The consequences of McDonaldization—at least as reflected in the prevalence of obesity and related matters—have been felt across the globe. The then conception of McDonaldization was predictive for the rest of the world, especially the Global South. Then, McDonaldization was emerging, but the world was not prepared for it. Alternatively, was it a process that should be resisted, controlled or managed? Most globalizing processes do not portend immediate risk (see Section 4.3 about risk society theory).

McDonaldization is a globalized and globalizing process of proliferation of fast-food, with its bureaucratic principles, which have broken the structures and walls, deepening across cultures and accommodating more individuals and households. Ritzer (2018:14) defined McDonaldization as "the process by which the principles of the fast-food restaurant are coming to dominate more and more sectors of American society as well as of the rest of the world". Ritzer called it the McDonaldization of society—of the world; of the globe and everything. The concept of McDonaldization originally comes from the consumption of fast-food, but now extends to everything and anything; it is more about the process of globalization and its related consequences. McDonaldization of society is about the rationalization of production, marketing, expansion drive and consumption of not only financial products but also social products, guided by bureaucratic culture. The boomerang effect is on global society as a whole. Societies are increasingly becoming one, developing similar characteristics, ethics and goals. Most societies are highly bureaucratic or organized. The principle of bureaucracy, from which the principles of McDonaldization emerged, was a brainchild of the German sociologist, Max Weber. At the core of the bureaucratic norm are rationalization and standardization. The world is dominated by rational action from an industrial perspective to individuals' conception of the world around them.

The digital world has further broken down the barriers to McDonaldization, leaving more possibilities and opportunities for societies to be co-opted. The online process has aided the compression of space and time, which globalization represents. Ritzer (2018: p. 14) observed that

> the height of McDonaldization is now to be found online". He further noted that "the digital world is important both on its own, as well as in how it interpenetrates with the material world … we now live in a world increasingly dominated by 'bricks-and-clicks' (or, 'atoms-and-bits').

The previous brick-and-mortar world is giving way to the digital world, which represents the idea of the McDonaldized or globalized world—of intense social connectivity. Ritzer's idea is not just about domination; individuals also participate (actively) in the McDonaldization process, especially in the digital world. Ritzer (2018:15) observed that, "in comparison to brick-and-mortar settings, the ability of digital settings to turn consumers into prosumers is almost unlimited". The digital world is less labor-intensive, it is a world of virtual interaction, not even with a human at the other end, but programmed technology through which individuals can "design and produce" what they want. Therefore, "consumers are largely on their own on the Internet to prosume—to "produce" that which they are interested in consuming" (Ritzer, 2018: p. 15). The enchantment of fast-food, by extension all McDonaldized systems, is based on four major principles:

1. **Efficiency:** A McDonaldized system finds the best possible and fastest way of satisfying a need or want. Without cooking, individuals can get fast-food, which somehow saves time and energy. By simple clicks, products can be ordered and delivered to the doorstep. This effortless method has been adopted in other spheres of life. A McDonaldized system is a series of interlinked and well-organized procedures or routines which facilitate the delivery of goods and services (including cultural products). For instance, efficiency has promoted fast-food culture around the world.
2. **Calculability:** A McDonaldized system involves calculable steps, mostly quantifiable steps that promote access to products or wants. Time is a major factor that is often quantified in a typical McDonaldized system. The calculable effort is about accuracy and precision, not only in the preparation of the goods but also in their delivery. Items can often be customized. While the desire is fulfilled, the crucial calculable aspect for the "providers" or "influencers" is to maximize returns from the process. For example, the tobacco industry is more interested in profits than in the "quality" of its product for human consumption.
3. **Predictability:** The output of a McDonaldized system is about the brands being similar from one country to the other, based on similar processes, rules and outcomes. The standardized system builds similar expectations: The products are the same from one country or continent to the next. Consumers have been consciously or unconsciously orientated to accept no surprises, like a scripted process, about which both the actors and the audience are already aware.
4. **Control:** Consumers have been orientated with certain expectations, thereby conforming to the system's specifications and regulations. Local culture is gradually under control, being westernized or McDonaldized or incorporated into the global (food and other commodities) culture. The local tastes and wants are steadily placed under the control of a McDonaldized system.

It is crucial to further relate the ongoing discussion with fast-food and other globalized or McDonaldized items. The digital world has not merely McDonaldized food but other *marketables* or *commodifiables*, especially in the realm of risk goods (including diet, tobacco and alcohol). Thinking of fast-food as a major indicator at the heart of McDonaldization of society, many scholars have acknowledged that the food market has surpassed other commodities. The non-western world sometimes focuses on movies and music as the major cultural trade within the global world. Waldfogel (2019) observed that the market for food at restaurants is up to ten times larger than that of films and music. The global food space is dominated by Italian, Japanese, Chinese, Indian and American food. Waldfogel (2019) used data, including fast-food expenditure, to calculate implicit trade patterns in global cuisines for 52 countries. Many nations are deeply involved in how to feed others and generate valuable foreign exchange. One major aspect of feeding others also includes the proliferation of fast-food restaurants (the data on fast-food include estimates from hamburgers, chicken and pizza, etc.). Waldfogel (2019) noted that Italy, Japan and Mexico dominated the international trade in cuisines, but the USA still has powerful dominance in the area of fast-food. While the general food trade reflects migration patterns (Waldfogel, 2019), the fast-food pattern still reflects hegemonic practices (from North to South).

Globalization (or McDonaldization) penetrates all ways of life, including diets. The process also promotes reliance on imported food, changing the relationship between income and fat consumption, thereby skyrocketing the rates of obesity and diabetes, among other NCDs (Brownell and Yach, 2006). Like previously mentioned, McDonaldization can also be extended to the major risk products, including cigarettes and alcohol. The global sale is increasing with the expansion of the market to the emerging economies of the Global South. It is through such expansion that profits can further be maximized. It is all about the quantity of sales, not the health implication of the products.

As previously mentioned, the fight against NCDs must emphasize the control of risk factors, including McDonaldization. A de-McDonaldization process can be achieved through food norms that "emphasize food quality and nutrient density over quantity and price" and discourage "foods known to contribute to poor diet and obesity" (Brownell and Yach, 2006). Ritzer (2018) acknowledged that "McDonaldization has swept across the social landscape" because of its principles, but not without uncertainties and disadvantages. Ritzer also noted severe health consequences, especially in terms of health dangers. Risks are manufactured and spread through globalization and McDonaldization. There are inherent dangers in the process: for example, globalized fast-food promotes the (global) consumption of more fat, cholesterol, salt and sugar. From the arguments so far, there are calculable positive associations between the rise of globalization and McDonaldization and increasing NCDs in the Global South. Hence, the WHO, with Member States, has developed some global NCDs control targets.

5.6 Global NCDs Control Targets for 2025

Most Member States of the WHO have endorsed 9 global voluntary targets meant to reduce premature death from the 4 major NCDs by 25% by 2025, which will save at least 37 million lives (WHO, 2019c). The global targets constitute the major policy health goals. The goals, according to the WHO (2019c), include:

1. A 25% relative reduction in the overall mortality from cardiovascular diseases, cancer, diabetes and chronic respiratory diseases.
2. At least 10% relative reduction in the harmful use of alcohol, as appropriate, within the national context. This targets a risk factor focusing more on the national or macro level.

3. A 10% relative reduction in the prevalence of insufficient physical activity. Reversing the increasing rate of physical inactivity will help to reduce related morbidity and mortality.
4. A 30% relative reduction in mean population intake of salt/sodium. High salt intake is correlated with high blood pressure and increased risk of stroke and health diseases.
5. A 30% relative reduction in the prevalence of current tobacco use (including smokeless tobacco) in persons aged 15+ years. Tobacco use is correlated with over 8 million deaths, especially among adults. The costs of the health burden surpass the revenue from tobacco.
6. A 25% relative reduction in the prevalence of raised blood pressure or a containment of the prevalence of raised blood pressure, according to national circumstances. This mainly targets a health condition, which influences the risk of other NCDs.
7. Halt the rise in diabetes and obesity. This is also targeting two health conditions, which are primary risk conditions for other NCDs.
8. Achieving that at least 50% of eligible people receive drug therapy and counseling (including glycemic control) to prevent heart attacks and strokes. This is because information and access to treatment will reduce the rate of mortality from NCDs.
9. An 80% availability of the necessary affordable technologies and essential medicines, including generics, required to treat major NCDs in both public and private facilities. This goal is also meant to improve access to treatment.

The extent to which nations have progressed toward and will achieve the set goals is another discussion. There is some mistrust in the control of NCDs. Some of the mistrust-generating issues include:

1. The major arguments from literature are that the significant risks are manufactured in the Global North and the major burden borne in the Global South, yet there are no drastic measures to control the risk manufacturing channels. A typical example is an unending debate about some countries of the Global North taking some responsibilities in climate control.
2. There is often a conflict of interest in many quarters. For example, halting McDonaldization is likely to hurt some economic, political interests and hegemony of the North. The world can democratically promote some drastic measures that will help to reduce risk factors, if it wants to.
3. Beyond health considerations, economic and political considerations are also involved in the control of diseases. In many cases, public health gains might be sacrificed for economic gains.
4. There is hesitancy from the global North to provide the required expertise and resources in the fights against NCDs. It is often treated as a national issue rather than global.
5. There is weak political capacity/will in the Global South to impose sanctions on certain (risk) products from the Global North. For example, how processed infant milk is promoted at the expense of breastmilk. There are no stiff measures against processed milk for newborns. Therefore, most low-income countries accept risk as a no-choice option.

5.7 Summary

- The rise of noncommunicable diseases (NCDs) is associated with increasing modernization and globalization. Many antecedents and emerging factors of development are fueling the rise of NCDs, which compounded the health situation in the Global South. The current health discourse is about epidemiologic transition involving a considerable pandemic of modern risks.

- Lifestyle often appears to exist only at the micro level, but emerging evidence has shown that lifestyle has a lot to do with macro and super-macro factors, which can coerce micro level behavior.
- The continuous process of industrialization, urbanization, global markets and media technologies have altered the realities of social existence beyond measure. Globalization is a factor of change, development and economic progress affecting all spheres of life, including nutrition, communication and human well-being.
- The Global South is experiencing some socio-economic transitions in line with the modernization agenda. The assimilation of modernization (globalization) recipes holds several implications (including health implications). For instance, tobacco usages have been globalized, spreading the risks and increasing related morbidity and mortality.
- This chapter also examines the behavioral factors in NCDs, with a focus on how globalization has accounted for the proliferation of these risk factors, which further increase the disease burden in the Global South.
- Globalization and its major drivers affect the prevalence of physical inactivity across the globe. Improvement in technology has led to a drastic reduction in physical activities; labor is technologically driven with less use of physical strength. The globalization era is that of digitalization and automation.
- Globalization also results in changing food patterns, which is another risk factor of NCDs. The increasing urbanization, modernization and the growth of global fast-food spell a common fate for the world in terms of a nutrition transition. One of the results is the hyper-increasing rate of obesity, which comes with related NCDs.
- This chapter strengthens its arguments using McDonaldization theory that the digital world has not merely McDonaldized food, but other *marketables* or *commodifiables* as well, especially in the realm of goods with high health risk (including tobacco and alcohol).
- Significant modern risks are manufactured in the Global North and the major adverse burden is borne in the Global South, yet there are no drastic measures to control the risk manufacturing channels. A typical example is an unending debate about some countries of the Global North taking adequate responsibilities in climate control.
- There is weak political capacity/will in the Global South to impose sanctions on certain (risk) products from the Global North. Therefore, most low-income countries accept risk products, such as e-waste, as a no-choice option.

Critical Thinking Questions

- Globalization has been implicated in the prevalence of noncommunicable diseases in the Global South. Reflecting on the realities of globalization, think deep about its roles in the prevalence of chronic diseases.
- With reference to any two specific noncommunicable diseases, reflect deeply on how globalization should be implicated in their spread. Can you mention some specific globalizing pathways responsible for the spread of such diseases?
- Noncommunicable diseases are associated with risk factors. Make specific arguments which situate globalization as a major context for the high prevalence of behavior risk factors for noncommunicable diseases in the Global South.
- With reference to the McDonaldization theory, do you think that enchantment of fast-food is influencing the prevalence of obesity. Why is it so and why not?
- How are the four major principles of McDonaldization theory influence globalization–health relationships?

- The realization of the global control targets of noncommunicable disease is sometimes impeded by mistrust between the Global North and South. Do you think that those mistrusts are valid? Why is it so and why not?

Suggested Readings

- Hanefeld, J. (2015). *Globalization and health.* New York: McGraw-Hill Education. Apart from other issues, the book presents a concise chapter on globalization and noncommunicable diseases.
- Ritzer, G. (2018). *McDonaldization of society: Into the digital age.* Ninth Edition. London: Sage. The book presents a sociological purview, through a historical lens, to show how the principles of fast-food influence people's lives, including both positive and negative consequences on individuals.
- MacGregor, H. (2019). Global public health, noncommunicable diseases, and ethics. In Mastroianni, A. C., Kahn, J. P. and Kass, N. E. (eds.), *The Oxford handbook of public health ethics.* Oxford: Oxford University Press. This chapter focuses on the framing of the "global" nature of noncommunicable diseases (NCDs) with reference to the implications of the growing burden in low- and middle-income countries. Oxford University Press.
- Fedacko, J., Takahashi, T., Singh, R. B., Pella, D., Chibisov, S., Hristova, K., Pella, D., Elkilany, G. N., Tomar, R. S. and Juneja, L. R. (2019). Globalization of diets and risk of noncommunicable diseases. In Singh, R. B., Watson, R. R. and Takahashi, T. (eds.), *The role of functional food security in global health* (pp. 87–107). Cambridge: Academic Press. The chapter supports the argument that the globalization of the Western diet is associated with the increasing burden noncommunicable diseases (NCDs) in the Global South.
- Labonté, R. and Arne Ruckert, A. (2019). The global diffusion of non-communicable diseases. In: *Health equity in a globalizing era: Past challenges, future prospects.* Oxford: Oxford University Press. DOI:10.1093/oso/9780198835356.003.0011. The chapter stresses the connection between globalization and the rise of noncommunicable diseases in the Global South.

References

Al-Ibrahim, M. S., & Gross, J. Y. (1990). Tobacco use. In Walker, H. K., Hall, W. D. & Hurst, J. W. (Eds.), *Clinical Methods: The History, Physical, and Laboratory Examinations* (pp. 214 –216, 3rd ed.). Boston, MA: Butterworth Publishers.

Alisi, A., Nobili, V. & Manco, M. (2019). Obesity and nonalcoholic fatty liver disease in children. In Bagchi, D. (Ed.), *Global Perspectives on Childhood Obesity: Current Status, Consequences and Prevention* (pp. 209–222). London: Academic Press.

Amzat J., & Razum, O. (2014). The interpretive perspective in medical sociology: Part II. In *Medical Sociology in Africa.* Cham, Switzerland: Springer International Publishing. doi: 10.1007/978-3-319-03986-2_8.

Barr, A. L., Young, E. H. & Sandhu, M. S. (2018). Objective measurement of physical activity: Improving the evidence base to address non-communicable diseases in Africa. *BMJ Global Health, 3,* e001044. doi: 10.1136/ bmjgh-2018-001044.

Brownell, K. D., & Yach, D. (2006). Lessons from a small country about the global obesity crisis. *Globalization and Health, 2,* 11. doi: 10.1186/1744-8603-2-11.

Chan, M. (2015). WHO Director-General commemorates 10th anniversary of historic tobacco treaty. Address at an event celebrating the 10th anniversary of the WHO Framework Convention on Tobacco Control, Geneva, 27 February.2015.

Cohen, L., & Swinnen, J. (2015). Economic growth, globalisation and beer consumption. *Journal of Agricultural Economics*, *67*(1), 186–207.

Donnelly, T. T., Fung, T. S. & Al-Thani, A. (2018). Fostering active living and healthy eating through understanding physical activity and dietary behaviours of Arabic-speaking adults: A cross-sectional study from the Middle East. *BMJ Open*, *8*(4), e019980. doi: 10.1136/bmjopen-2017-019980.

Dresden, D. (2019). How does smoking affect the body? *MedicalNewsToday*, www.medicalnewstoday.com/articles/324644.php. Accessed on August 22, 2019.

Fedacko, J., Takahashi, T., Singh, R. B., Pella, D., Chibisov, S., Hristova, K., Pella, D., Elkilany, G. N., Tomar, R. S. & Juneja, L. R. (2019). Globalization of diets and risk of noncommunicable diseases. In Singh, R. B., Watson, R. R. & Takahashi, T. (Eds.), *The Role of Functional Food Security in Global Health* (pp. 87–107). Cambridge: Academic Press.

Global Burden of Disease Study [GBDS] (2015). Risk factors collaborators (2016). Global, regional, and national comparative risk assessment of 79 behavioural, environmental and occupational, and metabolic risks or clusters of risks, 1990–2015: A systematic analysis for the Global Burden of Disease Study 2015. *Lancet*, *388*(10053), 1659–1724.

Guthold, R., Stevens, G. A., Riley, L. M. & Bull, F. C. (2018). Worldwide trends in insufficient physical activity from 2001 to 2016: A pooled analysis of 358 population-based surveys with 1·9 million participants. *Lancet Global Health*, *6*, e1077–86.

Haggblade, S., Duodu, K. G., Kabasa, J. D., Minnaar, A., Ojijo, N. K. O. & Taylor, JRN. (2016). Emerging early actions to bend the curve in sub-Saharan Africa's nutrition transition. *Food and Nutrition Bulletin*, *37*(2), 219–241.

Jernigan, D. H., Monteiro, M., Room, R. & Saxena, S. (2000). Towards a global alcohol policy: Alcohol, public health and the role of WHO. *Bulletin of the World Health Organization*, *78*(4). http://origin.who.int/bulletin/archives/78(4)491.pdf.

Juma, K., Juma, P. A., Mohamed, S. F., Owuor, J., Wanyoike, A., Mulabi, D. & Participants for the first Africa NCD research conference 2017 in Nairobi, Kenya (2019). First Africa non-communicable disease research conference 2017: Sharing evidence and identifying research priorities. *Journal of Global Health*, *8*(2), 020301. doi: 10.7189/jogh.09.010201.

Labonté, R., & Arne Ruckert, A. (2019). The global diffusion of non-communicable diseases. In *Health Equity in a Globalizing Era: Past Challenges, Future Prospects*. Oxford: Oxford University Press. doi: 10.1093/oso/9780198835356.003.0011.

Lee, K., Eckhardt, J. & Holden, C. (2016). Tobacco industry globalization and global health governance: Towards an interdisciplinary research agenda. *Palgrave Communications*, *2*, 16037.

Low, W. Y., Lee, Y. K. & Samy, A. L. (2015). Non-communicable diseases in the Asia-Pacific region: Prevalence, risk factors and community-based prevention. *International Journal of Occupational Medicine and Environmental Health*, *28*(1), 20–6.

Misra, A., Jayawardena, R. & Anoop, S. (2019). Obesity in South Asia: Phenotype, morbidities, and mitigation. *Currents Obesity Reports*, *8*, 43. doi: 10.1007/s13679-019-0328-0.

Misra, A., Nikhil, T., Shah, E., Naveed, S., Dewan, A., Usha, S. & Narayan, K. M. V. (2017). Diabetes, cardiovascular disease, and chronic kidney disease in South Asia: Current status and future directions. *BMJ*, 357, j1420.

Narain, J. P., Garg, R. & Fric, A. (2011). Non-communicable diseases in the South-East Asia region: Burden, strategies and opportunities. *National Medical Journal of India*, *24*(5), 280–287.

Ng, M., Fleming, T., Robinson, M., Thomsom, B., Graetz, N. & The Global Team (2014). Global, regional, and national prevalence of overweight and obesity in children and adults during 1980–2013: A systematic analysis for the Global Burden of Disease Study 2013. *Lancet*, *384*, 766–781.

Oyeyemi, A. L., Oyeyemi, A. Y., Omotara, B. A., Lawan, A., Akinroye, K. K., Adedoyin, R. A. & Ramírez, A. (2018). Physical activity profile of Nigeria: Implications for research, surveillance and policy. *The Pan African Medical Journal*, *30*, 175. doi: 10.11604/pamj.2018.30.175.12679.

Pang, T., & Guindon, G. E. (2004). Globalization and risks to health. *EMBO Reports*, *5*(Spec No, Suppl 1), S11–S16. doi: 10.1038/sj.embor.7400226.

Ritzer, G. (2018). *McDonaldization of Society: Into the Digital Age* (9th ed.). London: Sage.

Sharara, E., Akik, C., Ghattas, H. & Obermeyer, C. M. (2018). Physical inactivity, gender and culture in Arab countries: A systematic assessment of the literature. *BMC Public Health*, *18*(1), 639. doi: 10.1186/s12889-018-5472-z.

Siegel, K. R., Patel, S. A. & Ali, M. K. (2014). Non-communicable diseases in South Asia: Contemporary perspectives. *British Medical Bulletin*, *111*(1), 31–44. doi: 10.1093/bmb/ldu018.

Varela, A. R., Pratt, M., Powell, K., Lee, I., Bauman, A., Heath, G., Martins, R. C., Kohl, H. & Hallal, P. C. (2017). Worldwide surveillance, policy, and research on physical activity and health: The global observatory for physical activity. *Journal of Physical Activity and Health*, *14*, 701–709.

Waldfogel, J. (2019). Dining out as cultural trade. *Journal of Cultural Economics*, 1–30. doi: 10.1007/s10824-019-09360-5.

World Health Organization (WHO) (2002). Noncommunicable diseases in South-East Asia Region: A profile. WHO Regional Office for South-East Asia. https://apps.who.int/iris/handle/10665/205577.

WHO (2018a). Global health observatory data. www.who.int/gho/mortality_burden_disease/causes_death/top_10/en/. Accessed on August 20, 2019.

WHO (2018b). *Global Status Report on Alcohol and Health*. Geneva: WHO.

WHO (2018c). Noncommunicable Diseases (NCD) Country profiles, 2018. www.afro.who.int/health-topics/noncommunicable-diseases. Accessed on August 20, 2019.

WHO (2019a). Global strategy on diet, physical activity and health. www.who.int/dietphysicalactivity/pa/en/. Accessed on August 22, 2019.

WHO (2019b). Global strategy to reduce harmful use of alcohol. www.who.int/substance_abuse/activities/gsrhua/en/. Accessed on August 20, 2019.

WHO (2019c). Noncommunicable diseases: Campaign for action – meeting the NCD targets. www.who.int/beat-ncds/take-action/targets/en/. Accessed on August 26, 2019.

WHO (2019d). Tobacco: Key facts. www.who.int/news-room/fact-sheets/detail/tobacco. Accessed on August 22, 2019.

Wilson, T. (2004). Globalization, differentiation and drinking cultures, an anthropological perspective. *Anthropology of Food* [Online], *3*. http://journals.openedition.org/aof/261.

Yach, D., & Bettcher, D. (2000). Globalisation of tobacco industry influence and new global responses. *Tobacco Control*, *9*, 206–216.

6 Globalization and Infectious Diseases

6.1 Introduction

Chapter 5 discussed the links and related issues around globalization and noncommunicable diseases (NCDs). The current chapter focuses on infectious diseases. Unlike chronic diseases, infectious diseases tend to be acute, with an onset that is sudden or rapid and a lifespan that is usually short. Most infectious diseases (e.g., Apollo and catarrh) are self-limiting, i.e., may resolve on their own without medication. Infectious diseases tend to be non-degenerative; within a relatively brief period, they either resolve, are cured or result in disability or mortality. Although acute conditions are potentially treatable and curable, the burden of mortality from infectious diseases can be too high. For example, while malaria is curable, it was responsible for up to 435,000 deaths in 2017 (WHO, 2018a). Many acute diseases are also preventable, especially with the use of vaccines. Most childhood diseases (including whooping cough and polio) are vaccine-preventable. There are some vaccine trials for malaria and other acute diseases; the success of such trials will save millions of lives. The extent of the acceptability of vaccines is another debate. The categorization of infectious diseases is often grouped along with some health conditions, such as maternal and child mortality, which are not contagious.

As previously mentioned, the Global South faces the double burden of infectious and noncommunicable diseases. The burden of infectious diseases is very low in the Global North. Many parts of the Global South are still confronted with traditional risks, i.e., the risk of infectious diseases, while facing the rising threat of noncommunicable diseases (WHO, 2009). The burden from both diseases seems to be equal globally, up to 50% each. What should be understood is that the Global North has successfully won the battle against infectious diseases such as malaria, typhoid and cholera. Most infectious diseases are often regarded as diseases of poverty or underdevelopment. The state of development provides the context which explains the prevalence of infectious diseases. For example, the emergence of the Ebola virus disease (a zoonosis) has been traced to dietary behavior, specifically the hunting and consumption of bats (see Timothy et al., 2019). Why do people hunt and eat bats? One explanation is poverty—the search for food in the face of hunger for meat. Such (bush/wild) meats are not subject to any type of food test before consumption in most low-income countries. Even within a single country, the prevalence of infectious diseases is higher among the poorest residents, including waterborne and foodborne diseases. The biggest of all the infectious diseases that have attracted global attention over the years are malaria, tuberculosis (TB) and human immunodeficiency virus (HIV). While the three diseases have been effectively contained in the Global North, the burden (both morbidity and mortality) remains very high in the Global South—accounting for more than a million deaths annually.

DOI: 10.4324/9781003247975-6

The spread of infectious diseases is closely linked to globalization. The threat of infectious disease is constant, even in the North, because of the possible re-emergence of such diseases. Malaria has been eradicated in the Global North but could re-emerge because of the movement of people in and out of malarial regions. The emergence of some zoonoses have also prompted the study of globalization and health as diseases can travel across the globe within a few hours, leading to pandemics. The world is linked through world trade routes facilitated by development in the transportation system. The flow of goods and people also facilitates the flow of pathogens across the globe. The world is one big hub for all opportunities and uncertainties, including disease transmission. Before other arguments, it is vital to briefly examine the burden of infectious diseases, especially in the Global South.

6.2 Burden of Infectious Diseases in the Global South

As highlighted in Section 6.1, infectious diseases (often considered along with neonatal, maternal and nutritional diseases) are acute and responsible for millions of deaths. In the top 10 global burden of disease, 3 infectious diseases appear: Lower respiratory infections (with a crude death rate of 40 per 100,000), diarrhea (with a crude death rate of 16 per 100,000), and tuberculosis (with a crude death rate of 14 per 100,000) (WHO, 2018a). These three diseases are predominantly health problems of the Global South, with the most impoverished regions carrying the heaviest burden. The unequal burden accentuates that poverty is a fundamental cause of disease and a social determinant of health. Although many infectious diseases are curable, poverty and weak healthcare systems wane the control efforts. In the European region, for instance, the only infectious diseases in the top 10 causes of death are lower respiratory infections, accounting for a crude death rate of 27/100,000 as of 2016 (WHO, 2018b). The other nine diseases in the top ten are chronic diseases.

In the African region, seven of the leading ten causes of death were infectious diseases; others were accidents and two noncommunicable diseases (stroke and heart disease) (WHO, 2018b). Figure 6.1 shows the top five causes of death in the African region. In the top five causes of death, four were infectious, with only heart diseases as the fourth (see Figure 6.1). In the year 2000, HIV was the top killer disease in Africa, with no noncommunicable diseases among the top five causes of death. There was a slow but steady improvement in the control of infectious diseases between 2000 and 2016: Deaths from malaria were cut by almost 40%, while fatalities from measles went from fifth in the year 2000 to out of the top five in 2016. Roser and Ritchie (2019) reported that there was up to a 40% reduction in the rate of infectious

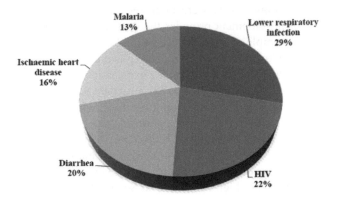

Figure 6.1 Top five causes of death in Africa (Source: WHO, 2018)

diseases between 1990 and 2016. Further decline is expected, with the increasing improvement in the condition and standard of living across the globe.

Africa also carries the burden of neglected tropical diseases, including dengue, trachoma, lymphatic filariasis, onchocerciasis, meningitis, trypanosomiasis and leishmaniasis. Different regions of Africa have some peculiar vectors that could lead to an occasional outbreak of specific diseases. The propensity to risk is often high when the environment is conducive to the breeding of the vector agents, as is the case with malaria and the proliferation of breeding sites for Anopheles mosquitoes. Many of the infectious diseases in sub-Saharan Africa (SSA) are zoonoses, and the human–animal interface increases the risk of transfer of such diseases to humans. Infectious diseases spread by air, water, climate, diet and general sanitary conditions, all of which are related to traditional risks of disease transmission. Germ theory is the basis for traditional risk, where pathogens move through some means from one person or place to another. Infectious diseases such as cholera and Lassa fever tend to become regional emergencies, while others, such as Ebola and TB, tend to become global emergencies.

Mortality data for Southeast Asia are different from those of the African region. In the top ten causes of death, the three infectious diseases on the list include lower respiratory infection (fourth), tuberculosis (fifth) and diarrhea (sixth) (WHO, 2018b). There has been a gradual shift in the burden of disease from infectious to NCDs in Southeast Asia, with NCDs accounting for the highest percentage of the burden of death. Overall, SSA, the Asian countries of India, Afghanistan, Pakistan, Nepal, Bangladesh, Myanmar, Laos and Papua New Guinea of the western Caribbean have the highest burden of infectious diseases (Roser and Ritchie, 2019). The eastern Mediterranean region also shares some burden of infectious diseases, with two among the top five causes of death, and four among the leading ten causes of death. The burden of infectious diseases in Europe and the Western Pacific region is low; only respiratory tract infections appear in the top ten (as the seventh) causes of death.

Historically, infectious diseases have constituted the highest burden of disease; only since the 1990s have NCDs become a significant challenge. Brachman (2003) noted that in the historical years (before the 18th century and shortly afterward), infectious diseases (such as yellow and typhoid fever, leprosy, plague, syphilis and smallpox) were dominant. Most efforts made at the beginning of medical development were toward detecting and treating such diseases and curtailing their spread. For infectious disease, the major obstacle has been the low adoption of preventive measures and poor socio-economic factors within the population. The epidemiologic transition indicates a change in disease burden over time: As the world can tackle infectious diseases, NCDs rise as a result of modern developments. Now, however, a new "science" is needed to tackle NCDs that will ensure curative therapy instead of just disease management.

While the list of infectious diseases is long, there is still the possibility of the emergence of new diseases and possibly re-emergence of old epidemics. The primary threat of infectious diseases in humans is from animal diseases (zoonosis). Zoonotic diseases often constitute a major medical challenge when transmitted to humans. For instance, Ebola virus disease (a zoonotic disease) wreaked severe havoc in some African countries before finally being put under control between 2014 and 2015. Infectious diseases tend to cause sudden epidemics. The cholera outbreak causes some deaths yearly in some low-income countries. Brachman (2003) noted that most epidemics are geographically localized but often cause global concerns because of their potential to escalate beyond confined locations. Fear of movement to and from endemic regions is one of the major problems because of infectious diseases transmitted through social contacts. For instance, HIV emerged in 1981 and became a pandemic for all time (Brachman, 2003), causing tremendous havoc (in terms of morbidity and mortality) on the general population, especially in SSA. The next section will examine some global health emergencies occasioned by infectious diseases.

6.3   Global Health Emergencies: The Case of Zika and Ebola

The next subsection will examine two major diseases of global concerns: Zika and Ebola. Incidentally, both are zoonoses, which have killed thousands of people in the last few years across several countries. The two diseases have the potential to spread across the globe due to globalization.

6.3.1   *Zika Virus in South America and the Caribbean*

Some infectious diseases have assumed magnitude of global emergency in the past decade (2009–2019). One such condition is Zika, a viral infection transmitted through the bite of an infected mosquito from the *Aedes* genus, mainly *Aedes aegypti*. Apart from an infected mosquito bite, the Zika virus also spreads from mother to fetus during pregnancy, through sexual contact, transfusion of blood and blood products and organ transplantation. Infection in pregnancy can result in fetal loss, stillbirth, congenital disabilities and preterm birth (WHO, 2019a). Zika is a zoonosis, first identified in monkeys in Uganda in 1947, and later in humans in 1952 in Uganda and Tanzania (WHO, 2019a). From 1960 to 2019, there have been reported outbreaks around the world, including Africa, the Americas, Asia and the Pacific Region. The WHO (2019b) reported that the Zika outbreak was recorded in the Island of Yap (Federated States of Micronesia) in 2007 and later in French Polynesia in 2013. As of 2019, a total of 86 countries had reported mosquito-transmitted Zika infections (WHO, 2019a).

The incubation period for infection with Zika ranges from 2 to 12 days. Because 80% of cases are asymptomatic (McNeil and Shetty, 2017), hidden outbreaks can circulate for an extended period before eventual manifestations. Collins (2019) reported the outbreak of Zika in Brazil in 2014 that went undetected for over a year. By then, it had spread to Honduras and Central American nations. In February 2016, the WHO declared a Public Health Emergency of International Concern, after a severe outbreak of Zika was reported in South America and the Caribbean (Cohen, 2019). From the onset of the epidemic in (February) 2015, up until (November) 2016, over 800,000 people were affected and close to 4,000 children were born with severe brain damage (Cohen, 2019). While it seemed the outbreak had wholly subsided, some cases were detected among US travelers returning from Cuba in mid-2017. The Zika outbreak also went undetected for about three months in the US until around 2016 and was later reported among those who had visited Cuba in 2017 (with 98% of 155 cases traced to Cuba) (Collins, 2019). Collins (2019) averred that the outbreak of Zika in Cuba was reported after infections had subsided elsewhere in the Caribbean. Zika portends a dangerous trend because of its late onset and mild manifestation. Even when contracted, it takes some time to manifest symptoms; therefore, the transmission might continue unknowingly for a long time before detection (Colins, 2019).

To date, there is no vaccine available for Zika, but it is preventable with some personal measures and vector control. The primary prevention of Zika is through the use of mosquito repellent or insecticides, mosquito protective screens and sanitation (to evacuate dumped standing water where mosquitoes breed) (Quintana-Domeque et al., 2018; Melo et al., 2019). Another major recommendation is that, during an outbreak, women should use contraceptives to postpone or delay pregnancy because of the severe effects of Zika on the fetus. Other preventive measures also include travel advice for pregnant women to avoid endemic areas and unprotected sexual intercourse with a partner with the travel history to endemic areas (McNeil and Shetty, 2017). It is also recommended that those returning from an endemic area should restrain from unprotected sex for at least six months.

Again, zoonoses continue to be a significant global threat to humans because of the ability to move from animals to humans. With the volume of air travel and general human mobility, any infectious disease tends to become a pandemic, affecting many countries of the world. In the case of Zika, some species of mosquito are responsible for its transmission. The vector was first identified in Uganda (1947 in monkeys); later outbreaks were reported South America (WHO, 2019b). The virus migrated with people to South and North America. HIV started the same way with a long incubation period, which delays the onset of symptoms. Like Zika, Ebola is another outbreak in recent times that warranted the declaration of a global health emergency.

6.3.2 Ebola Virus Disease in West Africa

In 1976, Ebola Virus Disease (EVD) joined the list of infectious diseases in humans when it was reported in Yambuku (Congo DR) and Nzara (South Sudan). It is another zoonosis, typically found in bats and porcupines, and transferred to humans through hunting and consumption of bats. Ebola is a deadly disease that spreads through contact with the bodily fluids (including blood, urine, sperm, feces, vomit and breastmilk) of an infected person. WHO (2019b) reported that the average EVD case fatality rate is around 50%, with past outbreak case fatality rates ranging from 25% to 90%. The incubation period is from 2 to 21 days. Ebola has a symptom complex manifesting like malaria, typhoid fever and meningitis. There have been several Ebola outbreaks since 1976, occurring in DR Congo, Gabon, South Sudan and Uganda. The first outbreak to affect multiple countries happened in 2014–2015, affecting Guinea, Liberia, Sierra Leone, Mali, Senegal and Nigeria, with international travel facilitating cases in Italy, Spain, the USA and the UK. The West African countries of Guinea (with 2,543 deaths), Liberia (4,809 deaths) and Sierra Leone (3,956 deaths) recorded the heaviest casualties, while 6 and 8 deaths were recorded in Mali and Nigeria, respectively (WHO, 2019a). Between 2018 and 2019, Ebola re-emerged in DR Congo, killing 33 people (WHO, 2019b).

The 2014–2015 outbreak started in Meliandou, Guinea, subsequently spreading to other West African countries. Timothy et al. (2019) conducted a study in Meliandou to understand the genesis of Ebola in the index site—the first case was a boy aged two years (S1) whose first contact with an Ebola virus reservoir was possibly from insectivorous bats. The disease then spread to the boy's sister and pregnant mother, then to a family caregiver, then to a local healthcare volunteer and the contact and spread continued (Timothy et al., 2019). Treatment of patients started prior to the identification of the disease; not until March 23, 2014 was EVD recognized as the cause of the death (Timothy et al., 2019). The delay in the case diagnosis was one of the significant factors in the immediate spread of the disease. Through traditional funeral practices, which required considerable physical contact with the dead bodies, the virus spread further.

From one index case in Meliandou (Guinea), Ebola spread thousands of miles away, with over 11,000 deaths recorded across 6 countries. The index case in Nigeria was a Liberian who flew into Nigeria on July 20, 2014 (Amzat and Razum, 2018). His diagnosis sent the entire country into a panic. The government started contact-tracing and quarantining all individuals who had had contact with the index case. In all, 20 cases were confirmed with a 40% fatality rate (8 deaths) (Amzat and Razum, 2018). In Sierra Leone, the first index case was a returnee from Guinea (in May, 2014), and later hundreds of people infected crossed the border from Guinea to Sierra Leone. Another significant event was the community funeral of a respected traditional healer who died of Ebola. The funeral and other events led to the spark of cases (over 14,000 cases), leading to more deaths (about 3,956), more burials and more cases (WHO, 2015). The case of the Ebola outbreak further buttresses the impact of globalization and health. It took several global measures to stop the spread of the disease. Richardson and Mosoka (2019) observed that the genesis of the Ebola outbreak could be traced to the weakness of the state and some unintended consequences of globalization, as reflected in the exploitative colonialism, structural adjustment, resource extraction, illicit financial flows, gender violence and poverty.

At the global level, Ebola outbreaks require a swift response and multisectoral collaborations. In general, the screening of travelers from affected countries is recommended. Anyone suspected of fever might be quarantined for proper monitoring. Also, within the community, contact tracing is essential to isolate and quarantine anyone who has contact with suspected Ebola patients. Although mandatory screening and quarantine pose serious ethical challenges, in the face of EVD, certain individual rights must be compromised for global health interests. Dead bodies (of Ebola victims) also need to be cremated (without traditional burial rites).

In terms of control, a vaccine that previously showed promise when used in the Guinea outbreak in 2015 (WHO, 2019b) brought hope in the 2018–2019 outbreak in DR Congo. The challenge, however, is how to ensure adequate vaccine coverage to those at risk of Ebola. This is particularly important as there is, to date, no licensed treatment or target cure for Ebola. The next section will examine some factors responsible for the emergence and re-emergence of infectious diseases.

6.4 Factors in the Emergence and Re-Emergence of Infectious Diseases

In addition to the social determinants of health (see Section 3.2.1), several factors are responsible for the emergence, re-emergence and burden of infectious diseases, especially in the Global South (see Morse, 1995). The emergence of most of the infectious diseases are dated in human history: They emerged at a point in time, and those that have been "eradicated" could re-emerge. For instance, Zika was first detected in 1947, Lassa fever in 1969, Ebola in 1976 and HIV in 1981. All the aforementioned diseases, generally zoonoses, are of global concern because they have the potential to escalate globally. The next subsection will explain some crucial factors which account for the burden of infectious diseases. One major factor, demographic change, serves as a base from which most other factors arise. For instance, increasing population (one of the indices of demographic change) in the South, is connected to expansive land use, increasing urbanization, human–animal interface, human mobility, increasing technology use and pressures on insufficient public health measures. The focus of this section is on the aforementioned factors linked to globalization concerning the emergence and re-emergence of infectious diseases. Figure 6.2 shows six crucial factors that will be discussed.

6.4.1 Land Use in Agriculture

Land use encompasses the areas of agriculture, deforestation, construction and economic activities (Gottdenker et al., 2014). It has been implicated as a factor underlying a range of human infectious disease risks (Shah et al., 2018). Land use is an integral aspect of the development of agriculture, both commercial and subsistence. From hunting and gathering to agrarian societies, cultivation, including cut-and-slash, has been the core practice in the human search for food, which leads to exposure to wildlife. However, increasing urban development necessitates the penetration into the thick forest for the cultivation of new land, leading to the disruption of wildlife and resulting in new stings and bites. Most parts of the Global South, particularly the low-income nations, are agrarian and need to cultivate land to ensure a sufficient supply of raw materials required in the Global North (see Section 4.4.1). Also, the process of adaptation requires economic production, especially with the use of land as a significant factor of production. Land use requires the extension or alteration of the local and regional environment on a global scale (Gottdenker et al., 2014).

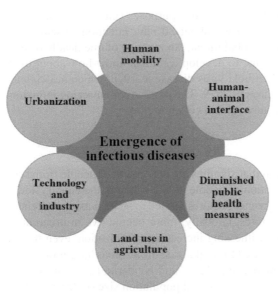

Figure 6.2 Factors in the emergence of infectious diseases

Morris et al. (2016) observed that the world is facing a rapid decline in biological diversity, which will result in "shifts in species community composition and severe disruption to established food webs, which are directly traceable to land-use change and deforestation". The major problem is that this shift is occurring in the Global South because of intensive land use and modification, population encroachment and deforestation. In developing nations, millions of people still rely on cutting trees for firewood used in cooking. The more the ecosystems are modified as a result of human land use, the higher the possibility of a new risk of infectious diseases. Like any other forest region, the tropical world harbors many hidden vectors of disease. Greater dependence on agriculture and deforestation, however, can dislodge some of these vectors in terms of habitation and food. Morris et al. write that land use changes are a significant predictor of emergence and re-emergence of infectious diseases.

Gottdenker et al. (2014: p. 626) also noted the altered niches for the vector, host, or pathogen and environment responsible for the transmission of infectious diseases. They argue that "anthropogenic change can alter food resources for hosts and vectors, and there are complex feedbacks between host nutrition and immunity". The primary issue is that land use facilitates contact between the host and vector. As people cultivate new land for agriculture, they move closer to some disease vectors. The emergence of malaria has been traced to the era of cut-and-slash agriculture in SSA (Wellcome, 2002). The human disruption, through agriculture, of forest regions (including pastoral nomadism) is a core factor in the emergence and spread of infectious diseases. The sleeping sickness (trypanosomiasis) is a typical example of how forest life facilitates the emergence of new infections. Trypanosomiasis is an insect-borne (tsetse fly) disease of rural areas among the agrarian population in SSA.

The scenario is similar in Southeast Asia, where agricultural land use exacerbates the risk of infectious diseases. More lands have been converted to human use, thereby "trespassing" beyond the usual human boundaries. Morand et al. (2014) observed that southeast Asia is gradually losing its biodiversity, which increases the risk of vector-borne and zoonotic diseases. The threat to wildlife and the reduction in forest cover make outbreaks more likely. The "encroachment" is a result of new economic activities, and the trend will likely continue as the human population increases; more land will be required for various purposes (including habitation). Mukherjee (2017) observed that in the last 30 years, about 30 new infectious diseases had emerged worldwide, potentially constituting a global threat. An average of one deadly disease emerges every year, and it often takes some time to develop technical know-how about treatment and control. Since the emergence of the Ebola virus disease in 1976, which has claimed thousands of lives, there is only hope of vaccines in 2019. The problem of emerging infectious diseases is a global challenge, which also requires global collaboration.

6.4.2 *Urbanization*

Urbanization is a process of demographic shift that signifies the movement of people from rural to urban areas; it results in a higher concentration of people in cities than in the countryside or rural areas. The search for opportunities and greener pastures has led to an increasing movement of people toward areas with better infrastructures. Globally, more people live in urban areas than in rural areas. The Global South is also witnessing increasing urbanization, even though most countries have fewer urban centers compared to rural areas; urban areas have more social amenities and economic opportunities. Morand et al. (2014) and Neiderud (2015) implicated increasing urbanization, i.e., changes in human behavior and population size or density, in the spread of infectious diseases. Urbanization leads to growth in terms of population. For example, there are several megacities (with population over 10 million) in the Global South, including Lagos (Nigeria), Kinshasa (DRC), Jakarta (Indonesia), Dhaka (Bangladesh), Beijing and Shanghai (China), Mumbai and Delhi (India) and Cairo (Egypt), among others. Urbanization is a continuous process, and the Global South is becoming more urbanized as more people move into the cities from rural areas.

Urbanization is a significant determinant of health in numerous ways. It is a significant factor in the event of an outbreak of infectious disease. Such diseases spread fast, where there is a high population density. In most cities of the Global South, intense competition for scarce amenities encourages movement to the urban areas, where some amenities are relatively available (compared to rural areas). Most quarters of urban centers end up as slums because of the shortage of necessary infrastructure. Major problems include indecent living conditions as a result of scarce amenities, such as water and electricity, and poor sanitation. For instance, diarrhea is correlated with the contamination of the environment and is the leading cause of death from infectious diseases. In typical situations, the increasing population is not supported by a commensurate increase in social amenities. Periodically, outbreaks of diarrhea and cholera, leptospirosis, lymphatic filariasis and leishmaniasis are likely due to poor sanitation (Loutan, 2012). Poor housing, including poor sanitation and waste management, can lead to the proliferation of insects and rodents, which can carry and transmit diseases (Neiderud, 2015).

Nevertheless, despite these disadvantages, urban areas are better equipped in terms of infrastructure than rural areas, and are often an improvement over what is obtainable in rural areas. Maternal health services, for example, in most urban areas are superior to those in rural areas. Due to urban bias in infrastructural development, there is a higher concentration of health services in urban centers. The increased availability of health services (although they may still be inadequate), improves health-seeking behavior. Child healthcare and immunization services are also better in urban centers. Despite the aforementioned relative benefits in urban areas, there are still many issues with the increasing urban population growth in the Global South. The services might be expensive and, therefore, not a realistic option for the urban poor. The high concentration of people is a major hub for contagious diseases. Loutan (2012) observed increasing transmission of dengue fever and chikungunya due to the adaptation of vector to urban conditions. Mukherjee (2017) also confirmed the increased risk of dengue fever due to rapid urbanization, deficient water supply and improper water storage, leading to the proliferation of mosquito breeding sites. Urban areas provide an opportunity for physical contact, touch and exchange of breath, which may facilitate the spread of diseases. For instance, TB is more prevalent in urban than in rural areas. Neiderud (2015) noted the high prevalence of TB in Dhaka (Bangladesh), which was above the national average. A typical contagious disease might spread rapidly in urban centers, and within a short period, become a global health challenge.

6.4.3 *Human–Animal Interface*

Human–animal interaction has been a significant factor in the emergence and re-emergence of infectious diseases. Some deadly infectious diseases, including brucellosis, bovine tuberculosis, rabies and anthrax, are zoonotic. The human–animal interface has enabled the transmission of animal diseases to humans through the consumption of meat, contact with an infected animal and direct contact with the vector. The fact that such diseases are zoonotic makes it challenging to control in humans. The world is, most times, not prepared for such disease outbreaks, and there might not be a known cure. A majority (up to 60%) of pathogenic infectious diseases in humans are zoonotic, and more of such diseases are emerging (Taylor et al., 2001). The primary threat is the characteristic of zoonotic diseases to emerge suddenly and re-emerge after some time. Taylor et al. (2001) observed that zoonotic diseases are twice as likely to be responsible for disease emergence than non-zoonotic species, and facts show that about three-quarters of new or emerging diseases are zoonotic, and are estimated to be responsible for over two million human deaths every year. The health of animals meant for consumption and those used for labor is essential because (animal) morbidity and mortality also have adverse effects on both household and national economy. In several countries, livestock sales offer substantial foreign exchange, which is used to provide social amenities.

In most cases, the initial transmission is from animal to human, with human–human transmission subsequently leading to outbreaks. Viral diseases are more likely (than other pathogens) to emerge and re-emerge, thereby leading to outbreaks. Cleaveland et al. (2001) observed that many domesticated animals are also reservoirs for pathogens that can be transmitted to humans. Therefore, there is increasing concern about the transmission of zoonotic diseases (from both domestic and wildlife) to humans (Daszak et al., 2000), which led to the notion of "One Health".

The concept of "One Health" has emerged to signify that the health of humans and other animals are interrelated and interdependent, especially concerning the transmission of deadly infectious diseases. Humans and other animals exist within the same environment and with a similar ecological support system. One Health is thus a fusion of human, animal and environmental health. In some cases, both humans and other animals share many resources, including living space, food and water. In typical rural areas of low-income countries, both share the same sources of water, and in urban areas, most animals are kept indoors with the opportunity to play within human space. Rabies, for instance, is transmitted through dog attacks, which are a common occurrence. Vaccinating dogs against rabies can, therefore, improve human health. Destoumieux-Garzón et al. (2018) observed that the increasing globalization of health risks is also related to the human–animal–ecosystem interface, which affects the emergence and re-emergence of pathogens. It is further observed that the understanding of global health strongly requires the integration of human health, animal health, plant health, ecosystem health and biodiversity. Destoumieux-Garzón et al. (2018) further reported that outbreaks of Ebola, avian flu and Zika are notable events that embody the concepts of globalization and One Health. It is often common to neglect the flow of animals and plants (and their products) when discussing that globalization enhances the flow of people. The three should be considered because of the likelihood of the flow of pathogens with them. So, globalization creates various flows and development that fosters the spread of infectious agents and other risks.

A "One Health" approach is important to control the emergence and re-emergence of infectious diseases. The Global South is known for nomadic pastoralist populations: these have close contact with animals and are highly mobile, traveling across boundaries and borders. The pastoralists produce a substantial amount of milk and meat consumed by the general population. Without adequate veterinary services, such consumables might not be hygienic for human consumption, resulting, ultimately, in the spread of disease across borders. Pastoral nomadism (the mobility of nomads with their animals) is another critical factor in the spread of infectious diseases. The fight against zoonoses will safeguard the spread of deadly infectious diseases in humans and will help to curtail the emergence and re-emergence of infectious diseases. The surveillance of domestic animals and wildlife populations has been intensified in some quarters, but more efforts are required in the Global South, the frontline of some outbreaks (such as Zika virus, Ebola virus and Coronavirus diseases).

6.4.4 *Human Mobility*

Human mobility is central to globalization and plays a paramount role in the spread of infectious diseases. Since the development of modern transportation systems, it has become easier to move within and between countries. In earlier times, mobility was tedious and slow, as humans were only able to cover relatively close distances or needed a long time to travel far. Limited mobility means low social contacts and activities. That is why, historically, infectious diseases could only spread within a confined area, to a few individuals in close proximity. With advancements in human mobility, the spatial limitations in the spread of infectious diseases no longer exist. Wesolowski et al. (2016) observed that the spread of infectious diseases depends on how, where and when people are moving. The "how" relates to the means of travel; air travel is a major concern in the spread of infectious disease because of the spatial coverage and volume of movement. "Where" is essential because it concerns whether someone is moving from an endemic area to a non-endemic area. "When" is about the period of epidemics or not. Wesolowski et al. (2016) noted that mobility affects pathogen dynamics through increased contact between susceptible and infected populations.

As mentioned in previous chapters, the compression of space is a significant outcome of globalization, not only concerning virtual messaging but also human mobility. Human mobility is the most discussed factor of globalization in the spread of communicable diseases. Mobility has expanded social networks and contacts in unimaginable ways. Air travel has facilitated the spread of infectious diseases because it is booming and the fastest; within a short time, passengers and goods can be delivered across the globe. A long distance can be covered within hours, allowing pathogens to travel as quickly as humans. Even movement within a country can cause the spread of infectious disease from rural to urban areas, and vice-versa. It is the same in international travel, as pathogens can travel fast via contacts who travel to different parts of the world. For instance, before people from an endemic area are even aware they have Ebola, their international air travel can lead to an outbreak within a few days in different countries. Findlater and Bogoch (2018) asserted that air travel extends the frequency and reach of infectious epidemics, which often pose a threat to global health security. Beyond the airport, Mangili et al. (2015) reported the possibility of contracting some infectious diseases in-flight, especially airborne diseases such as tuberculosis, severe acute respiratory syndrome, influenza, smallpox and measles. Mangili et al. (2015) noted that with the ease of transmission of infectious diseases and the increasing volume of air travel, global concerns are warranted, since the number of passengers amounts to nearly 42% of the world population in 2014 and might likely increase to approximately 70% by 2030. For instance, the pathogen of TB is quickly released into the air while talking, coughing, sneezing and vomiting, and can remain in the air for some time. Hence, there is a need for intensified efforts for global coordination. Early warning systems can potentially curtail the outbreaks of infectious diseases.

6.4.5 Technology and Industry

Continuous technological growth has enhanced industrialization, and it is a major driver of globalization. Modern technology has been deployed in all spheres of human life. Production processes are technologically driven. For instance, modernized food production and packaging allow goods to be transported to distant locations in a short time. Accidental contamination of food in one factory can spread quickly, amplifying the effects (Morse, 1995). A typical example is the E. coli outbreak in western USA, resulting from the consumption of hamburgers from a popular restaurant chain (CDC, 1993). The incidence indicated that a batch of pathogenic raw material might find its way into a large batch of the final product leading to contamination (Morse, 1995). In today's world of global production and distribution chains, the effects would be much more widespread. Additionally, there have been several cases of defects in automobiles that have caused accidents and injuries across some countries and prompted the withdrawal of specific vehicle models. Most of those automobiles were distributed globally; it took a series of like-patterned accidents to raise suspicion and confirm a defect (see Lucky and Takim, 2015).

Globalization of production and distribution of goods means that, in the case of accidental defects or contamination, the consequences can quickly become far-reaching. This also applies to medical products, including the global exchange of tissue and organs for transplantation, especially in the case of uncommon diseases for which the products might not have been screened. Perhaps in the early days of HIV and hepatitis B and C, there might have been some unintentional transmissions through blood products because of limited screening measures (Morse, 1995). In most cases, it takes time before an emerging infection is recognized and the mode of transmission understood. Before such recognition, there is always the possibility of hidden epidemics, especially for diseases with delayed onset. New technology might be required to recognize an emerging disease; advances in diagnostic technology have helped to identify new disease agents (some already widespread) (Morse, 1995). Morse cited Human herpesvirus 6 (HHV-6), *Helicobacter pylori* and some cancers as examples of diseases that must have been around long before being identified. Technological development must keep pace to cater to both known and unknown challenges.

6.4.6 Breakdown of Public Health Measures

Infectious diseases are (usually) preventable but do require the presence of strong public health measures. The measures must always be in place, not only during but, more importantly, before the outbreak. Infectious diseases require a swift response, without which severe damage can occur. In the Global South, the general problem is not only the weak health system but also the breakdown of public health measures. Infectious disease control requires public education in order to circulate necessary information to the population. There is a constant need for public engagement in terms of health education. Basic health education about the prevention of infectious disease can help to forestall any emergence or re-emergence. For instance, in affected areas, people need knowledge about the risk and transmission of malaria, TB and HIV, in order to take appropriate action against these diseases. The use of insecticide-treated bednets (ITN) has been propagated in the prevention of childhood malaria. Such a preventive measure can save thousands of lives. Beyond the use of ITN, sanitation could help to reduce mosquito breeding sites. For HIV, the "ABCDE" (**A**bstinence from sex; **B**e faithful to uninfected partner; **C**ondom use; **D**o HIV test; and **E**mpower women) of prevention has been the core preventive measure. TB preventive measures require an understanding of cough etiquettes and regular room ventilation. There is a constant need for public health education to strengthen the adoption and sustainability of such preventive measures further.

The role of primary healthcare personnel is not only to wait at the health facilities for patients, but to also meet people with information required to safeguard their health. Some health personnel work at the community level to engage community members, thereby saturating the community with health information. Public education is an essential public health measure. In instances where it is not adequate or not provided, there is a serious missing link which can manifest with severe consequences. Another essential measure is WASH (water, sanitation and hygiene). The emergence and re-emergence of infectious diseases, or the general epidemiology of most infectious diseases, are highly connected to WASH. Water is essential to life; access to clean water lowers or eliminates the risk of contracting some infectious diseases. As previously highlighted (see Section 3.3.4), there are still over 1.1 billion people (the majority of whom are in the Global South) without access to clean water, and about 2.5 billion also lack access to improved sanitation (Ritchie and Roser, 2019). Basic hygiene is essential for well-being as a fundamental health measure. Acute diarrheal diseases remain a leading cause of global morbidity and mortality, particularly among young children in the Global South largely in Africa and Southeast Asia) (Mokomane et al., 2018). As it is primarily a result of contaminated water and food, its control is strongly related to WASH. Children bear the burden of diarrhea, and most of the documented risk factors include malnutrition, early weaning, lack of piped water supply or treated water, poor water-storage practices, lack of careful handwashing and poor sanitation (Mokomane et al., 2018).

Vaccination has also been instituted as a significant public health measure. The early days of life must start with essential vaccinations, in order to avert morbidity, disability and mortality. Childhood immunizations are meant to safeguard children from both the risk of contracting and transmitting diseases such as including measles, polio, hepatitis B, yellow fever, whooping cough, tetanus and diphtheria, among others. Vaccination has significantly helped toward the total eradication of polio, but not without the possibility of re-emergence (Razum et al., 2019). Africa was declared polio-free on August 25, 2020 after four years without any case, leaving only two countries globally, Afghanistan and Pakistan, still with polio cases (WHO, 2020). The burden of infectious disease is compounded because of vaccine hesitancy or resistance in some countries of the Global South. Cooper et al. (2018) observed that, apart from the problem of unavailability in some quarters, there are still many parents who are hesitant about or refuse vaccination completely even when effective vaccines are available. Vaccine hesitancy or refusal is also a global problem, but it is highly prevalent in low-income countries. The widespread concerns about vaccines in the Global South are mainly due to misconceptions, rumors and conspiracy, and health system failures (Muñoz et al., 2015).

Public education, WASH and vaccination are three necessary public health measures, the breakdown of which could constitute a significant threat to population health, especially concerning the risk of infectious diseases. Depending on the type of outbreak, additional measures (such as social [or physical] distancing and use of face mask) can be recommended. Most infectious diseases can be brought under control using affordable procedures such as handwashing and the use of sanitizers in the case of COVID-19. The high prevalence of infectious diseases in the Global South, however, hints that more efforts are still required. The nature of infectious disease requires that there always be preparedness against sudden outbreaks. In practice, the WHO (2005) recommends five basic strategies, including "(1) epidemic preparedness and rapid response, (2) strengthening of public health infrastructure, (3) exchanging information with public and mass media through risk communication, (4) improving research and its utilization, and (5) continuing advocacy for political commitment and partnership building" (see also Mukherjee, 2017).

6.5 Summary

- Most parts of the Global South are still confronted with traditional risks, i.e., the risk of infectious diseases, while simultaneously facing the rising risk of noncommunicable diseases. Infectious epidemics constitute a significant threat to global health security because of their potential to escalate across boundaries.
- The threat of infectious disease is constant, even in the North, because of the possible re-emergence of such diseases. For instance, malaria has been eradicated in the Global North but could re-emerge because of movement of people in and out of malarial regions.
- The emergence of zoonosis has also prompted the study of globalization and health because they sometimes lead to pandemics. In the last few years, most public health emergencies have been declared because of zoonoses such as Zika virus, Ebola virus and Coronavirus.
- Extensive agricultural land use exacerbates the risk of infectious diseases. More lands have been converted to human use, thereby "trespassing" beyond the usual human boundaries; hence, the environment is gradually losing its biodiversity, which increases the risk of vector-borne and zoonotic diseases.
- Urbanization is a significant determinant of health in numerous ways. It is a significant factor in the event of an outbreak of infectious disease, which spread fast, where there is a high population density.
- Human–animal interaction has been a significant factor in the emergence and re-emergence of infectious diseases. Some deadly infectious diseases, including brucellosis, bovine tuberculosis, rabies and anthrax, are zoonotic. The human–animal interface has enabled the transmission of animal diseases to humans through the consumption of meat, contact with an infected animal and direct contact with the vector.
- The compression of space is a significant outcome of globalization because it facilitates the flow of people. Human mobility is the most discussed factor of globalization in the spread of communicable diseases.
- In the Global South, the general problem is not only the weak health system but also the breakdown of public health measures, such as WASH (water, sanitation and hygiene), vaccination, and public enlightenment programs, which intensify the spread of infectious diseases.

Critical Thinking Questions

- Urban life and urbanization mean that people are concentrated in specific places. Assess how concentration of people or urbanization influence the spread of infectious diseases in the Global South. How can the impacts of urbanization on infectious disease spread be mitigated?
- Zoonosis is a global health threat for humans, especially in the Global South. Reflect on specific ways that man–animal interface affects the emergence and re-emergence of infectious diseases. How can the man–animal interface be managed to curtain global health threats to humans?
- In what ways is the spread of Zika virus disease a typical representation of the impact of globalization on the spread of infectious diseases?

- Examine the critical global health measures that could help in controlling the spread of infectious disease like Ebola.
- What lessons can you deduce from the control of Zika and Ebola virus diseases for the control of future health emergencies?

Suggested Readings

- Amzat, J., and Razum, O. (2018). Healthcare emergencies in Africa: The case of Ebola in Nigeria. In: *Towards a sociology of health discourse in Africa.* Cham, Switzerland: Springer International Publishing. DOI 10.1007/978-3-319-61672-8_10. The chapter focuses on the spread and containment of Ebola in Nigeria to demonstrate the impact of the global flow of people on health and political resilience to contain a possible pandemic.
- Neiderud, C. J. (2015). How urbanization affects the epidemiology of emerging infectious diseases. *Infection Ecology and Epidemiology, 5,* 27060. doi:10.3402/iee.v5.27060. The article focuses on the many challenges of urbanization for global health and the epidemiology of infectious diseases.
- DeLaet, D. E., and DeLaet, D. L. (2012). Global health in the 21st century: The globalization of disease and wellness (1st ed.). New York: Routledge. https://doi.org/10.4324/9781315634425. The book provides a very good introduction to global health issues, including infectious diseases, with emphasis on the potentials of public health interventions.
- Vineis, P. (2017). *Health without borders: Epidemics in the era of globalization.* Cham, Switzerland: Springer International Publishing. The book discusses the relationships between economics, globalization and modern public health issues, especially infectious diseases.

References

Amzat, J., & Razum, O. (2018). Healthcare emergencies in Africa: The case of Ebola in Nigeria. In *Towards a Sociology of Health Discourse in Africa.* Cham, Switzerland: Springer International Publishing. doi: 10.1007/978-3-319-61672-8_10.

Brachman, P. S. (2003). Infectious diseases: Past, present, and future. *International Journal of Epidemiology, 32*(5), 684–686. doi: 10.1093/ije/dyg282.

Centers for Disease Control and Prevention (CDC) (1993). Update: Multistate outbreak of Escherichia coli O157:H7 infections from hamburgers western United States, 1992–1993. *Morbidity and Mortality Weekly Report, 42*(14), 258–263.

Cleaveland, S., Laurenson, M. K. & Taylor, L. H. (2001). Diseases of humans and their domestic mammals: Pathogen characteristics, host range and the risk of emergence. *Philosophical Transactions of the Royal Society of London. Series B, Biological Sciences, 356*(1411), 991–999. doi: 10.1098/rstb.2001.0889.

Cohen, J. (2019). Infected travelers reveal Cuba's 'hidden' Zika outbreak. *Science,* www.sciencemag.org/news/2019/08/infected-travelers-reveal-cuba-s-hidden-zika-outbreak. Accessed on September 6, 2019.

Collins, F. (2019). Uncovering a hidden Zika outbreak in Cuba. https://directorsblog.nih.gov/2019/09/03/uncovering-a-hidden-zika-outbreak-in-cuba/. Accessed on September 6, 2019.

Cooper, S., Betsch, C., Sambala, E. Z., Mchiza, N. & Wiysonge, C. S. (2018). Vaccine hesitancy: A potential threat to the achievements of vaccination programmes in Africa. *Human Vaccines & Immunotherapeutics, 10,* 2355–2357. doi: 10.1080/21645515.2018.1460987.

Daszak, P., Cunningham, A. A., & Hyatt, A. D. (2000). Emerging infectious diseases of wildlife: Threats to biodiversity and human health. *Science, 287* (5452), 443–449. doi: 10.1126/science.287.5452.443.

Destoumieux-Garzón, D., Mavingui, P., Boetsch, G., Boissier, J., Darriet, F., Duboz, P., Fritsch, C., Giraudoux, P., Le Roux, F., Morand, S., Paillard, C., Pontier, D., Sueur, C. & Voituron Y. (2018). The one health concept: 10 Years old and a long road ahead. *Frontiers in Veterinary Science*, *5*, 14. doi: 10.3389/fvets.2018.00014.

Findlater, A., & Bogoch, I. I. (2018). Human mobility and the global spread of infectious diseases: A focus on air travel. *Trends in Parasitology*, *34*(9), 772–783.

Gottdenker, N. L., Streicker, D. G., Faust, C. L. & Caroll, C. R. (2014). Anthropogenic land use change and infectious diseases: A review of the evidence. *EcoHealth*, *11*, 619. https://doi.org/10.1007/s10393-014-0941-z.

Loutan, L. (2012). Urbanization reshaping infectious diseases. *International Journal of Infectious Diseases*, *16*(S1), e20.

Lucky, B. O., & Takim, S. A. (2015). Manufacturing defects in the automobile industry, a case study of the remote causes and effects of Toyotas transmission malfunctions in cars. *International Journal of Engineering and Applied Sciences*, *2*(8), 15–29.

Mangili, A., Vindenes, T. & Gendreau, M. (2015). Infectious risks of air travel. *Microbiol Spectrum 3*(5), IOL5-0009-2015.

McNeil, C. J., & Shetty, A. K. (2017). Zika virus: A serious global health threat. *Journal of Tropical Pediatrics*, *63*(3), 242–248. doi: 10.1093/tropej/fmw080.

Melo, V. A. D., Silva, J. R. S. & Melo, C. R. (2019). Personal protective measures of pregnant women against Zika virus infection. *Rev Saude Publica*, *2*(53), 72, doi: 10.11606/s1518-8787.2019053001146.

Mokomane, M., Kasvosve, I., de Melo, E., Pernica, J. M. & Goldfarb, D. M. (2018). The global problem of childhood diarrhoeal diseases: Emerging strategies in prevention and management. *Therapeutic Advances in Infectious Disease*, *5*(1), 29–43. doi: 10.1177/2049936117744429.

Morand, S., Jittapalapong, S., Suputtamongkol, Y., Abdullah, M. T. & Huan, T. B. (2014). Infectious diseases and their outbreaks in Asia-Pacific: Biodiversity and its regulation loss matter. *PloS one*, *9*(2), e90032. doi: 10.1371/journal.pone.0090032.

Morris, A. L., Guégan, J., Andreou, D., Marsollier, L., Carolan, K., Croller, M., Sanhueza, D. & Gozlan, R. E. (2016). Deforestation-driven food-web collapse linked to emerging tropical infectious disease, *Mycobacterium ulcerans*. *Science Advance*, *2*(12), e1600387.

Morse, S. S. (1995). Factors in the emergence of infectious diseases. *Emerging Infectious Diseases*, *1*(1), 7–15. doi: 10.3201/eid0101.950102.

Mukherjee, S. (2017). Emerging infectious diseases: Epidemiological Perspective. *Indian Journal of Dermatology*, *62*(5), 459–467. doi: 10.4103/ijd.IJD_379_17.

Muñoz, D. C., Llamas, L. M. & Bosch-Capblanch, X. (2015). Exposing concerns about vaccination in low- and middle-income countries: A systematic review. *International Journal of Public Health*, *60*, 767. doi: 10.1007/s00038-015-0715-6.

Neiderud, C. J. (2015). How urbanization affects the epidemiology of emerging infectious diseases. *Infection Ecology & Epidemiology*, *5*, 27060. doi: 10.3402/iee.v5.27060.

Quintana-Domeque, C. Carvalho, J. R. & de Oliveira VH. (2018). Zika virus incidence, preventive and reproductive behaviors: Correlates from new survey data. *Economics & Human Biology*, *30*, 14–23. doi: 10.1016/j.ehb.2018.04.003.

Razum, O., Sridhar, D., Jahn, A., Zaidi, S., Ooms, G. & Müller, O. (2019). Polio: From eradication to systematic, sustained control. *BMJ Global Health*, *4*, e001633. doi: 10.1136/bmjgh-2019-001633.

Richardson, E. T., & Mosoka, M. P. (2019). The genesis of the Ebola virus outbreak in West Africa. *The Lancet Infectious Diseases*, *S1473-3099*(19), 30055–30056. doi: 10.1016/.

Ritchie, H., & Roser, M. (2019). Water use and sanitation. Published online at *OurWorldInData.org*. https://ourworldindata.org/water-use-sanitation [Online Resource]. Accessed on August 9, 2019.

Roser, M., & Ritchie, H. (2019). Burden of disease. Published online at *OurWorldInData.org*. Retrieved from: https://ourworldindata.org/burden-of-disease [Online Resource].

Shah, H., Huxley, P., Elmes, J. & Murray, K. (2018). Agricultural land use and infectious disease risks in southeast Asia: A systematic review and meta-analyses. *Lancet*, *2*(S20). doi: https://doi.org/10.1016/S2542-5196(18)30105-0.

Taylor, L. H., Latham, S. M. & Woolhouse, M. E. (2001). Risk factors for disease emergence. *Philosophical Transactions of the Royal Society of London: Biological Science*, *356*(1411), 983–989.

Timothy, J. W. S., Hall, Y. & Akoi-Boré, J. (2019). Early transmission and case fatality of Ebola virus at the index site of the 2013–16 west African Ebola outbreak: A cross-sectional seroprevalence survey. *Lancet Infectious Diseases, 19*(4), 429–438. doi: 10.1016/S1473-3099(18)30791-6.

Wellcome News (2002). *Research Directions in Malaria*. Supplement 6. London: Wellcome News.

Wesolowski, A., Buckee, C. O., Engø-Monsen, K. & Metcalf, C. J. E. (2016). Connecting mobility to infectious diseases: The promise and limits of mobile phone data. *The Journal of Infectious Diseases, 214*(4), S414–S420, doi: 10.1093/infdis/jiw273.

World Health Organization (WHO) (2005). *Regional Office for South-East Asia. Combating Emerging Infectious Diseases in the South-East Asia Region*. New Delhi: WHO-SEARO.

WHO (2009). *Global Health Risks: Mortality and Burden of Disease Attributable to Selected Major Risks*. Geneva: WHO.

WHO (2015). Ebola in Sierra Leone: A slow start to an outbreak that eventually outpaced all others. www .who.int/csr/disease/ebola/one-year-report/sierra-leone/en/. Accessed on August 12, 2020.

WHO (2018a). *World Malaria Report 2018*. Geneva: WHO.

WHO (2018b). Global health observatory data. www.who.int/gho/mortality_burden_disease/causes _death/top_10/en/. Accessed on September 2, 2019.

WHO (2019a). Zika virus. www.who.int/news-room/fact-sheets/detail/zika-virus. Accessed on September 6, 2019.

WHO (2019b). Ebola virus disease. www.who.int/news-room/fact-sheets/detail/ebola-virus-disease. Accessed on September 6, 2019.

WHO (2020). Global polio eradication initiative applauds WHO African region for wild polio-free certification. www.who.int/news-room/detail/25-08-2020-global-polio-eradication-initiative-applauds -who-african-region-for-wild-polio-free-certification. Accessed on August 29, 2020.

7 Globalization and Health

The Case of COVID-19

7.1 Introduction

The novel Coronavirus disease of 2019 (COVID-19) started early December 2019, became a pandemic, and overwhelmed the world. Before 2019, occasional disease outbreaks of global concern, including Black Death of 1348–1351, influenza of 1918–1920, the Asian flu of 1957–1958, severe acute respiratory syndrome (SARS) of 2002, Ebola of 2014–2015, Zika of 2015–2016, had occurred over the years, overriding the health infrastructures of various countries. On the other hand, Human Immunodeficiency Virus (HIV) disease was first diagnosed in 1981 but remains a significant global health challenge killing almost one million people in 2020 (UNAIDS, 2021). A global health emergency has been declared on many occasions—for instance, during the 2014–2015 Ebola crisis in West Africa. Between 1918 and 1920, influenza spread across the globe, which accounted for 50–100 million deaths globally, killing more people than the Black Death of 1348–1351, with about 62 million deaths (Mamelund, 2017). The pandemic started after the First World War (WWI), but it killed more people than the war (Stern et al., 2010; Oluwasegun, 2015). Influenza is generally referred to as the Spanish flu even though it did not originate from Spain. While Spain was one of the worst-hit countries, the flu's origin is still blurred, with some researchers pointing to France, China, Britain and the United States (Taubenberger and Morens, 2006). However, Texas in the United States recorded the early observation of the flu and fatalities. Many researchers believed that the virus moved with returning soldiers after WWI. In short, human mobility facilitated the spread of the flu. Despite the blurriness of the origin, the flu traveled with people worldwide, affecting over 500 million people, approximately 30% of the world population as of 1920 (Taubenberger and Morens, 2006).

As of 1918–1920, most African countries were under colonial rule during the pandemic; the colonies also participated in WWI. The movement of war returnees, primarily through the sea, was implicated in the flu spread. In short, war-related factors played a significant role as the first cases in Freetown (Sierra Leone), the sub-Saharan Africa (SSA) epicenter, were from England through the Royal Navy warship, which brought about 124 sick crew (Philips, 2014). Oluwasegun (2015) observed that the influenza pandemic started in phases, four sequential waves, but spread across the world through increasing human mobility, mainly through sea transportation. While the first wave was generally mild, the second was disastrous, with severe health consequences responsible for more than half of the total fatalities. The third and fourth waves were less lethal than the second. While the first wave affected North Africa, the lethal second wave affected SSA. The local populations were not that mobile, but the colonialists and sailors who were mobile were reckless, i.e., without observing isolation upon entering the colonized territories. Swiftly, the flu spread like wildfire, but during the early months of 1920,

DOI: 10.4324/9781003247975-7

slowly, the Spanish flu ended after taking its tolls. There were no global coordinating bodies then, as the League of Nations (LON) and its Health Organization (LONHO) were formed in 1920 after the pandemic (see Dubin, 1995). The Inter-Parliamentary Union (IPU), formed in 1889, a predecessor of LON, did not have a global outlook. The limited consensus about the causes of illness despite constant cholera threats and plagues (Dubin, 1995) could explain the lack of concerted centralized global health efforts despite the awareness of possible inter-border spread of contagious diseases. The Spanish flu control was a case of fragmented efforts with limited centralized coordination, although some best practices, including quarantines, self-isolation and use of facemasks, were widely embraced.

The human immune-deficiency virus (HIV) has been the worst pandemic of the modern era, with millions of deaths and still counting. HIV is a disease with a protracted course—even after its manifestation, people can live with it for several years. The emergence of zoonoses with a short course is a pressing concern in the 21st century and beyond. Unlike HIV, the emerging zoonoses, such as Ebola and SARS, kill their victims within some days. The incubation period of HIV could extend up to several years, but most virulent zoonoses only last 2–21 days. The novel Coronavirus disease of 2019 (COVID-19) emerged in early December 2019 in Wuhan, China. The initial impression was that like Ebola and SARS, it could be curtailed in no time. The past experiences would help stop the spread of COVID-19, but the world was wrong. Several challenges, in the form of delays (see Section 7.4), complicated the control efforts. Before and after 1918, Asia has been a significant source of the threats of contagious diseases, which could constitute a global health emergency (Taubenberger and Morens, 2006). Then COVID-19 emerged from China. The next sections will discuss some critical issues around the pandemic.

7.2 Globalization and the State of COVID-19 in the Global South

As it has been repeatedly observed, globalization is about the compression of time and space. Human mobility is facilitated through various modern means of transportation. Hence, an infection in Wuhan, China, became a global health problem (Amzat et al., 2020; Sohrabi et al., 2020). The human–animal interface (see Section 6.4.3) is another factor implicated in the origin of COVID-19, another zoonosis, which constitutes a threat to human health. Taylor et al. (2001) predicted that zoonoses would always constitute a significant threat to human health, including the emergence of a new human infection. Some animals are a reservoir of pathogens that could be introduced into a susceptible population (Wesolowski et al., 2016). Human dietary behavior is another crucial factor in the spread of zoonotic diseases. Consumption of wild animals has been linked to zoonotic infection in humans. Bats have been implicated in the spread of many infectious diseases in humans, including Ebola and COVID-19. Available evidence shows that COVID-19 emerged from Wuhan's Huanan Seafood Wholesale Market, specializing in aquatic animals and other live animals, such as bats, poultry, marmots and snakes (Lu et al., 2020; Sohrabi et al., 2020). Morens et al. (2020) observed that virologic, epidemiologic, veterinary and ecologic data indicates that "SARS-CoV-2 [severe acute respiratory syndrome-*coronavirus 2*], evolved directly or indirectly from a β-coronavirus in the sarbecovirus (SARS-like virus) group that naturally infect bats and pangolins in Asia and Southeast Asia". COVID-19 emerged from bats—the virus is a variant of a bat Coronavirus (Benvenuto et al., 2020).

Morens et al. (2020) observed that SARS-CoV-1 almost caused a near-pandemic in 2002–2003, but "neither SARS-CoV-2 nor its genetic sequences had ever been identified in viruses of humans or animals", hence it is a novel Coronavirus. The start of COVID-19 must be the infection of a person or group of persons in Wuhan, then the spread from person-to-person continues. Person-to-person transmission occurs predominantly through droplets spread by coughing or sneezing and through aerosols (produced e. g. by singing, shouting or strenuous physical exertion) from infected individuals. The virus may also remain infective on surfaces for several hours, but this indirect way of transmission is far less effective. A major challenge for pandemic control is that cases become infectious before they develop symptoms (Pennisi et al., 2020). Coronavirus presents with a dry cough, sore throat, fatigue, fever, loss of taste and smell, rhinorrhea, diarrhea and difficult breathing in infected persons (Chaplin, 2020). While every individual is at risk, those with the highest risk and severe outcome include those aged above 60 years old and those with underlying conditions, such as cancer, hypertension, diabetes and heart conditions.

The WHO declared the epidemic a public health emergency of international concern (PHEIC) on January 30, 2020, after noticing the virulent potentials of COVID-19. As of January 30, there were 7,711 confirmed cases, 12,167 suspected cases with 170 deaths and 124 people recovered in China (WHO, 2020a). The WHO also reported the situation in other countries with 83 cases in 18 countries, no deaths, but with 7 people without travel history to China, which suggested a possible start of person-to-person transmission. The first death outside China was recorded in the Philippines on February 2, 2020. The unprecedented spread of the COVID-19 continued with the first reported case outside China in Thailand on January 13, 2020—it was a returnee from Wuhan, the global epicenter. The case outside China sent a warning signal to the rest of the world to prepare for a possible pandemic. Perhaps, the virus's potentials were underrated and robust measures were not globally instituted to contain it at the earliest possible time.

Two nations, Italy and Iran, later joined China as the epicenters of COVID-19 and the primary sources of threats to other nations. Italy confirmed its first case on February 20, 2020, but in a month, Italy's cases jumped to over 22, 512 with 1,625 deaths (Livingston and Bucher, 2020). Iran joined the affected countries on February 19, 2020, when a returnee from China tested positive for COVID-19. The early response from Iran was inadequate as COVID-19 was considered as a hoax from the US. Wright (2020) reported that political laxity accounted for the pathetic COVID-19 situation in Iran. Unfortunately, Iran later became a COVID-19 epicenter in the Arab region, and transmission from returnees from Iran was recorded in several countries. By the end of March, the number of cases in Iran was over 35,000, with nearly 2,000 deaths. India also recorded its first case through a returnee from China on January 30, 2020. There was a sporadic increase in the number of cases in India, Pakistan, and Bangladesh passing the thousands mark very swiftly.

COVID-19 reached Africa on February 14, 2020, with the first case reported in Egypt (WHO, 2020b). The spread of COVID-19 in Africa was facilitated by returnees from hotspots in Europe, Asia and the United States (US). North Africa has close ties to Europe through migration, trade and tourism; it is not surprising that the first African COVID-19 case and death were recorded in North Africa. The second COVID-19 case was confirmed in Algeria on February 25—it was an Italian adult who arrived in the country some days earlier. The first death was a German tourist on March 8—as at which time, the number of cases in Egypt was barely 48. Nigeria recorded the first case of COVID-19 on February 27; it was an Italian on a business trip to the country (Amzat et al., 2020). On March 5, South Africa reported that a citizen who returned from Italy tested positive for COVID-19, and by March 27, two deaths were reported. By April 7, the number of cases in Africa had risen to over 10,000 with about 500 deaths (WHO, 2020b)

During the COVID-19 pre-pandemic period between December 31, 2019, and March 10, 2020, a study identified travel history to and from affected countries as a significant factor in the spread of COVID-19 (Dawood et al., 2020). The study examined the first 100 cases reported from 99 countries outside of China and reported that at least 76% had a recent travel history to an affected country, including China, Italy or Iran—the countries with the highest number of cases in the pre-pandemic period. Since the pandemic stage, COVID-19 has spread sporadically to all nations. Table 7.1 shows the cases of COVID-19 around the globe. As of September 2, 2020, there were slightly over 25.9 million cases, with over 860,000 deaths and over 18.2 million recoveries (Worldometer, 2020). Asia maintains the lowest death rate compared to the confirmed cases. The Global South region maintains the death rate below the global rate. The number of tests in the US relatively explains the total number of confirmed cases. For instance, India's total population triples that of the US, but its tests were near double that of India. The COVID-19 testing capacity influences the number of confirmed cases—cases can only be confirmed through tests. Within Africa, South Africa has 59 million people with about 186 COVID-19 testing sites, while Nigeria, with about 200 million people, has less than 84 testing sites, all with moderate test figures per day. Some nations, (e.g., the US and UK), commenced a general test of the entire population, but most developing nations restrict the tests because it gulps the limited national income, already badly affected by the pandemic. Specifically, as of September 2, 2020, the US has conducted COVID-19 tests for 25% of its citizens; Russia: 25.4%; India: 3.2%; Peru: 10%; South Africa: 6.2%; and Mexico: 1.1% (Worldometer, 2020).

Table 7.1 also shows that Mexico presents with a high death rate of over 10%. Spain is also not faring well with over 6%. The COVID-19 table is changing from time to time. For instance, Italy, Iran, France, Germany and the UK, were previously, around April 2020, in the top ten. In Asia, Iran, Bangladesh, Saudi Arabia and Pakistan have slightly above 300,000 cases and follow India on the top-10 list in the region. India recorded the highest single-day spike of 78,761 cases on August 30, 2020, signifying that that battle to bend or even flatten the curve should be intensified. Apart from Egypt, with 99,000 cases, Morocco, Nigeria, Ethiopia have about 50,000 cases and follow South Africa on the top-10 list in Africa. South America dominates the global top-ten list of COVID-19 cases with four countries, Brazil, Peru, Colombia and Argentina. For most of the countries, the curve bent downward as of early September 2020, but without adequate control measures, COVID-19 has the potential to re-emerge with a new wave like the Spanish flu of 1918–1920.

The WHO repeatedly warned Africa of a possible uncontrollable escalation of COVID-19. The warning was necessitated due to the poor health infrastructures and general low

Table 7.1 Burden of COVID-19 in selected regions and top 10 worst-hit countries

Country	Total Cases	Total Deaths	Total Tests	Fatality rate	Population
World	25,935,511	861,900	-	3.3	7,809,116,078
Selected Regions					
Asia	7,211,288	144,474	-	2.0	4,641,054,775
Africa	1,265,113	30,117	-	2.4	1,340,598,147
Europe	3,622,468	208,409		5.8	747,636,026
South America	6,389,282	204,669	-	3.2	653,962,331
Top ten Worst-Hit Countries					
USA	6,258,028	188,907	83,353,338	3.0	331,335,757
Brazil	3,952,790	122,681	14,352,484	3.1	212,817,864
India	3,773,483	66,491	44,337,201	1.8	1,382,308,045
Russia	1,005,000	17,414	37,100,000	1.7	145,945,354
Peru	657,129	29,068	3,233,034	4.4	33,048,955
South Africa	628,259	14,263	3,705,408	2.3	59,434,682
Colombia	624,069	20,052	2,777,107	3.2	50,974,767
Mexico	606,036	65,241	1,360,123	10.8	129,162,329
Spain	470,973	29,152	9,210,337	6.2	46,757,930
Argentina	428,239	8,919	1,277,751	2.1	45,266,317

Source: Worldometer, 2020: September 2, 2020, 11:42 GMT.

socio-economic capacity. Asia and Africa are characterized by communal social organization, crowded urban centers, large families in shared small spaces with little possibility for social or physical distancing (Harding, 2020). Such a social organization aids the spread of infectious diseases. Hence, the initial warning was that Africa could be the doom-land of COVID-19 with overpowering consequences. While it might be early to conclude about the burden of COVID-19 in Africa, the experience as of September 2, 2020, shows the opposite with a lower burden, without prejudice to the testing capacity and relatively lower death rate than initially feared (Harding, 2020). Experts' opinions relate that a youthful population and previous exposures to infectious diseases could explain Africa's relatively low infection rate (Harding, 2020), apart from the concerted efforts of the various African governments and disease control agencies (WHO-AFR, 2021). Meanwhile, as nations battle the health crisis, some conspiracy theories emerged generating an infodemic, i.e., widespread rumors and misinformation relating to the pandemic.

7.3 Infodemic and COVID-19 Conspiracy Theories

The rapid spread of information is a significant driver of globalization. The use of information and communication technology (ICT) has changed the patterns of communication in remarkable ways. Unlike the slow pace of information dissemination during the Spanish flu, information about COVID-19, both positive and negative, spread like wildfire. In no time, the information about COVID-19 gripped the world that there is a ravaging virus in China that could threaten global health. While some began to act, some wished away the information. The internet is a technological tool of the globalized era, which nourishes or breeds the global spread of information and misinformation. Therefore, infodemic, both accurate information and misinformation flourishes and spreads swiftly. Infodemic refers to the overabundance of information from numerous credible and questionable sources, which affect the public's judgment about a trending issue. An infodemic can also be defined as the existence of "a large increase in the volume of information associated with a specific topic and whose growth can occur exponentially in a short period due to a specific incident, such as the current pandemic" (PAHO, 2020: p. 1). The existence of social media is highly instrumental to the infodemic, with numerous self-acclaimed "experts" propagating all sorts of information. Infodemiology or information epidemiology emerged as a research area since 1996, focusing on the availability of health information (Eysenbach, 2002), but Eysenbach (2002) was the first to call it "infodemiology". Infodemiology is the "study [or science] of the determinants and distribution of health information and misinformation" (Eysenbach, 2002: p. 763) and their effects on the public and professionals.

An information pandemic is a reality because of extensive social networks and social media. Any conceived idea in any part of the world can easily be amplified across the globe. The popular social media amplify information and serve as data sources in infodemiology (Eysenbach, 2011; Zeraatkar and Ahmadi, 2018). The primary concern is an infodemic, which can be assessed through infodemiology and controlled through infoveillance, i.e., a matching method of information surveillance, which involves the monitoring and evaluating of health information available online (Eysenbach, 2011). Therefore, infoveillance measures "the pulse of public opinion, attention, behavior, knowledge, and attitudes by tracking what people do and write on the Internet" (Eysenbach, 2011).

Health information is vital in control efforts because gaps often exist between biomedical and lay explanations of diseases. The COVID-19 pandemic comes with many rumors and unfounded opinions circulated through social media such as WhatsApp, Twitter, TikTok, Instagram, Telegram, Facebook and various mobile apps, online platforms as well as blogs.

Twitter emerged as a significant source of information for COVID-19. Most COVID-19-related tweets had nonmedical frames (Park et al., 2020; Abd-Alrazaq et al., 2020). Hence, social media must be adequately monitored, especially during a pandemic, to ensure appropriate risk perception. There is a strong call for a "proactive and agile public health presence on social media to combat the spread of fake news" (Abd-Alrazaq et al., 2020), and to assist stakeholders "in their complex and fast-paced decision-making processes" (Park et al., 2020). During the pandemic and beyond, misinformation negatively impacts health and illness behavior, and it is a matter of life and death as people might resort to unproven drugs and disregard public health recommended measures (Ball and Maxmen, 2020). Therefore, infoveillance, including rumor surveillance, must be a routine to scrutinize different online platforms to capture public uncertainty about any trending issue.

An infodemic serves a double function, by providing both (accurate) information and misinformation concurrently. For instance, social media is characterized by limited quality control. Social media posts could get people informed, generate anxiety and circulate conspiracy theories or pseudoscience during a pandemic. Of utmost importance in this section are the COVID-19 related conspiracy theories. A conspiracy theory is about suspicion of intended or unintended malevolent goals (see Section 10.3.5). Amzat (2020, p. 210) described conspiracy theory as a practice of "describing ideas, actions, or events as heinous manipulations of another group, organization, or country despite proven evidence to the contrary". In such situations, hesitancy or resistance to scientific value is (rigorously) fostered. Such conspiracy theory breeds "repugnance to the adoption of evidence-based ideas, development agendas, and best practices" (Amzat, 2020, p. 210). Andrade (2020) asserted that conspiracy theories are historical, found among all social classes and could be harmful to disease control efforts. Some COVID-19 conspiracy theories developed around issues, including the virus's reality, origin and transmission, amid the pandemic.

7.3.1 Conspiracy Theory on the Reality of COVID-19

The first question is about the reality of COVID-19, which in this sense means whether COVID-19 exists or not. Belief in the reality of a disease is a significant step in taking preventive action. If an individual believes that a disease does not exist, they might not utilize any cautionary measures against such diseases. Amzat et al. (2020) described the emergence of "covidiots" who, despite millions of cases and deaths, do not believe in the reality of the virus and hence, would not take any recommended preventive measures. Millions of people across the globe and in different countries questioned the existence of COVID-19, claiming that it was a hoax or a trick by some interested groups to create anxiety to achieve certain ends. For instance, pharmaceutical companies could make money through such medical anxiety. It is not new that the reality of the disease is questioned. The campaign about "AIDS is real" emanated from such a belief. There must be intense risk communication for the remaining "covidiots" to admit that COVID-19 is real. The general low-risk perception of COVID-19 in Africa is significant and could result in more spread of the virus as many people still break COVID-19 protocols (Amzat et al., 2020).

A study in Bangladesh showed that a significant percentage of the respondents had poor knowledge of COVID-19 transmission and symptoms onset (Paul et al., 2020). A study in ten countries across Europe, America and Asia examined the risk perception of COVID-19 (Dryhurst et al., 2020). The study uncovered variation in risk perception in the different countries: It was highest in the UK compared with all other sampled countries. As previously argued, risk perception influenced the adoption of preventative health measures in all ten countries (Dryhurst et al., 2020). Risk perception is not automatically developed; it must be socially negotiated based on available information, personal experiences and trust in political and medical institutions handling the situation (Rickard, 2019). Due to the social nature of risk, appropriate risk communication is vital in disease control.

7.3.2 Conspiracy Theory on the Origin of COVID-19

Another major conspiracy theory is about the origin of COVID-19. It is widespread that COVID-19 was manufactured in a laboratory, then intentionally spread as a biological weapon, or mistakenly escaped from a laboratory in Wuhan, China. The belief in this laboratory-manufactured virus exists in the North and South (Freeman et al., 2020). The conspiracy assumes that COVID-19 was deliberately engineered to achieve certain ends, including population control and the development of biological and economic weapons. In a study in England, Stephen (2020) observed that many respondents believed in the bioweapon and lab-made conspiracy theories. Hence, more than half of the respondents blamed China for the spread of the virus. Almost 25% of Canadians believed in the lab-made conspiracy theory. About 20% believed that Bill Gates, the billionaire, deliberately created and spread the virus to microchip people or for population control (Ball and Maxmen, 2020). Up to 20% believed that the US military made the virus a biological weapon to fight other nations (Stecula et al., 2020). It is surprising that, although the US has one of the highest burden of COVID-19, the belief still prevails. This kind of infodemic affects public health efforts and, in many ways, global relations. Despite the fact that there is no evidence to support these claims, they linger for a long time.

The lab-made conspiracy theory exists because there are bioweapons, which constitute a significant global health challenge. After an extensive review about plague, biological weapons, biological terrorism and biological warfare, Inglesby et al. (2000) observed an aerosolized plague weapon with symptoms like severe pneumonia, including fever, cough, chest pain and hemoptysis. There are several potential agents of bioterrorism that could cause mass fatalities. In the real sense of the 21st century, bioterrorism, the purposeful release of toxic biological agents to claim casualties, is no longer a matter of uncertainty; it has happened several times in history (Gwerder et al., 2001; Riedel, 2004). Riedel (2004) documented the historical use of bioweapons, including the use of glanders and anthrax in WWI, plague and anthrax during WWII. The most significant global health threat is the fact that many countries, including Germany, Iran, China, France, Syria, North Korea, the US, Japan, the UK and Cuba, among others, continue to develop biological weapons for possible warfare or terrorism (NTI, 2015). Since China and the US have bioweapons, conspiracy theorists are not out of place to suspect a possibly lab-made COVID-19.

Many scientists have explained why COVID-19 is not a human-made, purposively manipulated or genetically modified virus (Cui et al., 2019; Andersen et al., 2020; Benvenuto et al., 2020; Zhou et al., 2020). The initial conclusion is that a zoonotic spillover is overwhelmingly more probable than a lab-made conspiracy theory. The most important reason is that the virus is novel; therefore, it is not a lab-cultivated variant of previously known SARS-CoV. Andersen et al. (2020) noted that "SARS-CoV-2 is the seventh coronavirus known to infect humans… if genetic manipulation had been performed, one of the several reverse-genetic systems available for betacoronaviruses would probably have been used". Despite this scientific assertion, the conspiracy theory will linger for a long time because beliefs are not readily amenable to change.

7.3.3 Conspiracy Theory on the Transmission of COVID-19

There is also a conspiracy theory about how Coronavirus spread to the rest of the globe. The insinuation is that the 5G network installed in Wuhan, China, is responsible for spreading the virus (Ahmed et al., 2020). The suspicion is that the virus is wirelessly transmitted, and therefore, places with the 5G network would bear a high burden of COVID-19. As stated earlier, the emergence of COVID-19 led to the proliferation of a complex mix of unverifiable, helpful and manipulated information, including misinformation and disinformation (Larson, 2020). Prominent among the messages were those implicating a 5G network. Larson observed that the Vaccine Confidence Project captured over 240 million online messages concerning COVID-19, an average of 3.08 million messages per day between the new year and mid-March 2020. The Project recorded over 113 million tweets about COVID-19, including the origin, mode of transmission and preventive guidelines (Larson, 2020). Many of the messages wrongfully implicated 5G network in COVID-19 transmission.

In addition, Ahmed et al. (2020) did a social network analysis and content analysis of Twitter data during the pandemic (April 2020) and captured the #5GCoronavirus hashtag trending on Twitter the UK. One-third of the posts linked 5G with the spread of COVID-19. The authors reported that the insinuation was spreading faster than any counterclaims. The respondents posted YouTube videos and fake news sites to support the 5G conspiracy. As a result of the theory, some 5G towers in the United Kingdom were burnt (Ahmed et al., 2020). The extent of the influence of such 5G misinformation is incalculable. The observed messages online signify a large volume of information available to the global population—some of which might also be shared among those who lack access to online platforms. Hence, it is astonishing that a wrong assumption about 5G, the latest advancement in the global system for mobile technology, infiltrated the globe. But countries such as Nigeria, Somalia, Ecuador, among others, without the so-called 5G network, also recorded a significant incidence of COVID-19, which triggered doubts about the toxic theory. Unfortunately, some countries halted or banned the installation of 5G networks, which in some way helped in propagating the conspiracy theory. Such misinformation also abetted the spread of the virus due to a negative attitude toward COVID-19 protocols.

7.3.4 Other COVID-19 Myths

There were controversies regarding the treatment of COVID-19. There were viral videos of preventive and curative measures, some of which have not been verified. Many online posts and visuals identified some natural ingredients in the early days, including garlic, lemon, apocalyptic leaves, ginger and Vit-C as home-brewed cures (Larson, 2020). These are safe ingredients that most people often use. The only problem is that it has not been ascertained whether these ingredients could solely cure or prevent COVID-19. The proliferation of the news made many people in the Global South trivialize COVID-19, hoping that the ingredients mentioned earlier could cure it. There were millions of messages, some with "authoritative" backings going viral. Ginger and lemon tea became a daily routine for COVID-19 prevention, with many gargling with apocalyptic hot water or ginger tea to ward off any suspected virus from the throat. Perhaps, the traditional prophylaxes must have helped in inestimable ways to reduce the burden of COVID-19 in many low-income countries; but despite the over-subscription to those natural ingredients, COVID-19 continues to ravage the globe.

Then, there were speculations about chloroquine, a malaria drug, as the primary cure for COVID-19, despite the fact that efficacy tests had not been completed. Incidentally in many countries, the treatment regime of COVID-19 included malaria drugs. Although some studies (Hashem et al., 2020; Li et al., 2020; White et al., 2020) showed some promises, they were not enough to conclude that hydroxychloroquine could cure COVID-19. In the twinkle of an eye, claims of efficacy of hydroxychloroquine were shared across the globe. Such misinformation stymies the control effort in many ways. First, it buttresses the conspiracy theory that there is a cure, but some stakeholders are "hiding" it for malevolent gains. It also signifies that COVID-19 data might not be real since there is a presumed cure. A particular viral video about the efficacy of hydroxychloroquine emanating from Washington DC shared by millions of people, including former President Trump (of the United States), made a mess of global health efforts in the face of the COVID-19 crisis. It was as if all efforts, including the figures and the death tolls, were politically motivated. Right from the pre-pandemic phase, former President Trump has been a subject of COVID-19 controversies. First, he called it a Chinese virus, assured Americans of high preparedness and later recommended ingesting some bleach to kill the virus.

In general, former President Trump was inconsistent in disseminating information as he downplayed the severity of the pandemic on many occasions despite the high COVID-19 fatality in the US. The inconsistency explained some of his actions that depicted low risk perception despite being in the high risk age group. For instance, he held some possible (COVID-19) superspreader events during his campaign, including a White House ceremony to unveil a Supreme Court nominee, held on September 26, 2020. A high rate of infection could be traced to any superspreader event, which is a mass gathering during the pandemic with very minimal adherence to preventive protocols such as use of facemasks and physical distancing. Sadly, former President Trump as well as his wife, personal assistant and six others who attended the White House ceremony, tested positive for COVID-19 on October 2, 2020, barely a month into the US presidential elections. It can be argued that Trump's handling of the COVID-19 crisis contributed, in no small measure, to his presidential election defeat in November, 2020. In general, an infodemic is a tremendous global health concern because the information from political figures could become global in seconds. When it is health misinformation, it increases the global risk of morbidity and mortality.

Due to the ocean of misinformation concerning hydroxychloroquine and the COVID-19 symptom complex, which presents like malaria and other respiratory conditions, there were also conspiracy insinuations of misdiagnosis in malaria-endemic areas that malaria or catarrh is being mistaken for COVID-19. The initial thought was that COVID-19 belonged to the other continents, not Africa. In other disturbing scenarios, many claimed that COVID-19 was meant for the elites who traveled by air. Most people heard of the big names who tested positive from the media. COVID-19 also ravaged the corridors of political power often in the global media radar. Many world leaders tested positive for COVID-19, including Boris Johnson (the UK Prime Minister), former President Donald Trump; Jair Bolsonaro (Brazilian President), Alexander Lukashenko, (Belarus' President), Nikol Pashinyan (Armenia's Prime Minister), Juan Orlando Hernandez, (Honduras' President), Prince Albert II of Monaco, Alejandro Giammattei (President of Guatemala) and many other political figures. The reports of their (i.e., the world leaders') positive status and treatment occupied the media space. The elite bias in the media report of the pandemic also projected the misconstrued elitist wave of COVID-19, especially in the early days of the pandemic in developing countries where air travel is seen as elitist.

In most low-income countries, air travel is still elitist, so the initial cases were returnees from the UK, China and Italy (Amzat et al., 2020). Therefore, COVID-19 was termed a disease of the rich. Dawood et al. (2020) confirmed that travel history was significant during the pre-pandemic period. It followed a similar pattern in the rest of the world when travel history was significant before the beginning of community transmission, which marked the declaration of a global health emergency. It took a long time before many people came to terms with the fact that travel history was no longer significant, especially during the pandemic stage. During the onset of transmission in many countries, the behavioral laxity accounted for the high burden of COVID worldwide. Most states faced the double burden of the pandemic and the infodemic, with the latter more lethal as it aided the spread of the former, thereby accounting for more cases and deaths.

The pandemic overwhelmed the health infrastructures of both high- and low-income countries—no country was adequately prepared for the pandemic. The situation in the Global South was exacerbated because of the already poor infrastructure. There were many permutations since, although the aforementioned traditional ingredients, garlic, lemon and ginger, could help, traditional medicine could not resolve COVID-19 complications. There was a scramble for traditional medicine. One major reference was the announcement of "COVID-Organic" by Madagascar President as the cure of COVID-19. As of March, during the announcement, Madagascar had less than 200 cases with 0 deaths, which made many think that the country had a magic wand against the virus. The country soon slipped into community transmission with 15,769 cases and 213 deaths (1.5% of the confirmed cases) as of September 14, 2020 (Worldometer, 2020). Whether COVID-Organic holds some curative promise or not, the announcement was not taken seriously. There has always been powerplay concerning any innovation from low-income countries. There were some pseudoscientific products, including herbal preparations and other unfounded claims from traditional healers and overzealous politicians, especially from the Global South. The notion of pseudoscience is not meant to denigrate all herbal products. In fact, it is advocated that some available herbal extracts from Africa and Asia that could inhibit viral replication and act against COVID-19-related opportunistic infections could be given further considerations in the form of clinical trials (Mirzaie et al., 2020; Ang et al., 2020).

7.4 Spread, Consequences and Control of COVID-19

In infectious disease control, any form of delay is always dangerous. The COVID-19 outbreak in Wuhan was initially concealed. The information was suppressed, but the condition was not adequately managed to prevent a pandemic. The information about the outbreak of COVID-19 came first as unofficial communication from Li Wenliang (who later died of COVID-19), a young ophthalmologist in Wuhan, China, who warned of a SARS-like outbreak (Larson, 2020). Unfortunately, the Chinese government suppressed the information for selfish national gains (Kynge and Hancock, 2020). The action of the Chinese government was a severe infraction of the global health protocol. The International Health Regulations (IHR of 2005) requires all Member States to notify the WHO within 24 hours of outbreaks of infectious diseases of international concern (Cash and Narasimhan, 2000; Sturtevant et al., 2007; WHO, 2016). Prompt reporting would have helped contain the spread in a specific location for effective control without constituting a national or international disaster. The delay or non-disclosure constituted a significant infraction on international efforts to curtail contagious diseases. Such failure to report in the earliest possible time, for which China is liable, is inimical to global disease surveillance regulation.

The pandemic should have been averted if China had followed IHR for surveillance systems, which is critical for identifying and preventing any emerging and re-emerging infectious diseases (see WHO, 2016). The WHO and other related bodies rely on every nation's cooperation within the global health governance to take responsibility in the case of any outbreak to curtail international or global vulnerability. The first level of the delay was the non-reporting of the outbreak when China accused the first reporter, Li Wenliang, of rumor-mongering. What was not clear was whether China was aware of the pandemic potential of COVID-19, but thought it could contain it, thereby secretly managing the crisis. The failure to report within the timeline triggered conspiracy that China was withholding some vital information from the global communities. It was one of the reasons that people manufactured the lab-made conspiracy.

Figure 7.1 shows that the delay in reporting and control efforts was significant in the progression of COVID-19 to the pandemic stage. The second level of delay also reflects the hesitancy

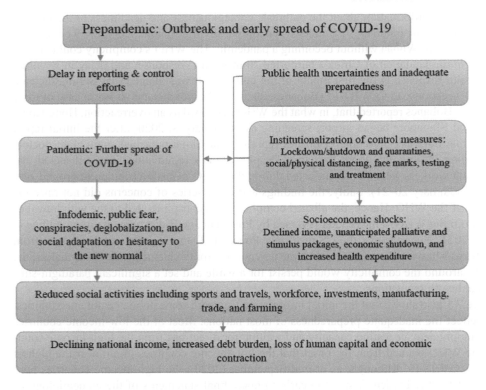

Figure 7.1 Consequences and control of COVID-19

before Wuhan's eventual lockdown, the global epicenter of COVID-19. Many people had traveled out of Wuhan after exposure to the virus. If Wuhan has been promptly locked down as a precautionary measure immediately after China's admittance of the outbreak, perhaps the pandemic potentials would have been curtailed. The lockdown of Wuhan was on January 23, 2020, more than 40 days after the outbreak. The lockdown was delayed for no apparent reason—to lock down a city would have been better than the resulting global lockdown. The WHO declared PHEIC on January 30, after the delayed lockdown of Wuhan. The emergency would have been declared as soon as human-to-human transmission was confirmed before the lockdown of Wuhan. WHO declared PHEIC much earlier during the Ebola outbreak of 2014–2015 in West Africa and 2019 in Democratic Republic of Congo (DRC) when the number of cases and countries affected are considered. The 2014 PHEIC declaration was made on August 8, 2014, with four countries (Guinea, Liberia, Nigeria and Sierra Leone) affected, accounting for about 1,711 confirmed and probable cases, including 932 deaths (WHO, 2014). The allegedly "delayed" 2019 PHEIC declaration was made on July 17 when there were 2,512 confirmed and probable cases, with 1,737 deaths in DR Congo, including two reported deaths in Uganda (Zarocostas, 2019). But that of COVID-19 was made after over 7,000 cases in 18 countries. Why was the case of COVID-19 so different that the WHO was sluggish in its declaration of PHEIC in the face of accelerated international transmission?

Global health delay in decision-making concerning the transmission of infectious disease is always pricey and lethal. Every minute counts—the declaration was 11 days after the confirmation of human-to-human transmission. China is a global traffic hub; it could have been estimated that, since the first reported case and death, many might have contracted the virus and moved out of China to other countries. Embedded mistakes and missteps could be observed in

China's delayed information about the outbreak, contagiousness and deadliness of the virus in the early days of the outbreak. If China was unequivocally transparent, COVID-19 could have been contained in Wuhan without becoming a pandemic. The WHO's complicity could also be observed in the laudation of China's purported "transparent" response, and delay in its initial public health response in the first month of the outbreak. It was alleged that Beijing dictated the WHO's response to COVID-19 (Bobanes, 2020), and if not dictated, it was a case of toxic negligence. Bobanes reported that, in what the WHO described as an overreaction, Hong Kong, Taiwan and Singapore began airport screening as of January 3, 2020, after the initial report of a possible outbreak in Wuhan. Bobanes reported that China punished some eight doctors for spreading information about the virus. Despite China's repudiation, it was detected that some health workers were already infected during the WHO's onsite visitation to ground zero in Wuhan (January 20–21). Sadly, the findings and other series of concerns did not raise the suspicion of the WHO. Hence, the alleged complicity and conspiracy led to the withdrawal of the US from the WHO; a move later reversed by President Joe Biden upon assuming Office in January, 2021. Nevertheless, the US or former President Trump's decision to withdraw from the WHO was hasty and mistimed—the time was not ripe for the blame game. Nevertheless, the questions around the complicity would persist for a while and set a significant paradigm-shift for global health regulations.

Figure 7.1 also shows that the initial information triggered some public health uncertainties, which reflect the inadequate preparedness of most nations. Most of the low-income countries were without adequate testing capacity and waiting for directions from the high-income countries. The WHO warned from the onset that the low-income countries might bear the highest brunt of COVID-19. Although, as of mid-September (2020), the high-income countries bore the highest fatality burden, it was too early to make final statements of the epidemiology of COVID-19 because of another possible wave in the light of hurriedly reopening of national economies. Three significant factors, an allegation of corruption or COVID-scam, dwindling political trust in the management of the pandemic and rushed reopening of the economy were responsible for the second wave in the Global South, despite the lower incidence compared to Europe and North America. For instance, the hardest-hit country in Africa, South Africa, reopened the economy after an extended total and partial lockdown of about 170 days without bending the COVID-19 curve.

Following the delay and ill-preparedness, COVID-19 became a pandemic, with the virus moving with the people due to global connectivity. This pandemic era also marked the period of infodemic, public fear and the beginning of a new normal, i.e., social alterations resulting from the pandemic. Initially, there was screening at the points of entry; later, most entry points, including airports, were shut. There was a ban on all international travel except for the movement of essential personnel and medical equipment. Between March and August, the world experienced deglobalization in the form of a drastic decline in the flow of people, goods and services, but information continued to flow virtually, primarily through social media.

After deglobalization, other control measures to reduce human mobility and contact were institutionalized including social restriction in the form of lockdowns and quarantines, social/physical distancing, use of facemasks, increased testing and treatment. The social measures were very vital because the virus does not move; it moves with the people. Hence, physical distancing, often called social distancing, was recommended and enforced in most countries. Sociologically, the concept of "physical distancing" is more appropriate than "social distancing" since other forms of interaction continued virtually. Caring for others does not stop, but an average of six-feet distance was recommended between two people. At the peak of the pandemic in Germany, the government banned all gatherings of more than two people. It was the same rule across all other continents, although the level of compliance varied.

All educational institutions were shut for months. More than 1.4 billion students in 186 countries were out of school due to the pandemic by the end of March 2020 (WEF, 2020). While educational activities continued online in high-income countries, more than 95% of students were stuck at home without any television or online educational activities in low-income countries. Inequality gaps reflect in the access to online learning, with 95% of students in Austria, Norway and Switzerland having a computer to use for their schoolwork, compared with only 34% in Indonesia (WEF, 2020), and a much lower percentage in Bolivia, Uganda, Sudan, Pakistan, Rwanda, Syria, Zambia, Zimbabwe and other low-income countries. Students from low-income backgrounds had little or no access to internet facilities. In Africa, South Africa was exceptional in facilitating online learning, especially for university students, through the provision of internet facilities for learners and instructors.

Figure 7.1 further shows that the world experienced overwhelming socio-economic shocks as a result of the pandemic. The four basic shocks include a sudden income decline, unanticipated palliative and economic stimulus budgets, economic shutdown and increased health expenditure. The shutdown of economic activities meant a decline in national income, with many national economies contrasting between 20% and 50% with an imminent economic recession worldwide. For low- and middle-income countries (LMICs), it was a complicated tragedy of depletion of already poor infrastructures and income. For oil-producing countries, both production and price fell by more than 50% than projected; for tourism-dependent economies, it was a complete shutdown. The debt burden increased as many nations borrowed more to alleviate the pandemic burden. Many economies could slump to pandemic debt, causing another global economic crisis. Since the people's welfare is always sacrosanct, most nations distributed palliatives to mitigate the effects of the lockdown (Yaya et al., 2020). For LMICs with high percentage of daily earners engaged in small and medium enterprises, including subsistence agriculture, the effects were extremely devastating and the so-called palliatives were grossly inadequate (Amzat et al., 2020). In general, the pandemic led to reduced social activities, including sports and travel, workforce, investments, manufacturing, trade and farming, not only within a country but also among nations. For instance, the Tokyo Olympics was postponed from summer 2020 to 2021; club soccer competitions, including Union of European Football Association (UEFA) Champions League, The English Premier League, Italian *Seria A* and Spanish *Laliga* were postponed and later remaining matches were played without spectators; and only about 1,000 resident pilgrims performed the 2020 annual Hajj in Saudi Arabia instead of the usual over 2 million pilgrims. In most LMICs, "COVID-hunger" was widespread—the choice between hunger and Coronavirus was not palatable.

Aside from palliatives for individuals and economic stimulus package for enterprises, the health expenditure skyrocketed due to the initiated public health measures, personal protective equipment (PPE) for health workers, COVID tests, and institutionalization of isolation centers and treatment of patients. For instance, the cost of a COVID-19 test per person is around US$130 in Nigeria, a country where the minimum wage is US$75 per month, and more than half of the population live below the poverty line of US$ 2 daily. Most African and Asian governments had to bear the costs of COVID-19 tests alongside other public health measures. The average cost of treatment per person in the US is around US$2,000. Treatment costs were also high in LMICs. There was global tussle for the few drugs with some promise in treating people with COVID-19. The US bought up the projected production of Remdesivir for three months, which showed some hope in the treatment of patients with COVID-19. The United Kingdom also earmarked about US$25 million to procure hydroxychloroquine, which has also been mentioned to have curative potentials for COVID-19. The US' and the UK's decisions could prevent other nations from having access to those drugs. There was also a "scramble" for vaccines when some promising vaccines were approved at the end of 2020. Despite warnings from the WHO, it was a game of power and vaccine nationalism (Eaton, 2021). Self-interest rather than a global coordinated approach will sustain unequal access to and allocation of vaccines which will prolong the burden of COVID-19. In the face of vaccine nationalism or inequity, the COVID threat will still be global because of the danger of further virus mutations or variants of concern (VoC), which could lead to a vaccine race (i.e., interminable need to develop a new vaccine for a new strain). The same scenarios will play out when a cure is discovered.

7.5 Looking Forward

COVID-19 resulted in socio-economic disruptions. The economies of nations significantly contracted, but hurried reopening will lead to more damages than projected. It is cost-effective to sacrifice economic resources that can be regained through prudent economic planning to avert human capital loss, which is not hastily reversible. The sustained human capital will restore the economy; thus, nations should prioritize public health gains over economic gains, or else, we lose everything. The world must avert a recurrence of the high fatality burden of the Black Death of 1348–1351 and the Spanish influenza of 1918–1920. Another notable dramatic and tragic development is global vaccine inequity. There is the need for a more equitable distribution of vaccines in order to save lives and avoid suffering among people in low-income countries, but also to prevent the emergence of new virus variants of concern (VoC), which would threaten population health world-wide.

The fundamental causes of the pandemic have been identified in the preceding sections. The first is the human–wildlife relations; the second is the series of delays in reporting to the appropriate agency that should issue global alert; and the third is a delay in implementing stringent measures to prevent the global spread of the viral disease. The aforementioned are only primary or fundamental issues, as there could be other explanations. Given the preceding, all relevant stakeholders need to redefine human–bat relations. This might be extended to wildlife, but that of bats needs urgent attention. Bats have been a reservoir of lethal viruses, including Ebola, SARS and Coronavirus, to humans. The case of bats causing a global health emergency is occurring too often, and there should be strict regulations to redefine human–bat interactions in a way that will preserve both wildlife and human health.

Lastly, the IHR should be strengthened by incorporating global sanctions in cases of delay in reporting diseases with pandemic potentials. Negligence concerning strict measures to curb the outbreak should also be sanctioned. While nations take responsibilities, the right to know is crucial in deciding appropriate lines of actions. If we do not redefine human–wildlife relations, strengthen the International Health Regulations and incorporate sanctions on negligence, the world will face the challenges of more global health emergencies in the near future.

7.6 Summary

- Coronavirus of 2019 (COVID-19) became a pandemic and overwhelmed the world. It is a major pandemic of the modern era with over 30 million cases and close to 1 million deaths within 10 months. Like the influenza pandemic of 1918–1920 with four sequential waves, COVID-19 also spread in waves.
- Before 2019, occasional disease outbreaks of global concern, including Black Death of 1348–1351, influenza of 1918–1920, the Asian flu of 1957–1958, severe acute respiratory syndrome (SARS) of 2002, Ebola of 2014–2015, Zika of 2015–2016, had occurred, overriding the health infrastructures of various countries.
- The spread of COVID-19 is a manifestation of a risk society, fueled by globalization or, specifically, human mobility. The index (first) case in most countries was a returnee from

an already affected country. Therefore, travel history to and from affected countries was a significant factor in the spread of COVID-19.

- The series of delays, insufficient preparedness, "complicity" of China and the World Health Organization accelerated the spread of the virus. Perhaps the pandemic could have been averted if China had followed International Health Regulations with prompt surveillance and reporting to the appropriate bodies. The pandemic overwhelmed the health infrastructures of both high- and low-income countries—no country was adequately prepared for the pandemic.
- Just as the COVID-19 pandemic was a global health emergency, so was the infodemic: The many rumors and unfounded opinions circulated through (online) social media which emerged as a significant source of information for COVID-19. During the pandemic and beyond, misinformation negatively impacts health and illness behavior, and it is a matter of life and death as people might resort to unproven drugs and disregard public health recommended measures.
- Conspiracy theories on the reality, origin, transmission, prevention and treatment of COVID-19 also became a significant global health concern because of their effects on risk perception, and subsequently, on global control efforts.
- There was a temporary deglobalization with the ban on all international travels except for the movement of essential personnel and medical equipment. Between March and August (2020), the world experienced deglobalization in the form of a drastic decline in the flow of people, goods and services, but information continued to flow virtually, primarily through social media.
- This chapter also looks at the global control efforts, socio-economic shocks of COVID-19 and how global health politics plays out as nations struggle to contain the virus. As nations reopen the economy, it is important to prioritize public health gains over economic gains.
- There is a significant power play between the South and the North in the "scramble" for vaccines since there are some approved vaccines since the end of 2020. Such power play or self-interest manifests in vaccine nationalism or inequity which will increase the danger of further virus mutations or variants of concern (VoC) that could prolong the global burden of COVID-19.
- Given that bats have been a reservoir of lethal viruses to humans, the relevant stakeholders need to redefine human–bat relations in a way that will preserve both wildlife and human health.
- Lastly, the International Health Regulations of 2005 should be strengthened by incorporating global sanctions in cases of delay in reporting diseases with pandemic potentials.

Critical Thinking Questions

- COVID-19 pandemic has shown that a health crisis has a wide range of consequences. With reference to your country, explain the global impacts of the pandemic from sociological, political, economic and medical perspectives.
- The social media is a space of information with impacts on disease control efforts. How was your experience of the infodemic during the pandemic? Assess the various ways that infodemics affect individual responses to COVID-19.
- There were real-time conspiracy theories during the COVID-19 pandemic. Highlight some of those theories, their impacts or implications for the global response to the pandemic.
- It was hard to imagine the world could be deglobalized due to a pandemic. Assess deglobalization and its social and health impacts on the global response to COVID-19.

- Health is politics and global health is more political. With reference to some political circumstances, assess whether your country was immersed in some internal and external politics of COVID-19. Identify and discuss the areas of crucial global politics in the response to COVID-19.
- With reference to the spread, control and consequences of COVID-19 pandemic, what sorts of global health mistrusts did you observe between the low- and high-income countries?

Suggested Readings

- Andersen, K. G., Rambaut, A., Lipkin, W. I., Holmes, E. C. and Garry, R. F. (2020). The proximal origin of SARS-CoV-2. *Nature Medicine, 26*, 450–452. https://doi.org/10.1038/s41591-020-0820-9. The article discusses the origin of COVID-19.
- Andrade, G. (2020). Medical conspiracy theories: Cognitive science and implications for ethics. *Medicine, Health Care, and Philosophy*, 1–14. Advance online publication. https://doi.org/10.1007/s11019-020-09951-6. The article is generally about health-related conspiracy theories.
- Ball, P., and Maxmen, A. (2020). The epic battle against Coronavirus misinformation and conspiracy theories. *Nature, 581*(7809), 371–374. https://doi.org/10.1038/d41586-020-01452-z. The article documents some important infodemic trends during the COVID-19 pandemic.
- Eysenbach, G. (2011). Infodemiology and infoveillance tracking online health information and cyberbehavior for public health. *American Journal of Preventive Medicine*, 40(5 Suppl, 2), S154-S158. The article details more information about health-related infodemic and infoveillance.
- Dawood, F. S., Ricks, P., Njie, G. J., et al. (2020). Observations of the global epidemiology of COVID-19 from the prepandemic period using web-based surveillance: A cross-sectional analysis. *The Lancet Infectious diseases*, S1473-3099(20)30581-8. Advance online publication. https://doi.org/10.1016/S1473-3099(20)30581-8. The article documents the pre-pandemic spread of Coronavirus in 2019.

References

Abd-Alrazaq, A., Alhuwail, D., Househ, M., Hamdi, M. & Shah, Z. (2020). Top concerns of tweeters during the COVID-19 pandemic: Infoveillance study. *Journal of Medical Internet Research*, *22*(4), e19016. doi: 10.2196/19016.

Ahmed, W., Vidal-Alaball, J., Downing, J. & Seguí, F. L. (2020). COVID-19 and the 5G conspiracy theory: Social network analysis of twitter data. *Journal of Medical Internet Research*, *22*(5), e19458. doi: 10.2196/19458.

Amzat, J. (2020). Beyond wishful thinking: The promise of science engagement at a community level in Africa. *Journal of Developing Societies*, *36*(2), 206–228. doi: 10.1177/0169796X20910600.

Amzat, J., Aminu, K., Kolo, V. I., Akinyele, A. A., Ogundairo, J. A. & Danjibo, C. M. (2020). Coronavirus outbreak in Nigeria: Burden and socio-medical response during the first 100 days. *International Journal of Infectious Diseases*, *98*, 218–224.doi: 10.1016/j.ijid.2020.06.067.

Andersen, K. G., Rambaut, A., Lipkin, W. I., Holmes, E. C. & Garry, R. F. (2020). The proximal origin of SARS-CoV-2. *Nature Medicine*, *26*, 450–452. doi: 10.1038/s41591-020-0820-9.

Andrade, G. (2020). Medical conspiracy theories: Cognitive science and implications for ethics. *Medicine, Health Care, and Philosophy*, 1–14. Advance online publication. doi: 10.1007/s11019-020-09951-6.

Ang, L., Song, E., Lee, H. W. & Lee, M. S. (2020). Herbal medicine for the treatment of coronavirus disease 2019 (COVID-19): A systematic review and meta-analysis of randomized controlled trials. *Journal of Clinical Medicine*, *9*(5), 1583. doi: 10.3390/jcm9051583.

Babones, S. (2020). Yes, blame WHO for its disastrous coronavirus response. *Foreign Policy*, https://foreignpolicy.com/2020/05/27/who-health-china-coronavirus-tedros/. Accessed on September 15, 2020.

Ball, P., & Maxmen, A. (2020). The epic battle against coronavirus misinformation and conspiracy theories. *Nature*, *581*(7809), 371–374. doi: 10.1038/d41586-020-01452-z.

Benvenuto, D., Giovanetti, M., Ciccozzi, A., Spoto, S., Angeletti, S. & Ciccozzi, M. (2020). The 2019-new coronavirus epidemic: Evidence for virus evolution. *Journal of Medical Virology*, *92*(4), 455–459. doi: 10.1002/jmv.25688.

Cash, R. A., & Narasimhan, V. (2000). Impediments to global surveillance of infectious diseases: Consequences of open reporting in a global economy. *Bulletin of the World Health Organization*, *78*(11), 1358–1367.

Chaplin, S. (2020). COVID-19: A brief history and treatments in development. *Prescriber*, *31*, 23–28. doi: 10.1002/psb.1843.

Cui, J., Li, F. & Shi, Z. (2019). Origin and evolution of pathogenic coronaviruses. *Nature Review Microbiology*, *17*, 181–192. doi: 10.1038/s41579-018-0118-9.

Dawood, F. S., Ricks, P., Njie, G. J., Daugherty, M., Davis, W., Fuller, J. A., Winstead, A., McCarron, M., Scott, L. C., Chen, D., Blain, A. E., Moolenaar, R., Li, C., Popoola, A., Jones, C., Anantharam, P., Olson, N., Marston, B. J. & Bennett, S. D. (2020). Observations of the global epidemiology of COVID-19 from the prepandemic period using web-based surveillance: A cross-sectional analysis. *The Lancet Infectious Diseases*, *S1473-3099*(20), 30581–30588. Advance online publication. doi: 10.1016/S1473-3099(20)30581-8.

Dryhurst, S., Schneider, C. R., Kerr, J., Freeman, A. L. J., Recchia, G., van der Bles, A. M., Spiegelhalter, D. & van der Linden, S. (2020). Risk perceptions of COVID-19 around the world. *Journal of Risk Research*, 23:7–8, 994–100. doi: 10.1080/13669877.2020.1758193.

Dubin, M. (1995). The league of nations health organisation. In P. Weindling (Ed.), *International Health Organisations and Movements, 1918–1939* (pp. 56-80). Cambridge Studies in the History of Medicine. Cambridge: Cambridge University Press. doi: 10.1017/CBO9780511599606.006.

Eaton, L. (2021). Covid-19: WHO warns against "vaccine nationalism" or face further virus mutations. *BMJ*, *372*, n292. doi: 10.1136/bmj.n292.

Eysenbach, G. (2002). Infodemiology: The epidemiology of (mis)information. *American Journal Medicine*, *113*(9), 763–765. doi: 10.1016/s0002-9343(02)01473-0.

Eysenbach, G. (2011). Infodemiology and infoveillance tracking online health information and cyberbehavior for public health. *American Journal of Preventive Medicine*, *40*(5, Suppl, 2), S154–S158.

Freeman, D., Waite, F., Rosebrock, L., Petit, A., Causier, C., East, A., Jenner, L., Teale, A. L., Carr, L., Mulhall, S., Bold, E. & Lambe, S. (2020). Coronavirus conspiracy beliefs, mistrust, and compliance with government guidelines in England. *Psychological Medicine*, 1–13. Advance online publication. doi: 10.1017/S0033291720001890.

Gwerder, L. J., Beaton, R. & Daniell, W. (2001). Bioterrorism. Implications for the occupational and environmental health nurse. *American Association of Occupational Health Nurses Journal*, *49*(11), 512–518.

Harding, A. (2020). Coronavirus in South Africa: Scientists explore surprise theory for low death rate. www.bbc.com/news/amp/world-africa-53998374?__twitter_impression=true&s=04&fbclid=IwAR2rsbqGvZNijEV6Qwcj-Ou12LG-lQ8y_XSrsgnzEXQ9oOaKVAi5gCFASOI. Accessed on September 4, 2020.

Hashem, A. M., Alghamdi, B. S., Algaissi, A. A., Alshehri, F. S., Bukhari, A., Alfaleh, M. A. & Memish, Z. A. (2020). Therapeutic use of chloroquine and hydroxychloroquine in COVID-19 and other viral infections: A narrative review. *Travel Medicine and Infectious Disease*, *35*, 101735. doi: 10.1016/j.tmaid.2020.101735.

Inglesby, T. V., Dennis, D. T., Henderson, D. A., Bartlett, J. G., Ascher, M. S., Eitzen, E., Fine, A. D., Friedlander, A. M., Hauer, J., Koerner, J. F., Layton, M., McDade, J., Osterholm, M. T., O'Toole, T., Parker, G., Perl, T. M., Russell, P. K., Schoch-Spana, M. & Tonat, K. (2000). Plague as a biological weapon: Medical and public health management. Working Group on Civilian Biodefense. *JAMA*, *283*(17), 2281–2290.

Kynge, J., & Hancock. T. (2020). Coronavirus: The cost of China's public health cover-up. www.ft.com/content/fa83463a-4737-11ea-aeb3-955839e06441. Accessed September, 23, 2020.

Larson H. J. (2020). Blocking information on COVID-19 can fuel the spread of misinformation. *Nature*, *580*(7803), 306. doi: 10.1038/d41586-020-00920-w.

Li, X., Wang, Y., Agostinis, P., Rabson, A., Melino, G., Carafoli, E., Shi, Y. & Sun, E. (2020). Is hydroxychloroquine beneficial for COVID-19 patients? *Cell Death & Disease*, *11*(7), 512. doi: 10.1038/s41419-020-2721-8.

Livingston, E., & Bucher, K. (2020). Coronavirus disease 2019 (COVID-19) in Italy. *JAMA*, *323*(14), 1335. doi:10.1001/jama.2020.4344.

Lu, H., Stratton, C. W. & Tang, Y. (2020). Outbreak of pneumonia of unknown etiology in Wuhan, China: The mystery and the miracle. *Journal Medical Virology*, *92*, 401–402.

Mamelund, S. (2017). Influenza, historical. In *International Encyclopedia of Public Health* (pp. 247–257, 2nd ed.). Amsterdam: Elsevier. doi: 10.1016/B978-0-12-803678-5.00232-0.

Mirzaie, A., Halaji, M., Dehkor, F. S., Ranjbar, R. & Noorbazargan, H. (2020). A narrative literature review on traditional medicine options for treatment of coronavirus disease 2019 (COVID-19). *Complementary Therapy in Clinical Practice*, *40* (101214): 1–8. doi: 10.1016/j.ctcp.2020.101214.

Morens, D. M., Breman, J. G., Calisher, C.H., Doherty, P.C., Hahn, B.H., Keusch, G. T., Kramer, L. D., LeDuc, J. W., Monath, T. P. & Taubenberger, J. K. (2020). The origin of COVID-19 and why it matters. *American Journal of Tropical Medicine and Hygiene*, 103(3): 955–959.

The Nuclear Threat Initiative (NTI) (2015). The biological threats. www.nti.org/learn/biological/. Accessed on September 9, 2020.

Oluwasegun, J. M. (2015). Managing epidemic: The British approach to 1918–1919 influenza in Lagos. *Journal of Asian and African Studies*, *52*(4):412–424. doi: 10.1177/0021909615587367.

Pan American Health Organization (PAHO) (2020). Understanding the infodemic and misinformation in the fight against COVID-19– Factsheet 5. https://iris.paho.org/bitstream/handle/10665.2/52052/Factsheet-infodemic_eng.pdf?sequence=14. Accessed on September 7, 2020.

Park, H. W., Park, S. & Chong, M. (2020). Conversations and medical news frames on Twitter: Infodemiological study on COVID-19 in South Korea. *Journal of Medical Internet Research*, *22*(5), e18897. doi: 10.2196/18897.

Paul, A., Sikdar, D., Hossain, M. M., Amin, M. R., Deeba, F., Mahanta, J., Jabed, M. A., Islam, M. M., Noon, S. J., & Nath, T. K. (2020). Knowledge, attitudes, and practices toward the novel coronavirus among Bangladeshis: Implications for mitigation measures. *PloS One*, *15*(9), e0238492. https://doi.org/10.1371/journal.pone.0238492.

Pennisi, M., Lanza, G., Falzone, L., Fisicaro, F., Ferri, R. & Bella, R. (2020). SARS-CoV-2 and the nervous system: From clinical features to molecular mechanisms. *International Journal of Molecular Sciences*, *21*, 5475.

Philips, H. (2014). Influenza pandemic (Africa). https://encyclopedia.1914-1918-online.net/article/influenza_pandemic_africa. Accessed on September 1, 2010.

Rickard, L. N. (2019). Pragmatic and (or) constitutive? On the foundations of contemporary risk communication research. *Risk Analysis*, *41*(3), 466–479. doi: 10.1111/risa.13415.

Riedel, S. (2004). Biological warfare and bioterrorism: A historical review. *Proceedings (Baylor University. Medical Center)*, *17*(4), 400–406.

Sohrabi, C., Alsafi, Z., O'Neill, N., Khan, M., Kerwan, A., Al-Jabir, A., Iosifidis, C. & Agha, R. (2020). World Health Organization declares global emergency: A review of the 2019 novel coronavirus (COVID-19). *International Journal of Surgery*, *76*, 71–76.

Stecula, D., Pickup, M. & van der Linden, C (2020). Who believes in COVID-19 conspiracies and why it matters? https://policyoptions.irpp.org/magazines/july-2020/who-believes-in-covid-19-conspiracies-and-why-it-matters/. Accessed on September 8, 2020.

Stephens, M. (2020). A geospatial infodemic: Mapping twitter conspiracy theories of COVID-19. *Dialogues in Human Geography*, *10*(2) 276–281. doi: 10.1177/2043820620935683.

Stern, A. M., Cetron, M. S. & Markel, H. (2010). The 1918–1919 influenza pandemic in the United States: Lessons learned and challenges exposed. *Public Health Reports*, *125*(Suppl 3), 6–8. doi: 10.1177/00333549101250S303.

Sturtevant, J. L., Anema, A. & Brownstein, J. S. (2007). The new International Health Regulations: Considerations for global public health surveillance. *Disaster Medicine and Public Health Preparedness*, *1*(2), 117–121. doi: 10.1097/DMP.0b013e318159cbae.

Taubenberger, J. K., & Morens, D. M. (2006). 1918 Influenza: The mother of all pandemics. *Emerging Infectious Diseases*, *12*(1), 15–22. doi: 10.3201/eid1201.050979

Taylor, L. H., Latham, S. M. & Woolhouse, M. E. (2001). Risk factors for disease emergence. *Philosophical Transactions of the Royal Society of London: Biological Science*, *356*(1411), 983–989.

UNAIDS [The Joint United Nations Program on HIV/AIDS]. (2021). *Global HIV/AIDS Ststistics—Fact Sheet*. Geneva: UNAIDS.

Wesolowski, A., Buckee, C. O., Engø-Monsen, K. & Metcalf, C. J. E. (2016). Connecting mobility to infectious diseases: The promise and limits of mobile phone data. *The Journal of Infectious Diseases*, *214*(4), S414–S420. doi: 10.1093/infdis/jiw273.

White, N. J., Watson, J. A., Hoglund, R. M., Chan, X. H. S., Cheah, P. Y. & Tarning, J. (2020). COVID-19 prevention and treatment: A critical analysis of chloroquine and hydroxychloroquine clinical pharmacology. *PLoS Medicine*, *17*(9), e1003252. doi: 10.1371/journal.pmed.1003252.

World Economic Forum (WEF) (2020). The COVID-19 pandemic has changed education forever. This is how. www.weforum.org/agenda/2020/04/coronavirus-education-global-covid19-online-digital -learning/. Accessed on September 16, 2020.

World Health Organization (WHO) (2014). Statement on the 1st meeting of the IHR Emergency Committee on the 2014 Ebola outbreak in West Africa. www.who.int/mediacentre/news/statements /2014/ebola-20140808/en/. Accessed on September 20, 2020.

WHO (2016). *International Health Regulation (2005)* (3rd ed.). Geneva: WHO.

WHO (2020a). COVID-19 cases top 10 000 in Africa. www.afro.who.int/news/covid-19-cases-top-10 -000-africa#:~:text=Reaching%20the%20continent%20through%20travellers,countries%20have %20reported%20cases. Accessed September 2, 2020.

WHO (2020b). Statement on the second meeting of the International Health Regulations (2005) emergency committee regarding the outbreak of novel coronavirus (2019-nCoV). www.who.int/news -room/detail/30-01-2020-statement-on-the-second-meeting-of-the-international-health-regulations- (2005)-emergency-committee-regarding-the-outbreak-of-novel-coronavirus-(2019-ncov). Accessed on September 1, 2020.

WHO-AFR [World Health Organization African Region] (2021) The Coronavirus Disease 2019 (COVID-19) Strategic Preparedness and Response Plan for the WHO African Region 1 February 2021 – 31 January 2022 (Update of 16 April 2021). Available at www.afro.who.int/sites/default/files/2021-04 /WHO%20AFR%20Covid-19%202021%20SRP_Final_16042021.pdf. Accessed on September 24, 2021.

Worldometers (2020). Coronavirus pandemic update. Reported cases and deaths by country, territory, or conveyance. www.worldometers.info/coronavirus/. Accessed on September 2, 2020.

Wright, R. (2020). How Iran became a new epicenter of the coronavirus outbreak. *The New Yorker*. www.newyorker.com/news/our-columnists/how-iran-became-a-new-epicenter-of-the-coronavirus -outbreak. Accessed on September 2, 2020.

Yaya, S., Otu, A. & Labonté, R. (2020). Globalisation in the time of COVID-19: Repositioning Africa to meet the immediate and remote challenges. *Global Health*, *16*, 51. doi: 10.1186/s12992-020-00581-4.

Zarocostas J. (2019). Ebola outbreak declared a PHEIC, world waits for next steps. *Lancet*, *394*(10195), 287–288. doi: 10.1016/S0140-6736(19)31712-X.

Zeraatkar, K., & Ahmadi, M. (2018). Trends of infodemiology studies: A scoping review. *Health Information and Libraries Journal*, *35*(2), 91–120. doi: 10.1111/hir.12216.

Zhou, P., Yang, X. L., Wang, X. G., Hu, B., Zhang, L., Zhang, W., Si, H. R., Zhu, Y., Li, B., Huang, C. L., Chen, H. D., Chen, J., Luo, Y., Guo, H., Jiang, R. D., Liu, M. Q., Chen, Y., Shen, X. R., Wang, X., Zheng, X. S., Zhao, K., Chen, Q., Deng, F., Liu, L., Yan, B., Zhan, F., Wang, Y., Xiao, G. & Shi, Z. L. (2020). A pneumonia outbreak associated with a new coronavirus of probable bat origin. *Nature*, *579*(7798), 270–273. doi: 10.1038/s41586-020-2012-7.

8 Global Health Politics and Diplomacy

8.1 Introduction

The global world must contend with the forces of globalization, and how it is shaping realities, including the epidemiology of health risks, risk factors, politics and policies of healthcare. The previous chapters examined how globalization is shaping the epidemiology of noncommunicable diseases (see Chapter 5) and infectious diseases (see Chapter 6). This chapter will examine the politics of global health or global disease control. While "politicking" should not overshadow the responsibility of healthcare provision, the reality is different because of particular profound interests in the face of limited resources and the need for priority setting. Most countries of the Global South are middle- or low-income countries. The inadequate income or level of development shows in all sectors, including healthcare infrastructure and disease burden. As previously noted, risk accumulates at the bottom of society, where, unfortunately, there is less capacity to deal with it. The Global South accounts for up to 70% of disease burden of both infections and noncommunicable diseases (WHO, 2018). The fundamental tragedy is, however, the inadequate capacity to reverse the trend. This is not to deny some improvement in health indicators in the last few decades, but it is good to acknowledge that there is still a lot to be done to improve health indicators further.

Since the argument is about global health or the realization that there are global forces shaping health realities, global collaboration is the pathway to ensure universal health coverage and reduce disease burden. Collaboration is about "give and take". Health politics is about what every nation is prepared to give, expect and implement toward the realization of key health goals. What nations need to give is not externally defined, but rather internally, to ensure health security within the country. The politics of healthcare starts internally: National policies, priorities and budgeting commensurate to the state of health of the country. Nations can expect to receive both material and non-material support, in the form of aid and policy guidelines or directions, respectively. Most policies must be tailored to domestic health needs and priority areas. Other critical areas are the sources of the policies and the level of involvement in drafting those policies and targets. It is often the criticisms that most policies are handed down without adequate consultations, thereby often serving only the interests of the powerful.

The critical issue is that globalization can be an un-equalizing process (see Giddens, 2002). As previously argued, the core nations (highly industrialized nations) (see Section 4.4.1) often decide the direction of events at the expense of the semi- and peripheral nations. Global politics is about the protection of interests, which is at the core of every global action. Interests are the dominant driver of the "policies" in global politics or international relations. In some instances, there are conflicting interests that set the regions apart. For instance, there have been contestations that most, if not all, conditionalities of grant or aid often contradict the initial interest of humanitarianism (if at all, it is disbursed on true humanitarian or altruistic grounds).

DOI: 10.4324/9781003247975-8

Sometimes, it is described as petting and robbing at the same time, a zero-sum argument about why humanitarian aid that flows from the North has not yielded much dividends in the South. Many countries of the South point accusing fingers in the direction of risk manufacturing from the Global North, which affects the health situation in the South. The bases of some policies, in particular neoliberal ones, are also controversial. Sometimes, it is a matter of blame-the-victims, that the South (i.e., the victim) is not doing enough to utilize available opportunities (despite constraints). Irrespective of the situation, the global circle is a hub of players with distinct interests and goals primarily meant to maximize benefits and avoid harm. The next few sections will examine critical issues in global health politics focusing on the division between the North and the South.

8.2 The What Is and Why of Politics in Global Health

Politics is embedded in most human activities, and global health action is no exception. One dimension of the macro aspects of politics is the division between the North and the South. Global health is a domain of power relations. McInnes et al. (2019) observed that global health politics is intimately concerned with power in at least two dimensions. First, power is unevenly distributed among and exercised by global health actors (or agents), but it is also embedded within global health structures. Second Within the global health networks, actors or agents, including national and global bodies, usually have specific (global health) interests, irrespective of the ultimate goal of achieving universal healthcare. Unfortunately, the power structure is not balanced; high-income countries have some "veto" power or a considerable advantage to influence the course of action. For the LMICs, the strategy is often to realign with powerful blocs in realizing some of their interests. McInnes et al. (2019) further noted that the interests and roles of global actors are within the so-called global health architecture, which is shaped by their relative power. The structures influence (both positively and negatively) the exercise of that power. The power structure is about rules (norms, regulations and ethics) and resources (both material and non-material) necessary to pursue a course of action. Global health action requires enormous resources, including financial, human capital and technologies, among others.

Beyond the global health diplomacy, which shape global health politics, there are many other critical issues relevant to the North–South divide. Despite diplomacy, the globalization of risks and vulnerabilities (see Section 2.3.1) is a major concern. Just as the world is socially, politically and economically connected, so it is also health-wise. There is a bi-directional flow of risk from North to South. Globalization comes with unprecedented manufacturing and distribution of modern risks—the uncertainties and consequences of modernity. Beyond the connectivity in terms of risk which has been examined in several aspects of this book, it is essential to briefly examine three issues in the context of global health politics before addressing the factors in global health diplomacy: Differential concern and priorities, differential capacity and resources, trickle-down science and weak health governance and political will.

8.2.1 Differential Concerns and Priorities

Population health (of different regions) is interlinked, but there are differential concerns and priorities across the regions. One of the major concerns of the Global South is that of medical exploitation, something often downplayed by the North (Kim et al., 2017). Kim et al. (2017) observed that modern medicine developed as a direct consequence of Western imperialism. The authors use the example of tropical diseases, which led to the development of tropical medicine as a part of the colonial agenda. The significant consequence of colonial medicine was the dislocation of indigenous medicine, leading ultimately to dependency. The neo-colonial trend continues with the South's dependence on health resources from the North. There have been some moves to develop indigenous medicine to cater to the needs of local populations who regularly rely on it, but modern medicine is still the mainstay of the healthcare system in global health (Amzat and Razum, 2018b). While a pharmaceutical breakthrough can hold some promise to resolve specific health problems, it also signifies medical dependence and the medical race to develop new drugs. The introduction of a malaria vaccine also means that nations must mobilize resources to make sure that all children under five years old are covered. In most countries of sub-Saharan Africa (SSA), the race to expand antiretroviral (ARV) treatment continues, with several people who need it yet to be covered.

The differences concerning the disease burden lead to some sophisticated politicking, which is shaping the state of global health. As will later be examined concerning global health security, the primary concern of the Global North is about the possible threat of infectious disease. This informs the over-emphasis on infectious diseases such as the human immunodeficiency virus (HIV), tuberculosis (TB), malaria, Ebola, Zika and severe acute respiratory syndrome (SARS). The concern and strategic power define what should be priority health goals, which affects the allocation of resources. In most interventions, the local concern might even be downplayed. Kim et al. (2017) observed that many of the US-funded Phase III clinical trials in the Global South were for allergic rhinitis and overactive bladder, which are not major local concerns. The most critical priorities in many parts of the Global South are: How to address the social determinants of health, especially poverty and other correlates of living conditions, which are generally poor.

The problem of agenda setting is still paramount in global health (see Section 7.3). Who are the actors responsible for setting the agenda and the solution? What interests do they protect? At whose expense? Do those actors consider global health inequalities? The imbalance of power explains the dissipating voice of the Global South in global health agenda setting such as SDG 3 and other prioritizations. It is not surprising that some diseases branded as neglected tropical diseases (NTDs) are most prevalent among the impoverished populations of the world. Even though the WHO is concerned about NTD-related morbidity and mortality, there is a grossly inadequate financial investment to address NTDs. Global health apartheid prevails, i.e., a focus on the dominant group (concerning health goals and allocation of resources) at the expense of the less-powerful group. Aginam (2019) observed that the prevalence of NTDs in low-income countries had perpetuated global health apartheid because about 90% of the global research and development (R&D) budget is devoted to the diseases of 10% of the world's population in high-income countries (of the North). The relative power in favor of the North permits the 10/90 gap in health-related R&D. The result is that several diseases of the relatively low-income regions will continue to be neglected (Aginam, 2019). For example, sleeping sickness (trypanosomiasis), Chagas disease or leishmaniasis continue to account for thousands of deaths annually, but still not prioritized in R&D as the neglected tropical diseases. Aginam (2019) also accused the global pharmaceuticals of prioritizing profit maximization as the primary motivation behind R&D. The differential interests, although inevitable, are responsible for the complexity of global politics. Global health politics should be humanitarian and altruistic—this will ensure more true collaboration and a reduction in the global disease burden.

8.2.2 Differential Capacity and Resources

The capacity and resources to pursue a specific course of action to achieve health goals also differ by country. Most countries in the Global South are described as low- or middle-income countries because they suffer from relatively inadequate capacity and resources. Globalization has further intensified the inequalities between the haves and have-nots. People in high-income countries are getting healthier, while others are confronted with poor health indicators. Kim et al. (2017) noted that the Global South is confronted with poor infrastructure, inadequate human resources for health and poor funding. Health interventions, including health research and development, require enormous resources that are frequently unavailable in many countries of the Global South. In many communities, there are no health facilities. Where they are available, the health workforce and equipment are grossly inadequate.

Health workers are continually migrating to high-income countries in search of better pay and work environment. There is a significant flow of health personnel from South East Asia to countries in Economic Co-operation and Development (OECD) countries (Tangcharoensathien et al., 2017; Yeates and Pillinger, 2018), which has further reduced the capacity of those Asian countries. This health workforce migration partly explains the reduced capacity in the Global South. Other complex issues must be considered in health workforce migration, including the right to movement, personal gains of migrants and some financial benefits (remittances) to home countries, among others, which make the control of such migration difficult (Buchan, 2015). What is not controversial, however, is that such migration exacerbates the challenges of a shortage of health workers in numerous countries of the Global South. Capacity is not only in terms of human resources, but it is also about technical know-how, including science, research and development.

8.2.3 Global Health and Trickle-Down Science

Beyond setting the agenda, the knowledge industry is the wellspring from which flow the solutions to the fundamental health problems confronting the world. However, the problems skew to the South, while the knowledge solutions skew to the North. "Science" or knowledge production becomes part of the politics of global health because of the fundamental questions regarding the flow of knowledge concerning major health problems. Reidpath and Allotey (2019) raise fundamental questions regarding this "trickle-down science" from the North to the South that is used to explain fundamental gaps in the science of global health. Trickle-down science is the "ideology" that the intellectual gravitas be concentrated in the Global North to produce the best science, then letting the methods, theories and insights trickle down to the Global South (Reidpath and Allotey, 2019).

Reidpath and Allotey (2019) made three fundamental points regarding trickle-down science. First, the ideology of western scientific medicine flows to the South, and in return, some of the few trained health workers find their way to the North. The health workforce migration further jeopardizes the health condition in a region already suffering from a shortage of a health workforce. There is a constant flow of nurses from the South to the North in search of better opportunities and higher income. Second, the North controls scientific research, and most medical institutions are oriented toward terminologies and problems defined by the West. Hence, most scientists from the Global South also end up focusing on the western agenda. For many health workers and researchers, a return to the South is often not desirable because of the poor work environment, including inadequate equipment and other supportive tools. Third, the North is less interested in the development of science in the South, resulting in science not being tailored to the needs of the South. Therefore, the knowledge-base or science that should drive valuable solutions is still grossly inadequate in the South. In general, the politics of science favors the North at the expense of the South.

The major institutes and journals of Global South studies are situated in the Global North. Therefore, the core experts on Global South studies are also in the Global North. The significant consequences of trickle-down science are glaring: Poor distribution of expertise and scientific capacity (Reidpath and Allotey, 2019). Therefore, it is challenging to raise adequate experts who would *un-neglect* the NTDs and tackle other disease conditions. The imbalance in knowledge production promotes a Northern gaze on Southern problems. However, the implementation of best practices needs to consider the context, adaptability and sustainability. Home-grown or glocalized solutions will define the future of healthcare interventions in the Global South.

8.2.4 Weak Health Governance and Political Will

One of the most pressing problems of the Global South is weak health governance and political will. Most global actors, including national actors, know an extensive amount about the health situation of the Global South. Some public policies and workable interventions do exist. However, in the face of weak political will, even the best solution becomes ineffectual. Best practices and policies are poorly pursued, and the government might not make use of the best opportunities available. The inadequate resolve to collectively influence the global health agenda is the first reflection of weak political will. The voice of the Global South within the global health network is often weak as well. This is partly why policy directions appear to be imposed; there is a need for the actors from the Global South to take more proactive steps and strategies to influence policy directions in ways that would be more beneficial to the region.

The meager available resources in the South need to be effectively utilized for better outcomes. Healthcare is not an optional need. Governments need to commit more resources and efforts to achieve better health outcomes. Some of the areas of need include balancing the distribution of health services between the rural and urban areas, improving the working condition of health workers, and providing more public health education, among others. Ensuring adequate healthcare is a major responsibility or obligation of a State. Taking such responsibility is a significant way of contributing to global health. There must be a fair distribution of concrete responsibilities regarding global health, and nations must be held accountable for fulfilling them. Barugahare and Lie (2015) observed that within global health circles, there must be a strong motive to achieve equity in global health financing. Therefore, all nations, especially those from the Global South, must meet their obligations to improve global health equity through intensified financial commitment with their budget allocations. Barugahare and Lie (2015) further observed that governments from the Global South should be required to allocate a satisfactory minimum percentage of their annual domestic budget resources to health, before receiving any external supplements. Barugahare and Lie (2016) noted that the inability of various countries to provide a certain threshold of healthcare reflects global distributive injustice due to a lack of political will to specify and enforce such obligations. Therefore, minimum obligations should be specified and enforced in the name of global health and distributive justice without infringing on national sovereignty.

8.3 Framing the Global Health Agenda

The first job of politics is about priority setting. What constitutes a global health problem that should be tackled? What resources should be allocated, and how would the resources be mobilized? Which government or organizations earmark what amount of resources and why? What are the global forces or interests that frame the global health agenda? In light of meager resources in every quarter, framing and setting the agenda is imperative to care for the most pressing health needs on a global scale. Health policies, like any other policies, exist within a frame; hence, global health policy should exist within a global frame. The frame is, however, a pool of interests, concerns, goals and processes, organized by different actors. Koon et al. (2016) described frames as "labels to describe a variety of ideas, packaged as values, social problems, metaphors or arguments", which aid priority setting. Koon et al. further observed that frames are sometimes ideological orientations and policy positions which guide global actions or collaboration. It is thus essential to note that the global health agenda is embedded within ideologies and interests, sometimes at the expense of other players. The global stage is a domain of power relations, and these unequal relationships are reflected in the global agenda. The frame, underlying context and interest should always be considered in the policy process since it affects the entire process and outcomes (Koon et al., 2016).

Additionally, frame signifies the structure and agency in the policy process—or in practical terms, the evolution (including the guiding principles) and implementation of policies. For instance, the concerns of each group would signify how health events are addressed. The concerns include the propensity of health risk, the organization of the healthcare system and the extent of involvement in global collaboration as prioritized within local politics. Therefore, Koon et al. (2016) noted that the context of health policy is embedded in highly charged ideological positions on numerous health matters. While the standard value that should frame the global health policy is the improvement of population health in general, every health goal is value-laden. Who or what defines a particular health goal? What is the set target, and for whom and how would it be achieved? Moreover, as previously mentioned, what resources are available and from where should one pursue a definite course of action toward the goal? So many questions surround the context of global health policy direction; the policy environment is rife with (political and economic) conflicts of interest.

Smith and Shiffman (2016) conducted a study on how the global health agenda is framed. Their primary argument was that contextual norms and expectations affect global health priorities. Using the case of maternal and newborn survival as a typical example, the authors observed that maternal health has a higher priority than newborn survival. They cited that the number of neonate mortality is six-fold the rate of maternal mortality, but the latter is more prioritized. For example, the main SDG health goals regarding newborn and maternal health are to reduce neonatal, under-five and maternal mortality to at least 12/1,000, 25/1,000 and 70/100,000 live births, respectively, by 2030. The authors noted that several factors accounted for the target setting, including favorable norms and concerned actors. It is reported that maternal and child health (MCH) has, for several years, made the issue of the newborn a secondary one after maternal health. The concern from various quarters, including scientific and ethical discourses, account for how health targets or policies are framed and financed. The principal argument is that political formulations and alignments are made to set a particular agenda irrespective of epidemiological concerns. The problem must be understood as requiring political action. The understanding, from some ideational lenses, is meant to attract attention and guide future action. The challenge is how to convey the problem epidemiology, severity, amenability to intervention and harm to at-risk individuals as a prerequisite for getting the required attention (Smith and Shiffman, 2016). The researchers further advanced that the first primary task is to mobilize coalitions (of donors, politicians, policy-makers, scientists and advocates) to engage in collective action against specific health challenges. Without such a coalition, a health problem might be neglected or under-prioritized.

The primary concerns as a result of ideological interests are the fundamental frames that shape global health policies. The starting point is the differential distribution of diseases leading to differential concerns. The particular interest here is more than just health; it concerns the global divide and unequal distribution of multiple factors occasioned by globalization, which affect health. As mentioned in previous chapters, the prevalence of both infectious and noncommunicable diseases are higher in the Global South. There are multiple factors to consider—risk, burden and resources, which are all unequally distributed. Moreover, the voices within the global health community are also unequally heard. Also, the commitment to specific policies or targets, significantly shaped by preferences and interests, is unequal. Smith and Shiffman

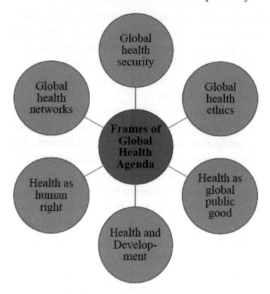

Figure 8.1 Factors in the diplomatic/political framing of global health agenda

(2016: p. 88) summarized that the divergence in global health priorities is "attributable to the differential in (1) network strategies and strength; (2) the construction and resonance of issue frames; and (3) alignment with strong and favorable norms". Concerning the divide (North/South), there are also differential concerns and policy frames shaping global health policies, some of which will be examined. Figure 8.1 shows factors in the diplomatic/political framing of global health agenda.

8.3.1 Global Health Security

The WHO (2019a) defines global health security as "the activities required to minimize the danger and impact of acute public health events that endanger the collective health of populations living across geographical regions and international boundaries". The condition of health in one place could have pandemic potentials (i.e., to spread to other places), especially in the case of infectious diseases (such as Zika, Ebola and Coronavirus diseases discussed in Chapters 6 and 7). In the case of noncommunicable diseases, the (manufactured) risk factors are also global (see Section 1.4.1.1). The typical instances are seen in the global burden of risk factors such as tobacco use, alcohol, diet and physical inactivity—all of which accumulate as a result of influences that transcend boundaries. Since the burden of infectious diseases is higher in the Global South, most countries in the North are concerned about the importation of infectious diseases. This concern becomes problematic when it translates to stigmatization and discriminatory practices. For instance, there are still some embassies demanding a medical certificate before granting visas to citizens of countries in the South. This would make it necessary for individuals with a migration-wish (from the Global South) to undergo mandatory screening for some diseases before being allowed to travel.

The primary concern in global health security is often on the threats of infectious diseases (Armstrong-Mensah and Ndiaye, 2018). Therefore, efforts are geared toward how to resist the spread from the "infested" region. This is a significant bias in the global health agenda occasioned by the frame of focusing on the region that is most vulnerable to infectious diseases.

The concern also assumes that the threat of diseases is uni-directional. The 2014–2015 Ebola outbreak has been the primary reference point in the framing of global health security. The death of thousands of people could have been prevented with adequate global preparedness. Previous outbreaks informed the promulgation of the International Health Regulation (IHR). Beyond infectious diseases, global health security is also concerned with human health in conflict situations, use of chemical or biological weapons and protection of (global) mass gatherings such as sports, festivals and religious migrations (WHO, 2019a). Global health security also incorporates issues or events concerning conflicts and wars, which often lead to deterioration of human conditions, including the destruction of infrastructures, increased epidemics and mortality.

WHO (2019a) observed that the duty of maintaining safety still rests on individual member countries, but that network organizations (including WHO) can provide support (where and when necessary) to help all countries fulfill their duty of safety and care for their citizens. The IHR, preceded by the International Sanitary Regulations of 1951, came into force in 1969, then revised in 1973, 1981 and lastly, 2005 to address the increasing global health threats and the need to respond with more effective surveillance and control practices (Baker and Forsyth, 2007; WHO, 2016). The collaboration requires that outbreak notification is sent to WHO following specific regulations. The IHR introduces a new instrument of the Public Health Emergency of International Concern (PHEIC) with guidelines on how such an emergency could be declared (Baker and Forsyth, 2007; WHO, 2016). The expectation is that, due to globalization and its aftermath, active collaboration is required to support greater global health security for all and build a safer future for humanity.

Furthermore, several nations and international organizations also launched the Global Health Security Agenda (GHSA) in 2014 to accelerate compliance with the WHO's International Health Regulations (Armstrong-Mensah and Ndiaye, 2018). The GHSA is designed to offer a robust collaborative approach to responding to any threat of (both human and animal) infectious diseases. Like the IHR, the GHSA agenda also covers other concerns, including biosafety and biosecurity, immunization, antimicrobial resistance, emergency coordination, medical countermeasures and deployment, among others.

8.3.2 Health and Development

The state of development of a nation is reflected in the state of health, and vice-versa. One of the underlying concerns is about how to ensure human progress in terms of overall development indicators; health is one of such significant indicators. It is only a healthy population that would drive the development agenda of a nation. Even when development is measured in terms of economic indicators, the healthy population drives the process. Health is instrumental to human functioning and is measured in terms of contributions to productive activities. As previously observed (see Chapter 1), diseases create vacuums in society. For instance, the death of a family breadwinner could mean that the children would be raised under challenging circumstances, which might prevent them from flourishing or achieving their life aspirations. Since the 18th century, there has been a causal relationship between economic development and the success recorded in the fight against morbidity and mortality, in both North and South (Thuilliez and Berthélemy, 2014). Improved health will always benefit development through an increase in productivity, and subsequently, the capacity to generate income. Most development efforts are directed toward helping poor and low-income nations to meet basic human needs (such as food and shelter). Health is a critical objective of development. Significantly, socio-economic development also leads to improvements in health sectors; as society advances, health institutions become stronger and responsive to health needs (Thuilliez and Berthélemy, 2014). Therefore, a nation should approach a development agenda as a way to increase individual and national productivity, not merely as a welfare services program (Grosse and Harkavy, 1980). Improvement in economic and social conditions will lead to an improvement in population health. Such improvement will rebound at national and global levels.

Beyond health matters, a low level of development has been correlated with security issues (human security in general), including terrorism and various conflicts/wars. The geography of conflict and war aligns with the conclusion that the level of development is related to civil unrest, terrorism and wars. There is also the expansion of global terrorism from the Eastern Mediterranean to other parts of the world in terms of operations and causalities. For instance, the *Boko Haram* terrorists in Nigeria claimed affiliation with the Islamic State (ISIS). Terrorism is a global security threat accounting for thousands of deaths and disabilities. For instance, up to 10,900 terror attacks and 26,445 deaths occurred in 2017, mostly in Iraq, Syria, Afghanistan, India and Nigeria (in the Global South) (Roser et al., 2019). Apart from actual causalities and other consequences (such as population displacement and homelessness), there are the hidden causalities concerning terrorism-related fear (including psychological, social and physical), and the opportunity costs (alternative development investments) of substantial security investment are inestimable. Globalization has latently aided the spread of terrorism and related consequences, thereby constituting a significant development challenge (including global health security).

In SSA, a substantial workforce has been lost to HIV (and various other diseases), leading to an emergency in various sectors due to a shortage of human resources. Impliedly, development cannot be achieved without an effective healthcare sector and appropriate threat control; a typical development agenda must consider investing in the health sector. For this reason, health issues have always appeared in the global development agendas, such as MDGs and SDGs. The development approach to global health policy directs the attention of development aid to vulnerable regions in terms of development needs. The critical areas of needs are often visible in the Global South as prioritized, most times, by the powerful development partners. While the significant burden of development also lies with individual nations, supportive aid should only be a catalyst; over-reliance on foreign aid could keep a nation perpetually poor unless it harnesses and mobilizes internal efforts to lift its citizens out of poverty.

The formation of a development agenda is a significant way of framing the global health agenda by setting health goals. Most development efforts will consider global health needs or priorities (Labonté and Gagnon, 2010). Priority is also accorded to infectious diseases because of their epidemic nature and rapid cause of casualties. Labonté and Gagnon (2010) observed that noncommunicable diseases are not as highly prioritized as infectious diseases in aid and development discourse, and are absent from the MDGs. The argument advanced is that noncommunicable diseases pose less risk to global (transborder) health security than do infectious diseases. Early detection and control would save many lives across national boundaries when epidemics are controlled before constituting global health emergencies. Based on these arguments, Malaria, HIV and tuberculosis (TB) are prioritized on the global health agenda. For global health security, international development agencies or partners often adopt a development approach, which is also a kind of modernization approach to global health policy. The approach is about the transformation from a traditional and agrarian society to a more industrialized and secular state. A few development partners considerably invest in improving the social determinants of health and social amenities (including water supply and education, among others). There have also been concerns about how to reduce global poverty, which is a development challenge. The aid flow to fighting poverty, and its consequent success, will also help to improve population health. Health signifies an investment in human capital, and therefore has an important place in the development agenda (Thuilliez and Berthélemy, 2014). Invariably, the health implications of development are crucial; hence, health is a significant priority in the global development agenda. Moreover, such prioritization is a vital frame shaping the global health agenda.

8.3.3 Health as Global Public Good

There are various necessary goods and services. While human needs are infinite, some needs are more urgent than others, i.e., required for survival. There are basic needs that constitute part of a human welfare package, ideally, but not necessarily, provided by the government. In sociology, there are imperative needs, not only at the societal level but also at the level of individuals, which must be fulfilled to ensure continued existence or survival. Health is one such need/good. Hazelkorn and Gibson (2019) discussed education extensively as a public good and related policy context. Healthcare is also relevant concerning the attributes of public goods that Hazelkorn and Gibson (2019) discussed, even though their focus was on higher education. The central premise of defining public good is that it should be non-excludable and non-rivalrous. The implication is that, as much as possible or in a strict sense, such goods should be all-inclusive in terms of coverage. The essence of this discussion is not to fall into the debate of whether health should or should not be a public good, but how the concept of health as a public good has shaped global health agendas or politics.

The provision and coverage of public goods have been the basis of the development index. Public goods are imperative because they translate to public benefits or values supporting human living conditions and, consequently, overall national development. The preceding subsection examined the relevance of health to development. It is through an inclusive development approach that population health can be improved. In the global context, health is a global public good with sustained global coloration to alleviate the adverse consequences of risk. Just as Hazelkorn and Gibson (2019) observed that the concept of public good has helped to reposition education policies to extinguish barriers as much as possible, so is it with the health sector. Perhaps, such conception forms the basis of "Health for All" or universal healthcare as the primary policy context of most nations. Therefore, there are endless questions regarding access to healthcare, including public health expenditures and policies.

Furthermore, the concept of health as a public good also fuels the humanitarian drive in global health, with the provision of technical know-how and related support to vulnerable regions, especially during infectious epidemics. One may argue that protecting others during infectious epidemics is purely humanitarian since it is also self-protection because of the possibility of global spread. However, just as the overall returns from education accrue not solely to the individual but the nations and, subsequently, the globe, so too can improved health status at the individual level ultimately benefit the larger society. For example, one case of TB is not only an individual problem, but it is ultimately a public problem or a social problem. One case of polio is not just a problem to the individual; it evokes a global response and signals that polio still exists as a global threat. The more the drive toward a humanitarian or global good concept, the more investment and interest in global health.

Perhaps, the "public" in public health should be replaced with "global"; health should be a global good or global public good because of social interconnectivity and the social boomerang of adverse effects of ill-health. Health helps in the production and reproduction of global goods and potential equity effects. It creates opportunities and social benefits. Lastly, it helps to reduce global inequalities. While the ripple effects of infection have been stressed, the condition of good health is incalculable. Referring to health as a global good raises a challenge about how to provide the resources (material, non-material and collaboration) required to sustain global health. The conception of health as a global good, however, remains a major ambition or vision, shaping policy drives and national actions. The argument of global public good tends to the massification of healthcare (used herein as): The massive extension of coverage of healthcare and elimination of barriers on a global scale with a consideration of the shared (social, political, economic) space, benefits and value. One profound implication not previously mentioned is that the world must also collaborate to ensure or protect other global public goods (such as peace and a healthy climate) that are requisites for good health. There should also be adherence to regulatory principles and policies concerning trade in products (such as tobacco and alcohol) that could adversely affect health as a global public good (Labonté and Gagnon, 2010).

8.3.4 Health and Human Rights

Human rights have evolved as a core value in human society. A previous section examined the globalization of health rights (see Section 2.3.8), which is also related to the arguments in this section. The human rights-based approach is dominant in healthcare and constitutes a significant frame, shaping the global health agenda. The human rights principle is often applied to healthcare to ensure universal coverage. As previously observed, the right to health is one of the fundamental human rights as enshrined in the WHO constitution. The significant advantage of this recognition of health as a right is the creation of legal obligations by the state to ensure adequate healthcare for all. It encourages states to view the provision of healthcare as a part of their duties, on which their performance can be assessed. Beyond the national level, the recognition of such rights in the constitution of global bodies also makes healthcare a global right. Human rights issues transcend boundaries—they are global issues. Any infraction on rights in one state is a global concern. Apart from the WHO, the right to health is also recognized in various international treaties including the Universal Declaration of Human Rights (UDHR), Article 25, the International Covenant on Economic, Social and Cultural Rights (Article 12), The African Charter on Human and People's Rights (Article 16), Organization of American States (OAS) as well as some national constitutions. Up to 70% of constitutions worldwide entrench health-related guarantees, and about 40% of constitutions include a justifiable right to health (Lamprea, 2017).

The right to health means that everyone has the right to the highest attainable standard of living adequate for health, which includes access to all health services and information, sanitation, balanced food, decent housing, good working conditions and a clean environment. The notion of the right to health includes the consideration of the determinants of health. Healthcare cannot be considered in isolation of human needs and conditions that would ensure quality health for all. Every government should provide human welfare and amenities that would support the attainment of health. It is also vital that the principles underlying human rights are applied in the understanding of the right to health. Such principles include equality and non-discrimination, the dignity of the human person, rights as a public good, public participation, entitlement and obligations and interdependence of rights, among others (see Amzat and Razum, 2018a). For instance, equality and non-discrimination imply that there should not be any form of bias in terms of personal attributes (such as gender, ethnicity, income and education) in the provision of healthcare. The principle of non-discrimination signifies that there should not be exclusion or inclusion criteria in healthcare. The principle also requires states to redress any discriminatory law, practice or policy.

The rights-based approach has led to a significant outcome described as judicialization—the right to seek redress or enforcement of the right to health in case of (perceived) injustice in the provision or access to healthcare. Lamprea (2017) described the judicialization of healthcare as the use of legal actions and rights-based injunctions to obtain medical treatments and pharmaceuticals. There have been some lawsuits seeking redress concerning discrimination in health systems and the allocation of scarce health resources in the countries of the Global

South. Lamprea (2017) observed that the emergence of health rights litigation in the 1990s and early 2000s, or what is described as a litigation epidemic, was bolstered by the increased burden of HIV/AIDS and by rights revolutions in South Africa and several Latin American countries (including Argentina, Brazil, Colombia and Costa Rica). Beyond country levels, the rights-based consideration has been applied to advocating for access to healthcare among undocumented migrants. Since the principle is non-discrimination, migration status should not determine access to healthcare. Also, and perhaps more importantly, global health signifies collective destiny, as the health of undocumented migrants would affect (documented) residents. Therefore, the legal or rights-based conception has significantly shaped the politics of global healthcare.

8.3.5 Global Health Networks

The memberships of global bodies or networks have also helped to shape global health policies and agendas. Such networks include both formal and informal institutions that help to shape the policy agenda of a country, provide support and monitor the progress of members. Shiffman (2017) described global health networks as webs of individuals and organizations with shared concerns for a specific condition. The number of such organizations is growing locally and globally. The networks help to define global health priorities based on specific interests. Shiffman (2017) noted that an effective organization could be highly influential in projecting particular health challenges as priorities. A reliable and effective network will facilitate the attention and allocation of resources. In every situation, there are competing interests and issues; thus, the first aspect of politics is framing the problem to become a significant priority. The power play within such organizations determines the flow of action. Most countries of the Global North have a stronger voice to project their priorities because such countries make more financial contributions to the fight against various diseases in different global networks.

Magnusson (2019) noted that the burden of NCDs was downplayed in various global health agendas, including the MDGs, thereby excluding them from priority funding areas. Perhaps, the priority is about health security from the purview of the North or to "rollback" infectious diseases. The "rollback" idea is most evident in Roll Back Malaria, with an emphasis on control rather than elimination; the biggest ambition was to "achieve malaria control across Africa by the year 2030" not the elimination of malaria (Feachem, 2018). In the beginning, the global bodies were aware that elimination was and is possible—so far, the malaria map continues to shrink, but the disease is still a major problem in SSA. The control efforts continue with the launch of a malaria vaccine in April 2019, meant to be used as a complementary malaria control tool (WHO, 2019b). In contrast (to malaria control efforts), HIV control receives considerably better attention. Magnusson (2019) observed that HIV/AIDS receives much attention because it has been framed as a public health, development, humanitarian and security crisis with profound consequences for the global community.

The global health network directs or influences national action mostly by presenting a pathway for collaboration required to achieve target health goals. Magnusson (2019) presented a framework for analyzing how global action in health may influence national actions (see Table 8.1). While Magnusson was referring specifically to noncommunicable diseases, the pathways generally present ways in which global networks help to frame a global health agenda. These pathways include the development of normative and legal instruments, including policy guidance; political accountability mechanisms by global institutions; the provision of economic and material support for implementation programs by globally significant donors; and capacity-building. The UN General Assembly, World Health Assembly (WHA) and other international non-governmental organizations (INGOs) set most targets, indicators

Table 8.1 How global health actions influence national action

Pathway	Global Actions, Activities, Processes	Intended Impact at National Level
Normative and legal instruments	Adoption of treaties, conventions Resolutions of international organizations (WHA, UNGA) Normative international instruments ("soft law"), including global strategies and action plans, recommendations, guidelines.	Legal and normative pressure for domestic policy change; better understanding of the case for policy action; better knowledge about policy options and policy priorities.
Political account ability mechanisms	Goals, targets, indicators, timelines, especially when supplemented by periodic reporting requirements (to the UN GA, WHA, etc.). Partnerships between key actors, including UN agencies, governments, private funders, INGOs. Accountability mechanisms used by civil society organizations (e.g., indexes, shadow reports).	Greater political commitment and pressure on national governments to implement effective policies Improved capacity for policy action at national level.
Economic support and incentives	Development assistance in health: Provision of direct economic and material support. Funding conditionalities.	Material resources for programs and initiatives Economic pressure for policy actions at national level.
Capacity-building	Coordination of training, mentoring and capacity building; sharing good practices and facilitating access to information.	Greater capacity for implementation of recommended policies and law.
Less formal path ways	Advocacy by champions in civil society and private sector. Popular movements in civil society Media campaigns mobilizing popular opinion.	Normative pressure for global and national policy change.

Source: Magnusson, R. (2019).

and timelines, which member countries then adopt as their control efforts. The previous MDGs (2000–2015) and SDGs (2016–2030) are typical illustrations of how global networks influence national action. There are WHO declarations (e.g., Control of NCDs 2013–2020, Ending Childhood Obesity, Physical Activity 2018–2030), INGOs (e.g., Save the Children, ActionAid, ChristianAid International, Bill and Melinda Gates Foundation, The Global Fund, CARE International, Comic Relief, Doctors without Borders and GAVI) and government agencies (USAID and DFID) shaping global health action.

The global health networks evoke global health actions with the aim of improving global population health. The networks involve the participation of and contribution from all stakeholders to monitor, respond, prevent and mitigate the global health crisis. Shiffman (2017) noted that four central problems are facing global health networks, including problem definition, positioning, coalition building and governance. Both problem identification and positioning have to do with agenda-setting and attracting critical attention and promulgation of solutions. Coalition building and governance relate to the formation and intensification of alliances at local, national and global levels to own and pursue the promulgated solutions. In most instances, countries sign into various conventions and declarations and then institute how to domesticate and facilitate the implementation to achieve the set goal. The major criticism is that such signatories are a significant way of bundling nations and agencies into some set agenda—sometimes ideological or political.

8.3.6 Global Health Ethics

The global health ethics movement is shaping the global health agenda. Ethics signifies the moral framework in the analysis of health and healthcare. Ethics is also a part of the global agenda involving moral obligations or responsibilities to ensure fairness and equity in addressing global health challenges. The WHO (2015: p. 10) defined health ethics with a broad focus, including

> ethical issues faced by health professionals, health policy-makers and health researchers, as well as by patients, families, and communities in a range of contexts related to health, including clinical care, health services and systems, public health, epidemiology, information technology and the use of animals in research.

Ethics is enmeshed in health-related perplexity concerning justice or equity in research, as well as preventive and curative activities. It is also concerned about the epidemiology of risk, service delivery and health governance. Global health ethics has emerged to focus on ethical concerns or issues that transcend national boundaries. Stapleton et al. (2014) defined global health ethics as the

> process of applying moral value to health issues that are typically characterized by a global level effect or require action coordinated at a global level … Global health ethics takes a predominantly geographic approach and may infer that the subject relates primarily to macro-level health phenomena,

but also with the consideration of micro effects. Codes of ethics moderated by some principles (such as autonomy, beneficence, non-maleficence, solidarity, distributive justice, liberty, egalitarianism, public good) govern ethical concerns at the global level.

In addition, Goldberg and Patz (2015) observed that global health ethics should imply that the health of anyone is linked to the health of all the rest. The health, illness or death of someone anywhere should be a concern to all of humanity. It is "One Health" in a very global sense. For instance, global health ethics should be defined by true partnerships and equity between the North and South, rather than as top-down or paternalistic modes which have characterized the fields of international health and tropical medicine (Myser, 2015). The ideals of global health ethics should be on how to resolve global inequalities and inequities in health-related matters within the global circle. The valid concern about humanity and the realization of the interconnectedness of various regions will project desirable global practice that would serve all. The true concern will demonstrate the importance of multisectoral and collaborative activities to share reflections and best practices on a global scale. It is important to note that bioethics in general, and health ethics in particular, is comprehensive and ambitious because it tends to raise ethical issues through moral reasoning about all aspects of health. The ambitious concerns have facilitated global health politics through the framing of health challenges and ethical principles of global concern.

The field of global health ethics is fast emerging because of the realization that there are ethical perplexities that are better addressed at the global level. The moral conundrum transcends boundaries relating to many areas: Health inequalities; health spending; distribution or allo-cation of global funding; prioritization of health challenges within global health networks; participation in global health research (who participates and where), including pharmaceutical trials; global innovations in research; global preventive or control activities, including access to vaccinations, access to information and quality of services; environmental health and cli-mate; global determinants of health; and nature of health partnerships and global governance, among others. With all the aforementioned concerns in mind, and admitting to the unequal vulnerabilities, global health ethics is one platform of bridging the gap between the North and South.

8.4 Summary

- The world must contend with the forces of globalization and how it is shaping reali-ties, including the epidemiology of health risks, risk factors, politics and policies of healthcare.
- This chapter examines the politics of health issues involved in the control of diseases or how to ensure functional health for all. There is intense "politicking" in healthcare because of profound interests in the face of limited resources and the need for priority setting.
- Global health is a domain of power relations: Power is distributed among and exercised by global health actors, but it is also embedded within global health structures. The global health networks and actors (including national and global bodies) are usually identified with specific interests irrespective of the ultimate goal of achieving universal healthcare.
- Global collaboration is the pathway to ensure universal health coverage and reduce dis-ease burden. Collaboration is about "give and take". Health politics is about what every nation is prepared to give, expect and implement toward the realization of key health goals. Irrespective of the situation, the global circle is a hub of players with distinct interests and goals primarily meant to maximize benefits and avoid harm.
- The differential disease burden often leads to some sophisticated politicking, which is shaping the state of global health. The concern and strategic power of a region define what should be priority health goals, which affects the allocation of resources.
- Global health apartheid prevails, i.e., a focus on the dominant group (concerning health goals and allocation of resources) at the expense of the less powerful group—about 90% of the global research and development (R&D) budget is devoted to the diseases of 10% of the world's population in high-income countries (of the North). The relative power in favor of the North permits the 10/90 gap in health-related R&D.
- There is a definite context of global health politics, including differential capacity and resources and trickle-down science. For instance, health interventions, including health research and development, require enormous resources rarely available in many countries of the Global South. The knowledge base or science that should drive valuable solutions is still grossly inadequate in the South. The imbalance in knowledge production promotes a Northern gaze on Southern problems.
- There are fundamental frames, a pool of interests, concerns, goals and processes, which influence global health agenda setting, including global health security, health as global public good, health as development, global health rights and ethics.
- Global health politics and ethics should be about true partnerships and equity between the North and South, rather than as top-down or paternalistic modes. The valid concern about humanity and the realization of the interconnectedness of various regions will project desirable global health practice that would serve all.

Critical Thinking Questions

- Why do you think global health is a domain of politics and politicking? It is possible to avoid politics for a more humanitarian stance?
- Should global health interventions be framed and executed as a public good? What factors could limit such framing?
- How are the differential concerns/priorities a significant impediment in the attainment of global health goals?
- Can political interest be separated in health prioritization among various governments? Which of political interest or health priority should prevail in global health, and why?
- There are always fundamental equity concerns in global health politics. In what ways is the Global South disadvantaged in global health politics?
- Assess the critical provisions of the International Health Regulations (IHR) as a tool in global health politics.

Suggested Readings

- Koon, A. D., Hawkins, B. and Mayhew, S. H. (2016). Framing and the health policy process: A scoping review. *Health Policy and Planning, 31*(6), 801–816, https://doi.org/10.1093/heapol/czv128. This is a comprehensive review about framing of health politics, the embedded interests and priorities.
- Labonté, R., and Gagnon, M. L. (2010). Framing health and foreign policy: Lessons for global health diplomacy. *Globalization and Health, 6*, 14, DOI: https://doi.org/10.1186/1744-8603-6-14. This article identifies and discusses six policy frames of global health diplomacy with global health equity concerns.
- Cohen, I. G. (2013). *The globalization of health care: Legal and ethical issues.* Oxford: Oxford University Press. The book discusses the legal and ethical analysis of the impacts of globalization on health.
- Brown, G. W., Yamey, G. and Wamala, S. (Eds.) (2014). *The handbook of global health policy.* Sussex: Wiley Blackwell. The book is very good in understanding the politics of global health cooperation, politics and policies.
- Youde, J. (2020). *Globalization and Health.* Maryland: Rowman and Littlefield Publishers. This book examines the various political dimensions of the intersections between globalization and health.
- Kay, A., and Williams, O. (Eds.) (2009). Global Health Governance: Crisis, institutions and political economy. London: Palgrave Macmillan. The various chapters discuss the challenges to global health governance and the contradictory and ineffective responses to them.
- Birn, A., Pillay, Y. and Holtz, T. H. (2017). *Textbook of Global Health* (4th Edition). Oxford: Oxford University Press. An introductory book that draws from political economy considerations at community, national, and transnational levels to discuss global health and its politics.

References

Aginam, O. (2019). Global politics of neglected tropical diseases. In McInnes, C., Lee, K. & Youde, J. (Eds.), *The Oxford Handbook of Global Health Policy.* Oxford: Oxford University Press.

Amzat, J., & Razum, O. (2018a). The right to health in Africa. In *Towards a Sociology of Health Discourse in Africa.* Springer International Publishing. doi: 10.1007/978-3-319-61672-8_2.

Amzat, J., & Razum, O. (2018b). Traditional medicine in Africa. In *Towards a Sociology of Health Discourse in Africa*. Springer International Publishing. doi: 10.1007/978-3-319-61672-8_6.

Armstrong-Mensah, E., & Ndiaye, S. M. (2018). Global health security agenda implementation: A case for community engagement. *Health Security*, *16*(4), 217-223. doi: 10.1089/hs.2017.0097.

Baker, M. G., & Forsyth, A. M. (2007). The new International Health Regulations: A revolutionary change in global health security. *The New Zealand Medical Journal*, *14*;*120*(1267), U2872.

Barugahare, J., & Lie, R. K. (2015). Obligations of low-income countries in ensuring equity in global health financing. *BMC Medical Ethics*, *8*(16), 59. doi: 10.1186/s12910-015-0055-3.

Barugahare, J., & Lie, R. K. (2016). Understanding the futility of countries' obligations for health rights: realising justice for the global poor. *BMC International Health and Human Rights*, *16*(1), 15. doi: 10.1186/s12914-016-0090-2.

Buchan, J. (2015). Health worker migration in context. In Kuhlmann E., Blank, R. H., Bourgeault, I. L., & Wendt, C. (Eds.), *The Palgrave International Handbook of Healthcare Policy and Governance*. London: Palgrave Macmillan.

Feachem, R. (2018). Roll back malaria: A historical footnote. *Malaria Journal*, *17*. doi: 10.1186/s12936-018-2582-0

Goldberg, T. L., & Patz, J. A. (2015). The need for global health ethics. *The Lancet*, *386*(10007), PE37–PE39. doi: 10.1016/S0140-6736(15)60757-7.

Giddens, A. (2002). *Runaway World: How Globalization is Shaping the World*. Profile Books.

Grosse R. N., & Harkavy, O. (1980). The role of health in development. *Social Science and Medicine*, *14*(2), 165–169.

Hazelkorn, E., & Gibson, A. (2019). Public goods and public policy: What is public good, and who and what decides? *Higher Education*, *78*(2), 257–271. doi: 10.1007/s10734-018-0341-3.

Kim, J. U., Oleribe, O., Njie, R. & Taylor-Robinson, S. D. (2017). A time for new north-south relationships in global health. *International Journal of General Medicine*, *10*, 401–408. doi:10.2147/IJGM.S146475.

Koon, A. D., Hawkins, B. & Mayhew, S. H. (2016). Framing and the health policy process: A scoping review. *Health Policy and Planning*, *31*(6), 801–816. doi: 10.1093/heapol/czv128.

Labonté, R., & Gagnon, M. L. (2010). Framing health and foreign policy: lessons for global health diplomacy. *Globalization and Health*, *6*, 14. doi: 10.1186/1744-8603-6-14.

Lamprea, E. (2017). The judicialization of health care: A global south perspective. *Annual Review of Law and Social Science*, *13*(1), 431–449.

Magnusson, R. (2019). Noncommunicable diseases and global health politics. McInnes, C., Lee, K., & Youde, J. (Eds.), *The Oxford Handbook of Global Health Policy*. Oxford: Oxford University Press. doi: 10.1093/oxfordhb/9780190456818.013.35.

McInnes, C., Lee, K. & Youde, J. (2019). Global health politics: An introduction. In McInnes, C., Lee, K. & Youde, J. (Eds.), *The Oxford Handbook of Global Health Policy*. Oxford University Press.

Myser, C. (2015). Defining "Global Health Ethics". *Bioethical Inquiry*, *12*(5). Doi: 10.1007/s11673-015-9626-8.

Reidpath, D. D., & Allotey, P. (2019). The problem of 'trickle-down science' from the Global North to the Global South. *BMJ Global Health*, *4*(4), e001719. doi: 10.1136/bmjgh-2019-001719.

Roser, M., Nagdy, M. & Ritchie, H. (2019). Terrorism. Published online at *OurWorldInData.org*. Retrieved from: https://ourworldindata.org/terrorism [Online Resource].

Shiffman, J. (2017). Four challenges that global health networks face. *International Journal of Health Policy Management*, *6*(4), 183–189. doi: 10.15171/ijhpm.2017.14.

Smith, S. L., & Shiffman, J. (2016). Setting the global health agenda: The influence of advocates and ideas on political priority for maternal and newborn survival. *Social Science & Medicine*, *166*, 86–93. doi: 10.1016/j.socscimed.2016.08.013.

Stapleton, G., Schröder-Bäck, P., Laaser, U., Meershoek, A. & Popa, D. (2014). Global health ethics: An introduction to prominent theories and relevant topics. *Global Health Action*, *7*, 23569. doi: 10.3402/gha.v7.23569.

Tangcharoensathien, V., Travis, P., Tancarino, A. S., Sawaengdee, K., Chhoedon, Y., Hassan, S. & Pudpong, N. (2017). Managing in- and out-migration of health workforce in selected countries in South East Asia region. *International Journal of Health Policy and Management*, *7*(2), 137–143. doi: 10.15171/ijhpm.2017.49.

Thuilliez, J., & Berthélemy, J. (2014). Health and development: A circular causality. *Revue d'économie du Développement*, *22*(HS01), 109–137. doi: 10.3917/edd.hs01.0109.

World Health Organization (WHO) (2015). *Global Health Ethics: Key Issues*. Luxemburg: Global Network of WHO Collaborating Centres for Bioethics.

WHO (2016). *International Health Regulation (2005)* (3rd ed.). Geneva: WHO.

WHO (2018). Noncommunicable Diseases (NCD) Country profiles, 2018. www.afro.who.int/health-topics/noncommunicable-diseases. Accessed on August 20, 2019.

WHO (2019a). Health security. www.who.int/health-security/en/. Accessed on September 12, 2019.

WHO (2019b). Malaria vaccine pilot launched in Malawi. www.who.int/news-room/detail/23-04-2019-malaria-vaccine-pilot-launched-in-malawi. Accessed on September 14, 2019.

Yeates, N., & Pillinger, J. (2018). International healthcare worker migration in Asia Pacific: International policy responses. *Asian Pacific Viewpoint*, *59*(1), 92–106.

9 Globalization and Migrants' Health

A Global South Perspective

9.1 Introduction

Migration plays a significant role in the discussion of globalization and health because the flow of people is a substantial driver of globalization. Migration has been implicated in the emergence and spread of infectious diseases, including cholera, human immunodeficiency virus (HIV), and tuberculosis (TB), among others (see Chapter 6). It is a significant factor in the globalization of health risks and vulnerabilities of infectious diseases (see Sections 2.3.1 and 6.4.4). This chapter will examine migration as a determinant of health by looking at the dimensions of migration in the global era. Examining migration patterns caused by globalization can help us to understand how migration has become a public or global health issue and how it is responsible for the various health challenges. Migration is a form of historical human behavior or activity involving the movement of people from one location to another. One dimension of migration is the duration; it might be for a short time, a long time or permanent. Migration can be within a country; the most common form is rural–urban migration. The world is becoming more urbanized. As at 2015, the world urban population (54%) has slightly outgrown the rural population; if the trend continues, more than two-thirds of the world's population will reside in urban areas by 2050 (Ritchie, 2018). In most low-income countries, more people still live in rural areas; up to 60% of the African population live in rural areas (Ritchie, 2018). There are health consequences of the demographic shift of urbanization (see Section 6.4.2). Continuous urbanization puts pressure on urban infrastructures, which often aids in the transmission of infectious diseases (Neiderud, 2015).

Migration can also occur internationally, with the movement of people from one country to another. From the 1990s, there has been an increasing voluntary flow of people from the Global South to the Global North, with countless people still wishing to migrate. A survey in 31 countries, mostly in the Global South, indicated that three out of ten people wish to relocate permanently to another country, with the most preferred destinations including the USA, Germany, Canada, the UK, France and Australia (WEF, 2019). Saudi Arabia is the only state of the Global South in the top ten possible migrant destinations. While movement between the North and South is bi-directional, the wish for a long-term migration is higher in the South than in the North. In some countries of the South (including Sierra Leone, Haiti, Liberia, Congo [Kinshasa] and the Dominican Republic), up to half of the population wish to move to another country (WEF, 2019). In general, migration-wish is defined by the availability of food, work and safety, apart from other infrastructures. In most instances, there are push factors, conditions that instigate people to leave a place, and pull factors, conditions that attract individuals to other places.

Unequal levels of development between the North and South constitute the basis for the pull and push. Pull factors in the North often stem from media representation; the North is portrayed as the Eldorado or Gold Coast. Hence, migration becomes a wish or dream for many people

DOI: 10.4324/9781003247975-9

to gain access to the beauties of the North. The media representation of most countries in the South is usually opposite of the North, often portrayed as a place of minimal opportunities, including poverty and conflicts. The signals in such media representation cultivate migration-wish and eventual push, or sometimes desperation, to migrate out of certain quarters. In general, globalization, and particularly advancements in modern transportation, have eased the process of migration, leading to a cohort of people called migrants (local or international) in every city of the world. Migrants are often forced to live in difficult circumstances that are detrimental to health. The health of migrants is a significant discourse in global health since migration is a strong determinant of health (see Razum and Wenner, 2016; Wickramage et al., 2018; Legido-Quigley et al., 2019). Before discussing the nexus between migration and health, it is essential to consider the most worrisome dimension of migration that is of global health importance: Forced migration.

9.2 Forced Migration: A Global Health Issue

Forced migration or displacement or involuntary migration is a major tragedy of the modern world. Tragic circumstances often surround migration, including war, environmental disasters and trafficking. Gostin and Roberts (2015) described forced migration as the human face of a health crisis. They further observed that the situation is truly tragic because each stage of the forced migration journey is fraught with tremendous health risks. In the case of conflict, infrastructures are destroyed, leaving minimal access to essential amenities of life (such as water and sanitation).

Forced migration (sometimes called deracination) is the act of moving from one place to another due to events beyond an individual's control. Forced migration refers to the movements of refugees and internally displaced people by conflicts, natural or environmental disasters, chemical or nuclear disasters, famine or development projects (IOM, 2019). Unfortunately, many people have been forced to move due to unpleasant circumstances such as conflict, famine, development projects or persecution in their home countries. Zetter (2014, p. 21) observed that conflict and forced displacement might "erupt spontaneously from unpredictable and multiple triggers, leading to a state of radical uncertainty and high levels of livelihood vulnerability for those affected". Apart from tragedies, involuntary migrants also include people forced out of their homes because of deception or coercion. These two categories can be found within the Global South countries. Some categories of forced migration, will be described in the subsequent subsections.

9.2.1 Human Smuggling

The first type of involuntary migrant is one who is a victim of human smuggling. Migrant smuggling and trafficking (see Section 9.2.2) are different from each other, but they are both of global concern. The UN (2000) defined migrant smuggling as "a crime involving the procurement for financial or other material benefits of illegal entry of a person into a country of which that person is not a national or resident". Both migrant smuggling and trafficking occur in inhumane circumstances, often resulting in morbidity or mortality. In smuggling, an individual wants to use every means possible, including paying agents or smugglers, to enter another country without proper documentation. This is the case of several travelers from various African countries traveling (by road) through Libya to Europe daily. Many migrants from the Eastern Mediterranean (including Syria, Jordan and Yemen) also follow through Libya. Such migrants pay agents who arrange boats (usually overloaded) to travel across the "deadliest stretch of the Mediterranean Sea" (Sakuma, 2019). Shipwreck happens too frequently because of overloading, resulting in thousands of deaths every year. Sakuma (2019) observed that smuggling routes across the central Mediterranean Sea mark the deadliest point of all migration in Africa. The desert is a massive arena for human smuggling. Many migrants travel great distances, but Libya is the primary entry point to Europe. A smuggling business has been firmly established, whereby desperate migrants pay hundreds of US dollars to ride in a single boat not designed for extended sailing for an approximately 200-mile trip between Libya and Europe. Subsequently, the Mediterranean is now a vast unmarked grave to thousands of migrants who have capsized at sea (Sakuma, 2019). The desperation is a result of both the pull and push factors previously mentioned. The UNODC (2018b) estimated that around 2.5 million migrants are smuggled yearly for an economic return of up to US$5–7 billion.

Several migrants face serious risks, both from the journey and from potential trafficking or being sold or captured as slaves. Most parts of Libya are war-torn; thousands of Libyans have been displaced, and several migrants have been brought down in crossfire or captured for other purposes. Conditions inside Libya have deteriorated since the citizens' uprising against Gaddafi and the government's collapse in 2011. The NATO (North Atlantic Treaty Organization) incursion in Libya (in support of the anti-government movement) is a typical example of western amplification of crisis in the Global South, which has led to the protracted destruction of lives and properties. The incursion generated a severe humanitarian crisis of global concern (including a health crisis) beyond Libya. The development of several militia groups and the proliferation of arms have also aided insurgency and terrorism in other countries (see Pedde, 2017). A 2019 report documented that Libya's crisis has spurred terrorism in 13 different countries, including Nigeria, Burkina Faso, Niger, Algeria, Mali, Tunisia, Egypt, Syria, Italy, France, Germany, Belgium and the United Kingdom (Curtis, 2019). Armed conflict between various rivaling factions has engulfed Libya as they fight for legitimacy, thereby causing a massive displacement of thousands of Libyans who have been left without work or a place to call home. Thousands of non-Libyan migrants are used as pawns in the power struggle while thousands languish in overcrowded detention centers, experiencing torture and unsanitary conditions, among other human rights violations (Sakuma, 2019). Libya's migrant crisis is severely affecting the Eastern Mediterranean and extends deep into Europe.

Other parts of the Global South are experiencing similar situations, as there are thousands of individuals in Latin America and the Caribbean risking often deadly passage to the US or Canada through dangerous routes (see IOM, 2016; Greenfield et al., 2019), where smuggling, rape, extortion and kidnappings are not uncommon (IOM, 2016). Other crimes linked to migrant smuggling include human trafficking, identity fraud, corruption and money laundering. UNODC (2018b) observed that Asia and the Pacific Region are also experiencing the real costs of human smuggling in terms of considerable suffering and death of the smuggled migrants. The UN Agency reported the discovery of mass graves containing the bodies of migrants from Myanmar and Bangladesh in Southern Thailand. UNODC (2018b) noted that some countries in the Asia-Pacific Region simultaneously serve as a source, transit, and destination for smuggled migrants. Human smuggling constitutes a real global danger to the health of migrants in both transit and destination countries. Smuggled migrants are highly vulnerable to abuse or assaults, exploitation and trafficking.

9.2.2 *Human Trafficking*

The UN (2000) defined trafficking in persons as

> [T]he recruitment, transportation, transfer, harboring or receipt of persons, by means of the
> threat or use of force or other forms of coercion, of abduction, of fraud, of deception, of the

abuse of power or of a position of vulnerability or of the giving or receiving of payments or benefits to achieve the consent of a person having control over another person, for the purpose of exploitation.

In human smuggling, the individual pays to be smuggled, meaning that he/she consents to the action. In human trafficking, there is no consent, or "consent" is only obtained through deception and coercion. In this case, an individual is moved or smuggled without his/her consent. This is a gross violation of human rights and a major global health concern. Because a trafficked person is an individual who is coerced or tricked into situations in which their bodies or labor are exploited, which may occur across international borders or within their countries, trafficking is a form of abduction and exploitation of people to enslave them (Amzat and Magaji, 2019).

The UNODC (2018a) reported that there over 30 million trafficked persons and the dangerous trend might continue if there is no stiff control measure. Some primary origins of trafficked persons from the Global South include Mauretania, Uzbekistan, Haiti, Qatar, India, Pakistan, Congo (DR), Nigeria, South Africa and Sudan. Women and children constitute up to 49% and 30% victims of human trafficking, respectively, and more than 70% of trafficked women face sexual exploitation (including forced commercial sex work). Apart from sexual exploitation, other reasons for trafficking include forced labor, organ removal and child soldiers, among others (UNODC, 2018a). Although human trafficking is a global problem, the pattern of movement is usually from less developed countries in Africa, Asia and Latin America to more developed countries in Europe, North America and some developing countries (UNODC, 2018a). Individual countries may serve as origin, destination or transit, or a combination of all of these (Amzat and Magaji, 2019).

Human trafficking is a denigration or mortification of the human person. Sexual exploitation is a defilement of sexual health and rights and leads to vulnerability to all sorts of sexual infections, including HIV/AIDS. Within the context of coercion, protective sexual behavior might not be consistently practiced. Greenbaum and Stoklosa (2019) observed that trafficked persons often experience a multiple burden of health problems, including traumatic and physical injury from hazardous work, physical and sexual assault, sexually transmitted infections, "chronic untreated medical conditions, pregnancy and related complications, malnutrition, complications of substance use disorders, post-traumatic stress disorder, major depression, and suicidality". Unfortunately, due to the coercive context of the problem, most trafficked persons might not have access to healthcare, even when they require it. Survivors also require medical attention as part of rehabilitation from the mental, social and traumatic experiences.

9.2.3 *Refugees, Asylum Seekers and Internally Displaced Persons (IDPs)*

One category of migrants is refugees: Persons who have been displaced and have traveled across international boundaries. As of 2019, there are up to 25.9 million refugees worldwide, more than half of which are below the age of 18 (UNHCR, 2019a). Children are the worst hit by the global refugee crisis. While a majority of refugees live in a neighboring country, many of them travel a long distance for a more comfortable zone. For instance, there are numerous refugees from Syria seeking a place in Germany and other European countries. Up to 57% of global refugees flow from the three countries of Syria, South Sudan and Afghanistan (UNHCR, 2019a). These are all war-torn areas with collapsed infrastructures and poor health indicators. Without discrimination, refugees from war-torn areas, with the breakdown of public health measures (such as sanitation and water), often pose a public health threat in terms of communicable diseases, because such refugees are exposed to health risks throughout their survival migration.

Another category of migrants is asylum seekers. An asylum seeker is a person who applies for international protection from domestic persecution. The primary reason 3.5 million people seek asylum annually (UNHCR, 2019a) is persecution based on their ethnicity, religion, sexual orientation or identity, alleged witchcraft, or for their work or politics (including journalists, academics and activists). A further group of migrants is internally displaced persons (IDPs); nationals who are migrants within their own country, due to domestic crises. IDPs are a global concern in general and a global health concern in particular, albeit a more urgent concern for some countries of the Global South. There are three major categories of IDPs based on the causes of displacement: Conflict-, disaster- and development-induced displacement. Wars/conflict and violence due to religious and ethnopolitical conflicts are responsible for slightly more than half of the displacement, while the remaining IDPs are fleeing natural disasters, such as famine and floods in Africa (Owoaje et al., 2016), volcanic eruptions, wildfires and storms. As of the end of 2018, there were over 41 million people internally displaced worldwide. In the first half of 2019, about 10.8 million new IDPs were added (3.8 million due to conflict and 7 million due to disasters) (IDMC, 2019). The countries with a high burden of refugees and IDPs include Syria, Congo (DR), Somalia, Nigeria, Ethiopia, Afghanistan, Yemen, South Sudan, Sudan, Iraq and Colombia (IDMC, 2019). Each of these countries has slightly over 2 million IDPs, except Syria and Colombia, with over 5 million IDPs. Syria has been in civil war since 2011, while Colombia is facing an internal conflict since 1964.

Displacement is a global problem with severe health implications. The first major problem of displacement is the forceful removal from a comfort zone into a place devoid of the basic amenities of life. Displacement is marked by grossly inadequate access to shelter, sanitation, food and safe water. The deprivation of basic needs exposes displaced persons and refugees to health risks, including violence and diseases such as measles, diarrhea, malaria and acute respiratory infections (Connolly et al., 2004; Owoaje et al., 2016; UNHCR, 2019b). Owoaje et al. (2016) reported a range of additional health problems, including malnutrition in children (stunting and wasting) and adults, and mental health problems, especially post-traumatic stress disorder (range: 42%–54%) and depression (31%–67%). The more general problem is a diminished quality of life and less resistance to disease. IDPs are also susceptible to negative behavioral changes, including increased substance abuse, aggression and higher levels of sexual and domestic violence (UNHCR, 2019a).

The UNHCR (2019b) also reported several problems associated with sexual and reproductive health. Sexual violence increases as a result of displacement, in addition to the associated problems of forced and early pregnancies, unsafe abortions, obstructed labor, sterility, incontinence, vaginal fistulae and sexually transmitted infections (UNHCR, 2019b). The risks are exceptionally high because of the breakdown of public health measures (such as WASH). Refugees from most developing countries of Asia and Africa are characterized in their health profile by acute-onset severe malnutrition and outbreaks of infectious diseases (Burkle, 2006). Where there is humanitarian assistance, the delivery of services is often problematic in most instances due to on-going conflict or overwhelming disaster. Connolly et al. (2004) observed that service delivery mechanisms are often unreliable during crises due to loss of health staff, damaged infrastructures, insecurity and poor coordination.

A complex emergency requires more technical and sophisticated measures in terms of security and flow of aid materials. Lam et al. (2015) observed that population displacement is a significant threat to some global eradication programs of vaccine-preventable diseases because of the instability of the population and difficulty in reaching them promptly. Complex emergencies do not only affect those who migrate; persons left behind who are unable or unwilling to relocate, including the disabled, women, children and the elderly, may suffer from violence (Burkle, 2006). Civilians suffer most during conflict situations; only a few become refugees, while some remain stranded without alternatives (Burkle, 2006). Kang et al. (2019) observed that the displaced population often finds it challenging to navigate and negotiate health services. Other problems include language barriers and inadequate interpretation services, lack of awareness of the structure and lack of insurance, difficulty meeting the costs of services, and perceived discrimination relating to race, religion, and immigration status.

9.3 Migration–Health Nexus

The process of migration and the state of being a migrant have health implications. Many studies have examined health and migration to affirm that the health of migrants is an essential concern in public and global health (Razum and Wenner, 2016; Wickramage et al., 2018; Legido-Quigley et al., 2019). The concepts of "universal health" and "right to health" signify that every individual must be included in healthcare coverage, irrespective of their migration status and other personal attributes. The process of migration is complex, and the outcome often uncertain. The factors that push people out of a particular place are determinants of health, as are the factors that pull people to another location. Many people migrate to escape poverty without any assurance of aid at the host countries. Most people who migrate are healthy young adults who provide additional manpower to the host nations, mostly in the Global North, at the detriment of the countries of origin, most LMICs. The additional manpower includes the critical sectors such as education, healthcare and defense (see Section 10.3.2 on migration of health workers), but not all migrants are skilled labor who could easily fill a space in the destination countries. Therefore, the realities or experience of migration sometimes reflect some gaps between expectations and reality. The new setting (to which a migrant moves) might only provide a minimal improvement over their place of origin. The potential impacts of migration on health, in terms of health consequences and vulnerabilities, are essential issues that need researching. As previously mentioned, there are dangerous migration trends in the form of smuggling and trafficking for illicit purposes (including forced labor and sex), which are global health concerns. The next few subsections will examine some specific factors explaining the increased health vulnerability of migrants, including living and working conditions, particular health risks and lifestyle factors, and social integration and well-being (see Figure 9.1).

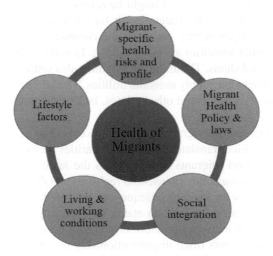

Figure 9.1 Factors determining the health of migrants

9.3.1 Migrant Living Conditions

Living conditions, including the living environment and available supportive amenities, constitute a major social determinant of health. Whether within local or international migration, the living conditions of migrants are often relatively poor. Most migrants live at the margins of the host societies. In internal migration, such as rural–urban migration, most migrants concentrate on the margins of the communities. Long ago, Park and Burgess (1925) observed that migrants are always in the concentration zone, where there is a minimal infrastructure to support decent living. Park and Burgess (1925) examined the growth of the city and developed the concentric ring model, which depicts urban land usage in concentric rings with migrants at the edge of the outer ring (described as the concentration or commuter zone). Even when migrants live in large cities, they tend to stay off the city center or the business zone, where they only visit for some job opportunities. Since Park and Burgess developed their model, many developments and changes have come to modern society. However, the fact remains that migrants are often segregated, even in high-income host countries. The disadvantaged groups, including migrants, often reside in particular districts or neighborhoods. The Peckham district in South London, England, for example, is home to more than 70% of people of African and Asian descent. There are several "Peckhams" around the world (in major cities); they begin as designated places for migrants, and may later be transformed into permanent residences.

Residential segregation of migrants is a feature in most countries. In the Global North, irregular, sometimes called undocumented, migration has become common. An irregular or undocumented migrant is one not entitled by law to enter or stay in another country but still stays or enters without valid legal requirements. Specifically, irregular migration breaches the legal condition of residence and movement of a particular country. Being irregular presents a significant challenge on its own because it signifies limited legal rights. Irregular migrants are mostly unwanted in the host communities and might risk prosecution or deportation, depending on the legal framework of the host country. For instance, legislation in Russia is very hostile toward undocumented migrants; migrants often face ethnoracial harassment, profiling, wage discrimination and other forms of maltreatment (including physical abuse) (Agadjanian et al., 2017; Vakulenko and Leukhin, 2017; HRW, 2019a). During former President Donald Trump's presidency (January 2017–January 2021), the USA instigated antagonistic regulations toward irregular migrants, including different forms of inhuman subjugation (Legido-Quigley et al., 2019). In terms of residential infrastructure for migrants, while it might be relatively good in high-income countries, in the Global South, where most of the states already have limited infrastructures, migrant quarters are generally poor. Migrants may dominate the commuter zone, slums and relatively cheap quarters, where essential amenities are often lacking. In many cities in the Global South, migrants live in the streets and slums. Thousands of migrants also settle in an informal settlement where local authorities might not supply essential utilities. The informal settlement is also characterized by high levels of violence and other crimes, lack of financial services and safety nets, poor sanitation and health services.

Razum and Wenner (2016) described the German immigration policy as exclusionist and observed differential access to social facilities, which translates to health disparities between the immigrants and non-immigrants. In China, most migrants cannot access the same local social welfare system as residents because of the *hukou* policy (household registration) (Zhang, 2017). Most migrants live in adverse conditions, with severe consequences to their health. Zhang noted that the results often manifest in disparities in health status between migrants and local residents. The influx of immigrants often increases pressure on existing resources, including housing. It has been observed that immigrants often disproportionately occupy the lowest-quality accommodation. Therefore, the underlying housing problems facing immigrants include homeownership, affordability, crowding and low housing quality (Schill et al., 1998). It is further observed that immigrants in the US—especially Puerto Ricans, Dominicans, Caribbeans, Africans and Latin Americans—are more likely to live in poorly maintained units (Schill et al., 1998).

Irregular migrants live in the shadows of society with limited legal rights, fear of arrest, prosecution and deportation. They are often denied fundamental rights and freedoms, and are disproportionately vulnerable to discrimination and marginalization (UN, 2014). The common assumption in most host communities is often to equate being irregular with being illegal. Such migrants are even regarded as criminals out to cheat the social security system or misuse the services of the country of destination without paying the required taxes (UN, 2014). The psychological trauma of being irregular is enormous. Therefore, there have been some movements to recognize the fundamental rights of all migrants (including the irregular or undocumented).

9.3.2 *Working Conditions*

One of the primary purposes of migration is to find better job opportunities. The movement of migrant workers between the North and South divide is often mutually beneficial, especially the movement of skilled workers. While the South often complains of a brain drain or a shortage of professionals, some countries in the North need to fill vacancies in critical sectors of their economies. The main concern in this subsection is not about the gains and losses from the movement of workers but how working condition is a significant factor in migrant health. Hargreaves et al. (2019) estimated that there are currently about 150 million international migrant workers (employed outside of their home countries). Relative to their non-migrant counterparts, migrant workers tend to work under more challenging conditions and unsafe environments. Irrespective of the level of safety equipment and measures provided, although grossly deficient in most cases, migrants work in hazardous and exploitative environments with considerable risk of injury and ill-health (Hargreaves et al., 2019). People migrate with high expectations of better jobs and income without first considering the rate of unemployment in the destination countries. For most migrants, the first significant challenge is how to get a job. Hence, many of them face inadequate or unstable incomes and risks associated with illness as a result of no or low incomes, and the inability to pay for healthcare.

A systematic review of the working condition of migrants in Europe and Canada show the poorer working conditions and occupational health compared to non-migrants (Sterud et al., 2018). The report found that work injuries, perceived bullying and discrimination and risks of physical or chemical hazards were consistently higher among immigrants than among native workers (Sterud et al., 2018). The study also reported more sick days or disability pensions among immigrants compared to residents. Sweileh (2018) reviewed documents from the year 2000 to 2017 on the conditions of migrant workers. The findings highlighted serious global health concerns, which might sometimes be under-reported because of potential adverse effects on the political and human rights reputation of various governments.

The flow of migrants is not only South to North; increasingly, migration occurs within the Global South. Some countries in the Global South host millions of migrant workers. For instance, a report found that nearly 22 million, or 84%, of all refugees and asylum seekers live in the low- and middle-income countries in Asia and Africa (Khattab and Mahmud, 2019). The ILO (2016) observed that the Arab States host up to 17.6 million migrant workers, representing 35.6% of all workers in the region and 1.7% of the global migrant worker population. The HRW (2019b) noted that Qatar has an exploitative labor system that accommodates forced labor and unfair conditions, such as low wages, excessive overtime, poor housing and grossly inadequate access to legal services. The existing *kafala* system in many Arab countries (including Bahrain,

Jordan, Kuwait, Lebanon, Oman, Saudi Arabia and the United Arab Emirates) undermines workers' rights and freedom by tying migrant workers' visas to their employer and severely restricting their ability to change employers (HRW, 2019b).

There are still migrant workers who live on work conditions that can best be described as modern slavery. Many of them face physical, psychological, sexual and other forms of abuse daily. Some workers are forced into commercial sex work and other menial jobs without safety equipment. For instance, the growing "maid trade" or domestic workers trade is becoming more lucrative; workers are commodified and sold, more or less, as slaves, and must endure low wages, exploitation and abuses from employers (see ILO, 2018). Worldwide, immigrants often find themselves employed in sectors that expose them to hazards or risks, putting them at increased risk of injury, morbidity and mortality. Despite these poor work conditions, there is little or ineffective regulation affirming the rights of migrant workers in several countries.

9.3.3 Migrant-Specific Health Risks and Lifestyle Factors

Health risks specific to migrants at various phases of their journey deserve a closer examination. The first phase is the pre-departure condition and context. The health profile of different nations shows the burden of both communicable and noncommunicable diseases. The health situation in the place of origin holds implications for the health profile of migrants. Zimmerman et al. (2011) observed that at the pre-departure phase, migrant health is influenced by personal characteristics, including genetics, environment and personal circumstances. Smuggled migrants and refugees face some pathetic circumstances as the journey itself is highly risky. Many migrants die in the Mediterranean Sea while attempting to cross to Europe. Also, because the journey is usually on irregular routes and can take several days, months or even years), substantial risks stem from inadequate access to social amenities and healthcare (during the journey. Irregular migrants often experience violence, including physical and sexual abuse along the route (see Section 8.2), apart from other traumatic experiences that may affect their well-being (Zimmerman et al., 2011).

Many migrants traveling through illegal routes suffer from diminished immunity as a result of inadequate basic needs (such as shortages of food and material for basic hygiene). Irregular migration is often a story of horrors and vulnerabilities for those that manage to cross over to the desired destination. The stopovers or interceptions in transit locations further exacerbate the vulnerabilities. According to Zimmerman et al. (2011), the transit sites are points where local pathogens could be carried from one place to another. Zimmerman et al. (2011) further explained that transition often involves vulnerability to local health and environmental conditions. For example, the malaria deaths of Burmese refugees fleeing through malaria-endemic areas, and Mexican migrants who die from heat exposure on treks across the desert toward the United States. The transition phase is also the time of exposure to criminal activity, including kidnapping and rape.

The lifestyle of migrant is often different in terms of risk behavior. The circumstances of migration, socio-political environment, and migration status determine several lifestyle issues that influence migrant health. Migration is a social correlate of sexually transmitted diseases (including HIV), because of the increased risk behavior among migrant population (Amzat, 2010; Abdulkader et al., 2015; Zhang et al., 2017). In most instances, migrants might be single or separated from their spouses. Abdulkader et al. (2015) reported that unprotected, recent non-spousal sex was common among male migrants, which could increase their HIV/AIDS vulnerability. Zhang et al. (2017) observed increased HIV vulnerability among Mexican migrants varies across migration phases (pre-departure, transit, destination, interception and return). The authors reported increased substance use before sex, unprotected sex and sex with casual partners and sex workers. The study concluded that sexual behaviors and risk vary significantly among migrants at different migration phases.

Although migration is a correlate of the risk of HIV transmission, migration does not equate to HIV vulnerability in absolute terms. Studies have documented that migration is selective toward healthy individuals, i.e., mainly healthy persons migrate (Vearey, 2012). In this case of the selective theory of migration and health, the receiving nations benefit immensely, and might even be the source of health risk to migrants. It is not only people living in poverty that migrate or wish to migrate; there is an increasing number of well-educated migrants, including doctors, lecturers and other professionals. For instance, forced migration as a result of natural disasters might not correlate to social standing; in fact, those from the upper- and middle-class wealth quantiles constitute early escapees from conflict or disaster regions. Therefore, it amounts to discrimination and stigmatization to assume that all migrants constitute health risks. In most cases, it is the discrimination and stigmatization manifesting in limited social acceptance and access to healthcare that even increase the vulnerability of migrants to specific disease conditions and social ills (see Fernandez, 1998).

In general, it is incontrovertible that lifestyle change is associated with migration; a migrant in a new social environment must acculturate to the new social space. For example, among those who move to the Global North, increased weight gain may result from the adoption of western diets. The extent of change is a function of individual socio-economic circumstances in the place of destination. Spadea et al. (2018) observed that unhealthy behaviors are exacerbated by the sense of loneliness and low levels of integration in the host country.

9.3.4 Social Integration and Well-Being

Another challenge that migrants often face is social integration. Most migrants face culture shock in destination countries, in addition to uncertainties, anxieties, social tensions and new, sometimes disorienting, encounters. A migrant is confronted with new beliefs and social etiquettes. Hence, one major challenge is to learn and unlearn specific social processes and decorum to fit into the new environment. Fox et al. (2017) observed that such acculturation is an essential construct in the analysis of health disparities in minority populations. The process of acculturation enables the internationalization of host cultural traits and orientations, which may minimize the initial stress and lead to the adoption of new lifestyles, which are also consequential for health. While acculturation might help to reduce discrimination in the long run, the relationship between acculturation and health is complex and multilevel. Fox et al. (2017) noted that acculturation influences patterns of minority health and disease risk.

Migrants experience a new set of health risks, behaviors and a new set of constraints and opportunities which are consequential for their health. The new place comes with new diets, health systems, environmental and social risks. While migrants need to be selective in social integration, hard choices must be made in all efforts toward social inclusion. Abraído-Lanza et al. (2016) studied the Latino immigrants in the US and observed that the relationship between acculturation and health exhibits a mixture of negative and positive consequences. Greater acculturation both improved and worsened some health indicators. The authors observed several risky health behaviors and outcomes associated with acculturation, including alcohol use, increased smoking, high Body Mass Index (BMI), decreased consumption of low-fat foods, but increased physical activity. Dahlan et al. (2019) observed that migration involves changes in health-related lifestyle often associated with noncommunicable diseases such as heart disease, diabetes and hypertension.

In terms of social conditions, migrants often experience reduced social support or capital and increased social isolation; for example, due to language barriers, which can worsen mental health. Abraído-Lanza et al. (2016) reported that differences in social networks or levels of support might explain differential health profiles between immigrants and non-migrants. More often than not, social network size shrinks significantly following migration, impacting social well-being. Most highly industrialized countries are more individualistic than middle- and low-income countries (in the Global South). The reduced social networks and encounters can have adverse consequences on health. Marginalization or isolation is often experienced when migrants struggle to maintain their original cultural identity by resisting host culture (Dahlan et al., 2019). In most instances, the higher the level of social integration (measured by adaption to the new culture including the length of stay, language proficiency and social networks), the better the health status and utilization of health services (Fassaert et al., 2009; Dahlan et al., 2019). There is a positive correlation between the level of social integration and the utilization of primary healthcare services, including improved timing of consultations for curative services.

Beyond the issue of the level of integration, another dimension is that being in a new place signifies the sharing of social space, which means increased social contacts. Migrants also contribute to the population health of a particular place, not only in terms of health data but also through mutual vulnerability and risks. Shared social space implies that new migrants could spread and acquire health risks. The possibility of mutual vulnerability is a primary global health justification for genuine attention to migrant health—both the host and migrant populations benefit.

9.3.5 Access to Healthcare

The particular circumstances of migration affect migrants' access to healthcare. Access to healthcare is the ease with which individuals can utilize healthcare services. Chiarenza et al. (2019) observed that barriers to access healthcare among migrants include legislative, financial, administrative, cultural and inadequate information. Migrants on the move are often unaware of the health system of the destination country. Out-of-pocket payment is still common in the Global South, while in the Global North, the reverse is the case. This is compounded by the fact that a majority of migrants might not have adequate funds to cover healthcare costs. The irregular migrants (mainly the smuggled or trafficked), for instance, might arrive at their destination without any means of livelihood. Also, because they are undocumented, they might not have access to funds to cover healthcare costs (see Chiarenza et al., 2019). In typical circumstances, migrants are at the lower cadre of the society. In some European countries (Cyprus, Greece, Sweden, etc.), emergency care requires payment, while in other countries (Spain, Germany, Demark and the UK), it is free. Where it is not free, and there is no ability to pay (the case for most migrants), increased morbidity and mortality are expected. Many countries of the Global North set some financial barriers, which a majority of the undocumented or irregular migrants might not be able to meet (O'Donnell, 2019). Poverty is a significant factor pushing most people out of their countries of origin; hence, for the majority, the capacity to cover healthcare costs is low. Such exclusionist policy questions the right to health and universal healthcare, which constitute global health justification to provide healthcare coverage to the migrants.

Cultural barriers also limit access to healthcare. One prominent aspect is the language barrier. Many people move without mastering the language of their destination country. Most refugees and smuggled migrants often face the difficulty of even communicating in the language of the destination country. While language problems can be eased through the use of interpreters, cultural mediation services are often inadequate, which often limits access to care

(Chiarenza et al., 2019; O'Donnell, 2019). There are also cultural sensitivities that should be considered. Understanding cultural sensitivities or ensuring cultural competence is problematic because of the diverse background of most migrants. Beyond the language and other cultural issues, a majority of migrants lack proper understating of the structure and organization of the new health system (O'Donnell, 2019). The required procedure of accessing a health facility differs from country to country; lack of understanding of such procedures might limit access to healthcare.

Another complicated issue is the lack of knowledge of the health profile of migrants. Migrants arrive at their destination country with a distinct health profile. In typical instances, migrants might be suffering from conditions not prevalent in the destination countries. Chiarenza et al. (2019) noted that immigrants are exposed to multiple health risks and often have different disease profiles than residents of the host population. Some of those health conditions might constitute emergencies, which sometimes require the immigrant to be quarantined. For instance, a total of 267 imported cases of *Plasmodium vivax* malaria from western Africa were reported in the Russian Federation from 1984–2017 (Baranova et al., 2019).

9.3.6 Governance and Migration Policy

Different legislations also regulate the health of migrants. The first legal issue is establishing the status of a migrant as either irregular, undocumented or regular. Normally, regular migrants are required to obtain health insurance coverage before departure from their country of origin. In most instances, a refugee status must be recognized in order to access certain health services. The WHO (2018) reported that the recognition of the legal status is the crucial factor determining access among refugees. On the other hand, for labor migrants, access to healthcare is determined by both legal status (whether irregular or not) and official employment status. The WHO has often encouraged nations to provide healthcare as a fundamental right without any form of discrimination. In this sense, migration status should not be a yardstick in accessing healthcare. The principle of universal healthcare implies that migrants should also be comprehensively covered. Unfortunately, even where there are some entitlements to healthcare, most migrants are unaware of these (WHO, 2018).

As previously mentioned, many countries of the Global South also accommodate migrants and refugees. For instance, South Africa is home to an estimated four million migrants, including a high percentage that are irregular migrants from neighboring countries in search of greener pastures (SAHRC, 2018). The initial public/global health challenge is minimizing the hostility toward migrants in South Africa. While mild hostility is an everyday issue, deadly xenophobic attacks on African migrants to South Africa have occurred in recent years (Mabera, 2017; Amusan and Mchunu, 2017). Beyond physical attacks, there are also policy discriminations against migrants. For instance, the South African Immigration Act does not explicitly recognize the right to health of migrants (SAHRC, 2018). Consequently, migrants are systematically exempted from some public services (including healthcare). In most circumstances, migrants live in a highly vulnerable situation as a result of legal or systematic exclusion from the public health system (SAHRC, 2018). The South African Constitution recognizes the right to health for its citizens but fails to admit that the non-inclusion of migrants, irrespective of their status, is a violation of internationally recognized efforts toward universal healthcare coverage.

China's internal migrant population is now massive; up to 245 million in 2017 (see NHCPRC, 2017). Internal migrants, frequently from rural to urban areas, face poor living conditions and poor long-term health outcomes (Hesketh et al., 2008; Shao et al., 2018). Most migrants in China who are responsible for the production of China's urbanization process are exempted from urban social welfare and security systems (Shao et al. 2018). Rural–urban migrants face barriers to enrolment in the health insurance system of China. This is especially problematic, as the health of internal migrants can easily impact the health of the host urban population. Considering the high population of urban centers in China, and the vulnerability of other countries as a result of global movements, a small infectious disease outbreak could rapidly become a global health emergency. Therefore, predictably, the COVID-19 outbreak in Wuhan, China became a pandemic killing millions of people (Amzat et al., 2020) (see also Chapter 7).

Migration is a reality that affects people worldwide. Migrants are vulnerable and face limited access to healthcare services. The situation is often worse for undocumented or irregular migrants, given their insecure legal status. Extending healthcare coverage to migrants is still a major global health challenge because the current healthcare delivery system and migrant health policies are not conducive for migrants to seek appropriate health services. Governments worldwide, particularly of high-income nations, need to appreciate the global health reasons for providing appropriate health services to migrants (whether documented or not).

9.4 Summary

- This chapter examines migration patterns made possible through globalization and how migration has become a public or global health issue, and therefore responsible for various health challenges.
- The health of migrants is a global health discourse because migration status is a significant determinant of health. The most worrisome dimension of migration of global health importance is forced migration. The dimension includes human smuggling, trafficking and displacement, with their accompanying severe humanitarian and health crises.
- The "push factors" in the Global South, especially conflict and other development challenges, have a lot to do with globalization through economic interests and military activities of the Global North.
- There is a strong migration–health nexus. Migrants face (difficult) circumstances that impact on their health. Health risks concerning migration are bi-directional between the migrants and the hosts.
- There are global health reasons to provide appropriate health services to all migrants. In the face of mutual vulnerability between the host and migrant population, any exclusionist policy questions the right to health and universal healthcare, which, among other reasons, constitutes a global health justification to provide healthcare coverage to the migrants.

Critical Thinking Questions

- How does migration (think separately of voluntary and involuntary migration) affect health?
- Why are migration and health hotly debated and contentious issues in global health?
- Is the Global North complicit in conflict-related forced migration from the Global South? Evaluate the health consequences of such conflict-related forced migration.
- Are there adequate global health reasons to provide appropriate health services to all migrants? What limitations do host countries face?
- Critically describe the health condition of migrants in your locality/country.
- How can migration-related health challenges/concerns be mitigated?

Suggested Readings

- Gostin, L. O. and Roberts, A. E. (2015). Forced migration: The human face of a health crisis. *JAMA, 314*(20), 2125–2126. The article documents the various dimensions of global migration crisis and the incommensurate global response.
- Razum, O., and Wenner, J. (2016). Social and health epidemiology of immigrants in Germany: Past, present and future. *Public Health Reviews, 37*, 4. doi:10.1186/s40985-016-0019-2. The article provides a full understanding of health inequalities related to migration in Germany.
- Sterud, T., Tynes, T., Mehlum, I. S., Veiersted, K. B., Bergbom, B., Airila, A., Johansson B., Brendler-Lindqvist, M., Hviid K. and Flyvholm, M. A. (2018). A systematic review of working conditions and occupational health among immigrants in Europe and Canada. *BMC Public Health, 18*(1), 770. doi:10.1186/s12889-018-5703-3. This is a good article about the working conditions and occupational health among immigrants in Europe and Canada.
- Zimmerman, C., Kiss, L. and Hossain, M. (2011). Migration and health: A framework for 21st century policy-making. *PLoS Medicine 8*(5), e1001034. doi:10.1371/journal. pmed.1001034. This is a classical article about the migration–health nexus.
- Illingworth, P. and Parmet, W. E. (2017). *The health of newcomers: Immigration, health policy, and the case for global solidarity*. New York: NYU Press. The book reflects on the misimpressions about immigrants, and their impact on healthcare systems.

References

Abdulkader, R. S., Goswami, K., Rai, S. K., Misra, P. & Kant, S. (2015). HIV-risk behavior among the male migrant factory workers in a north Indian City. *Indian Journal of Community Medicine, 40*(2), 108–115. doi: 10.4103/0970-0218.153874.

Abraído-Lanza, A. F., Echeverría, S. E. & Flórez, K. R. (2016). Latino immigrants, acculturation, and health: Promising new direction in research. *Annual Review of Public Health, 37*(1), 219–236.

Agadjanian, V., Menjívar, C. & Zotova, N. (2017). Legality, racialization, and immigrants' experience of ethnoracial harassment in Russia. *Social Problems, 64*(4), 558–576.

Amusan, L., & Mchunu, S. (2017). An assessment of xenophobic/afrophobic attacks in South Africa (2008–2015): Whither *Batho Pele* and *Ubuntu* principles? *South African Review of Sociology, 48*(4), 1–18. doi: 10.1080/21528586.2017.1411744.

Amzat, J. (2010). Social correlates of HIV among youths in Nigeria. *Hemispheres: Studies on Cultures and Societies, 25*, 1–13.

Amzat, J., & Magaji, A. M. (2019). Sociology of social problems: An introduction. In A. A. Abdullahi & Ajala, E. M. (Eds.), *Contemporary Issues in Sociology and Social Work: An Africanist Perspective* (pp. 45–60). Ibadan: College Press, Lead City University.

Amzat, J., Aminu, K., Kolo, V. I., Akinyele, A. A., Ogundairo, J. A. & Danjibo, C. M. (2020). Coronavirus outbreak in Nigeria: Burden and socio-medical response during the first 100 days. *International Journal of Infectious Diseases, 98*, 218–224. doi: 10.1016/j.ijid.2020.06.067.

Baranova, A., Sergiev, V., Morozova, L., Turbabina, N. & Morozov, E. (2019). Imported *Plasmodium vivax* malaria in the Russian Federation from western sub-Saharan Africa. *Hindawi Journal of Tropical Medicine, 26*, 4610498. doi: 10.1155/2019/4610498.

Burkle, F. M. (2006). Complex humanitarian emergencies: A review of epidemiological and response models. *Journal of Postgraduate Medicine, 52*, 110–115.

Chiarenza, A., Dauvrin, M., Chiesa, V., Baatout, S. & Verrept, H. (2019). Supporting access to healthcare for refugees and migrants in European countries under particular migratory pressure. *BMC Health Services Research, 19*, 513.

Connolly, M. A., Gayer, M., Ryan, M. J., Salama, P., Spiegel, P. & Heymann, D. L. (2004). Communicable diseases in complex emergencies: Impact and challenges. *Lancet, 364*, 1974–1983.

Curtis, M. (2019). How the West's war in Libya has spurred terrorism in 14 countries. *Middle East Eye*. www.middleeasteye.net/opinion/how-wests-war-libya-has-spurred-terrorism-14-countries. Accessed on October 24, 2019.

Dahlan, R., Badri, P., Saltaji, H. & Amin, M. (2019). Impact of acculturation on oral health among immigrants and ethnic minorities: A systematic review. *PLoS ONE 14*(2), e0212891. doi: 10.1371/journal.pone.0212891.

Fassaert, T., Hesselink, A. E. & Verhoeff, A. P. (2009) Acculturation and use of health care services by Turkish and Moroccan migrants: A cross-sectional population-based study. *BMC Public Health, 9,* 332. doi: 10.1186/1471-2458-9-332.

Fernandez, I. (1998). Vulnerable to HIV/AIDS. Migration. *Integration, 57,* 36–42.

Fox, M., Thayer, Z. & Wadhwa, P. D. (2017). Acculturation and health: The moderating role of socio-cultural context. *American Anthropologist, 119*(3), 405–421. doi: 10.1111/aman.12867.

Gostin, L. O., & Roberts, A. E. (2015). Forced migration: The human face of a health crisis. *JAMA, 314*(20), 2125–2126.

Greenbaum, J., & Stoklosa, H. (2019). The healthcare response to human trafficking: A need for globally harmonized ICD codes. *PLoS Medicine, 16*(5), e1002799. doi: 10.1371/journal.pmed.1002799.

Greenfield, V. A., Nunez-Neto, B., Mitch, I., Chang, J. C. & Rosas, E. (2019). Human smuggling from Central America to the United States: What is known or knowable about smugglers' operations and revenues? Homeland Security Operational Analysis Center operated by the RAND corporation. www.rand.org/pubs/research_briefs/RB10057.html.

Hargreaves, S. Rustage, K., Nellums, L. B., McAlpine, A., Pocock, N., Devakumar, D., Aldridge, R. W., Abubakar, I., Kristensen, K. L., Himmels, J. W., Friedland, J. S. & Zimmerman, C. (2019). Occupational health outcomes among international migrant workers: A systematic review and meta-analysis. *Lancet Global Health, 7,* e872–e882.

Hesketh, T., Ye, X. J., Li, L. & Wang, H. M. (2008). Health status and access to health care of migrant workers in China. *Public Health Reports, 123*(2), 189–197. doi: 10.1177/003335490812300211.

Human Rights Watch [HRW] (2019a). Russia: Police round up migrant workers. www.hrw.org/news/2019/12/24/russia-police-round-migrant-workers.

Human Rights Watch (HRW) (2019b). Qatar: Migrant workers strike over work conditions: Defy ban under labor law. www.hrw.org/news/2019/08/08/qatar-migrant-workers-strike-over-work-conditions. Accessed on October 10, 2019.

Internal Displacement Management Center (IDMC) (2019). Global internal displacement database. http://www.internal-displacement.org/database/displacement-data. Accessed on September 24, 2019.

International Labor Organization (ILO) (2016). *Migrant Domestic Workers across the World: Global and Regional Estimates*. Geneva: ILO.

ILO (2018). Domestic work: Recognizing the rights of domestic workers. www.ilo.org/global/about-the-ilo/newsroom/features/WCMS_641738/lang--en/index.htm. Accessed July 25, 2019.

International Organization for Migration (IOM) (2016). Migrant smuggling. https://rosanjose.iom.int/site/en/migrant-smuggling. Accessed on September 23, 2019.

IOM (2019). International migration law: Glossary on migration. No. 34. https://publications.iom.int/system/files/pdf/iml_34_glossary.pdf. Accessed October 16, 2019.

Kang, C., Tomkow, L. & Farrington, R. (2019). Access to primary health care for asylum seekers and refugees: A qualitative study of service user experiences in the UK. *British Journal of General Practice, 69*(685), e537–e545. doi: 10.3399/bjgp19X701309.

Khattab, N., & Mahmud, H. (2019). Migration in a turbulent time: perspectives from the global South. *Migration and Development, 8*(1), 1–6. doi: 10.1080/21632324.2019.1552501.

Lam, E., McCarthy, A. & Brennan, M. (2015). Vaccine-preventable diseases in humanitarian emergencies among refugee and internally-displaced populations. *Human Vaccines & Immunotherapeutics, 11*(11), 2627–36. doi: 10.1080/21645515.2015.1096457.

Legido-Quigley, H., Nicola, P., SokTeng, T., Leire, P., Suphanchaimat, R., Wickramage K., McKee, M. & Pottie, K. (2019). Healthcare is not universal if undocumented migrants are excluded. *BMJ, 366,* l4160.

Mabera, F. (2017). The impact of xenophobia and xenophobic violence on South Africa's developmental partnership agenda. *Africa Review, 9*(1), 28–42. doi: 10.1080/09744053.2016.1239711.

National Health Commission of the People's Republic of China (NHCPRC) (2017). *Report on China's Migrant Population Development*. Beijing, China: China Population Publishing House.

Neiderud, C. J. (2015). How urbanization affects the epidemiology of emerging infectious diseases. *Infection Ecology & Epidemiology*, *5*, 27060. doi: 10.3402/iee.v5.27060.

O'Donnell, C. A. (2019). *Health Care Access to Migrants in Europe*. Oxford Research Encyclopedia, Global Public Health Series. Oxford: Oxford University Press. doi: 10.1093/acrefore/9780190632366.013.6

Owoaje, E. T., Uchendu, O. C., Ajayi, T. O. & Canmus, E. O. (2016). A review of the health problems of the internally displaced persons in Africa. *Nigerian Postgraduate Medical Journal*, *23*(4), 161–171. doi: 10.4103/1117-1936.196242.

Park, R. E., & Burgess, E. W. (1925). The Growth of the city: An introduction to a research project. *The City* (pp. 47–62). Chicago, IL: University of Chicago Press.

Pedde, N. (2017). The Libyan conflict and its controversial roots. *European View*, *16*, 93. doi: 10.1007/s12290-017-0447-5.

Razum, O., & Wenner, J. (2016). Social and health epidemiology of immigrants in Germany: past, present and future. *Public Health Reviews*, *37*, 4. doi: 10.1186/s40985-016-0019-2.

Ritchie, H. (2018). Urbanization. Published online at *OurWorldInData.org*. Retrieved from: https://ourworldindata.org/urbanization [Online Resource]. Accessed on July 25, 2020.

Sakuma, A. (2019). Damned for trying. www.msnbc.com/specials/migrant-crisis/libya. Accessed on September 23, 2019.

South African Human Rights Commission (SAHRC) (2018). Ensuring health and access to health care for migrants: A right and good public health practice. www.sahrc.org.za/index.php/sahrc-media/opinion -pieces/item/1422-ensuring-health-and-access-to-health-care-for-migrants-a-right-and-good-public -health-practice. Accessed October 15, 2019.

Schill, M. H., Friedman, S. & Rosenbaum, E. (1998). The housing conditions of immigrants in New York City. *Journal of Housing Research*, *9*(2), 201–235.

Shao, S., Wang, M., Jin, G., Zhao, Y., Lu, X. & Du, J. (2018). Analysis of health service utilization of migrants in Beijing using Anderson health service utilization model. *BMC Health Services Research*, *18*(1), 462. doi: 10.1186/s12913-018-3271-y.

Spadea, T., Rusciani, R., Mondo, L. & Costa, G. (2018). Health-related lifestyle among migrants in Europe. In Rosano, A. (Ed.), *Access to Primary Care and Preventative Health Services of Migrants* (pp. 57 –64). Cham, Switzerland: Springer International Publishing.

Sterud, T., Tynes, T., Mehlum, I. S., Veiersted, K. B., Bergbom, B., Airila, A., Johansson B., Brendler-Lindqvist, M., Hviid K. & Flyvholm, M. A. (2018). A systematic review of working conditions and occupational health among immigrants in Europe and Canada. *BMC Public Health*, *18*(1), 770. doi: 10.1186/s12889-018-5703-3.

Sweileh, W. M. (2018). Global output of research on the health of international migrant workers from 2000 to 2017. *Globalization and Health*, *14*(1), 105. doi: 10.1186/s12992-018-0419-9.

UN (2000). United Nations convention against transnational organized crime and the protocols thereto. www.unodc.org/unodc/en/organized-crime/intro/UNTOC.html#Fulltext. Accessed on September 23, 2019.

UN (2014). The economic, social and cultural rights of migrants in an irregular situation. www.ohchr.org /Documents/Publications/HR-PUB-14-1_en.pdf. Accessed on October 9, 2019.

United Nations High Commissioner for Refugees (UNHCR) (2019a). Figures at a glance. www.unhcr.org /figures-at-a-glance.html. Accessed on September 25, 2019.

UNHCR (2019b). Health: Fact sheet 15. www.unhcr.org/en-lk/4794b5d32.pdf. Accessed on September 25, 2019.

United Nations Office on Drugs and Crime (UNODC) (2018a). *Global Report on Trafficking in Persons 2018*. United Nations.

UNODC (2018b). *Migrant Smuggling in Asia and the Pacific: Current Trends and Challenges Volume II*. Regional Office for Southeast Asia and the Pacific.

Vakulenko, E., & Leukhin, R. (2017). Wage discrimination against foreign workers in Russia. *Russian Journal of Economics*, *3*(1), 83–100.

Vearey, J. (2012). Learning from HIV: Exploring migration and health in South Africa. *Global Public Health*, *7*(1), 58–70. doi: 10.1080/17441692.2010.549494.

Wickramage, K., Vearey, J., Zwi, A. B., Robinson, C. & Knipper, M. (2018). Migration and health: A global public health research priority. *BMC Public Health*, *18*(1), 987. doi: 10.1186/s12889-018-5932-5.

World Economic Forum (WEF) (2019). Which countries do migrants want to move to? www.weforum .org/agenda/2017/11/these-are-the-countries-migrants-want-to-move-to/. Accessed on September 23, 2019.

World Health Organization (WHO) (2018). *Health of Refugees and Migrants: Regional Situation Analysis, Practices, Experiences, Lessons Learned and Ways Forward*. Geneva: WHO European Regional Office.

Zetter, R. (2014). *Protecting Forced Migrants: A State of the Art Report of Concepts, Challenges and Ways Forward*. Federal Commission on Migration FCM.

Zhang, X., Rhoads, N., Rangel, M. G., Hovell, M. F., Magis-Rodriguez, C., Sipan, C. L., Gonzales-Fagoaga, H. E. & Martínez-Donate, A. P. (2017). Understanding the impact of migration on HIV risk: An analysis of Mexican migrants' sexual practices, partners, and contexts by migration phase. *AIDS and Behavior*, *21*(3), 935–948. doi: 10.1007/s10461-016-1622-4.

Zhang, Y. (2017). Unequal living conditions between urban migrants and local residents in China. *Procedia Engineering*, *198*, 728–735.

Zimmerman, C., Kiss, L. & Hossain, M. (2011). Migration and health: A framework for 21st century policy-making. *PLoS Medicine*, *8*(5), e1001034. doi: 10.1371/journal.pmed.1001034.

10 Global Health Targets and the Global South

10.1 Introduction

Globalization is a force shaping the organization of healthcare in various ways. As previously discussed, globalization influences some global determinants of health (see Chapter 3). Beyond that, globalization affects the structure and organization of health in various countries. The second chapter of this book focuses on the various faces of globalization, which include globalization of healthcare (itself), healthcare targets and health technology, among others. These faces shape the structure of health, considering some global health goals. The concept of "universal healthcare" helps to frame health goals in various countries. The idea is that every country must drive toward the elimination of barriers to healthcare. Ideally, no individual should experience any barrier to accessing healthcare; in reality, billions of people still have limited access to quality healthcare. Globalization is promoting enchantments in terms of ideas that are shaping healthcare across the world. Global bodies manage the direction of healthcare organizations through agenda setting or health goals, which are expected to be met within a specific timeline. Although some previously set goals have not been met, the emergence of new strategies and targets are essential landmarks in the organization of healthcare.

Globalization is continuously expanding the concept and practice of modern healthcare into one of a globally created major product that caters to the well-being of the people. While the initial view is to consider modern healthcare as a solely western product, the reality often signifies that it is now beyond such lopsided attribution. What is, however, the reality is that the western world is more advanced in terms of modern healthcare, and is leading the initiative, science and innovation in modern healthcare. But with globalization, some science and innovations trickle-down as much as possible, but not without some limitations. The limitations manifest in the unequal development or situation of healthcare. Beyond the enchantments of globalization, there are also physical medicinal products promoted by globalization and its drivers, which are also shaping healthcare. Innovations and technologies are an essential consideration in healthcare. The world is witnessing what (Nye, 2002) described as globalism. Invariably, modern healthcare is the hallmark or mainstay of healthcare services all over the world. The global voice about healthcare is about modern healthcare. There is a limited appreciation of alternative or traditional medicine in the global health agenda.

A fundamental argument about globalization and healthcare is about the inequality of its distribution, especially between the North and South. In the process of globalization, there are winners and losers; some populations benefit more than others. Despite the hope that globalization is unifying the world and closing the inequality gap, globalization is, in fact, widening that gap. It is in this context, therefore, that globalization is exploitative, perhaps as a new possibility for capitalist exploitation or capital accumulation, subjugating the weaker nations. It is a

DOI: 10.4324/9781003247975-10

world system (relations) (Wallerstein, 2004) described in this context as a global health system (see Section 4.4.1). A system of unequal relations, dependence and exploitation, which has further denigrated already weakened structures. Beyond the Wallersteinian or historical materialist arguments, every nation is gradually developing the capacity to rise above limitations and ensure appropriate healthcare to its citizens. There is another angle of self-responsibility to escape the exploitative trap and effect a more proactive system that works despite limitations. Some, however, have argued that globalization and its attendant consequences are inescapable. Globalization is now like the oxygen that humans breathe, espoused by Ritzer (2003) as the globalization of *nothing* and *something*. Irrespective of the argument, the ultimate truth remains: Globalization affects healthcare. To further the foregoing arguments, the next section will examine global health targets.

10.2 Global Health Targets

A previous chapter (see Section 2.3.5) highlighted the globalization of health targets, which signifies the gradual harmonization of health goals. Most parts of the world, especially the Member States of the World Health Organization (WHO), are moving in the same direction to achieve set health goals. The harmonization of the targets is a means of ensuring accountability in the management of the health sector. The epidemiology and burden of health problems often shape the agenda setting of world bodies. Therefore, some diseases are termed "neglected" because of their relatively low burden and their geographic limitations. Priority setting is vital to allocate appropriate resources in order to maximize benefits. Most health issues accounting for a high burden of morbidity and mortality around the world have always attracted some attention, though sometimes not adequate. In the Global South, the primary targets have always been around maternal and child health (MCH) (including child immunization), human immunodeficiency virus (HIV), malaria, tuberculosis and access to healthcare. In general, resolving health issues in the Global South moves at a snail's pace; with more improved and consistent efforts, health crises can be tamed. The efforts, however, must be geared toward set global targets.

There are embedded frames and politics (power relations) involved in agenda setting (see Section 8.2). Beyond politics, the foundation of global health targets is epidemiology and global threat. As previously examined, there is a double burden of noncommunicable diseases (NCDs) (see Chapter 5) and infectious diseases (see Chapter 6) in the Global South. The fundamental reality is that, despite the burden, the capacity to control, anticipate and react to the health situation is low in most countries of the Global South, even as the contribution to the count of morbidity and mortality is high. Despite this epidemiologic imbalance, drawing up a health target has helped in several ways.

Global health targets help as a means to a common end or goal. The organizational set-up often requires some set objectives, which every member aims to achieve. A policy direction helps in structuring the movement or activities of states; a policy direction serves as a constant reminder of the need to do more and more to achieve the set goals. In most cases, periodic monitoring and evaluation reports document the progress made and what needs to be done to meet goals or achieve more. The common goal is a healthier globe. Setting up goals ensures that efforts are systematic and consciously purposeful. The target creates ambition for states within the limits of their resources and sometimes complement the resources (through global partnerships). It is important to note that many states often agree with global health targets, although the strategies sometimes vary. The agreement is often on the basis that healthcare is a major priority for every state. There is a budget-line for health at all levels, which signifies some form of commitment to ensuring improved population health. The question of whether in some regions such a budget is adequate or commensurate with need is a prominent debate. There is also a budget benchmark that every state is required to meet.

The global health target is an effort to frame a collective journey for stakeholders through a participatory approach. The primary collective efforts include the identification of the existing gaps and disadvantaged regions. It is a collective effort to set policy direction to improve human health. The ultimate goal of agenda setting is to bring nations together by establishing a legitimate role for each nation. Therefore, global agenda setting in healthcare is also meant to promote local "responsibilization". Since it is a global agenda, and the periodic evaluation will expose whether the state is faring above or below the benchmark, most nations view the promotion of healthcare as a legitimate political role, the basis on which political performance could be assessed. Despite the truism that health is everybody's business, it is also every nation's business. Improvement in population health is both a function of the individual and the government. The nation can perform a more protective role by ensuring basic primary public health measures, such as the supply of water and health services. For instance, in many countries of the Global South, free child immunization is a responsibility of the government. The state can also do a lot to stimulate demand for such free services to meet up with the supply.

The state is justified in intervening to improve population health. The commercial regulatory role on some harmful substances or products is an example of such interventions. For instance, monitoring commercial activities of the tobacco industry has been a protective role of the state. Irrespective of the rights of individuals, the state could consistently limit the marketing and advertisement of (potentially) harmful products that could jeopardize the health of the population. Among other efforts, the imposition of hefty tax has also been used to limit the marketability of such products. The macro efforts have the potential to complement those at the micro level. The power of self-protection might be undermined if the state does not complement it. State intervention mobilizes citizens toward a common goal. When the state takes on the role of mobilizing its citizens, in the aggregate, global citizens are mobilized to achieve global targets.

The global agenda is concerned with global health security as it relates to the globalization of health risks (see Sections 2.3.1 and 6.3). Global processes influence the spread of risks (see Section 6.4). Collective efforts are understandable and mandatory to curtail global risks, both for traditional risks (of infectious diseases) facilitated by human mobility and trade on a global scale and for the modern risks of NCDs (see Section 5.3). For instance, the global food trade has played a significant role in the risk of NCDs, especially diet-related diseases such as heart disease and diabetic conditions (see Section 5.4) (see Brownell and Yach, 2006). The world has become McDonaldized, with overwhelming consequences (see Ritzer, 2018). Beyond the transmission of risk, many diseases (such as chronic diseases and HIV) are endemic in every country. Such a common disease burden also necessitates global targets and efforts. Moreover, in the case of infectious diseases, human mobility might still affect the prevalence and transmission from one place to another.

Global health targets facilitate the globalization of health policies and partnerships (see Section 2.3.6) and help mobilize global actors in the actualization of the goal. Lorenz (2007) observed that individual global health partnerships had a positive impact on some settings and target programs. Global health partnerships help to strengthen planning expertise in several areas. In most cases, the capacities of the partnerships then spread to remote or underserved areas. Lorenz also noted that performance-based funding (adopted by many partners) has dramatically improved administrative transparency and monitoring capacities. Lorenz (2007) observed further that global health partnerships created awareness of some critical health problems (including HIV, malaria and poliomyelitis). The partnerships, in turn, significantly helped in providing funds, workforce and expertise in the fight against many diseases. Different countries have provided partnerships through their international agencies, such as

GIZ [German Corporation for International Cooperation], DFID [Department for International Development, UK], USAID [the United States for International Development], SIDA [Swedish International Development Cooperation Agency], among others. This is in addition to some international non-governmental organizations (such as GAVI [the Global Alliance for Vaccines and Immunizations] and the Bill and Melinda Gates Foundation), which have also contributed immensely to setting policy directions and provision of required resources to curtail diseases around the world.

10.2.1 The Unmet Previous Targets: "Health for all" by the Year 2000

Health targets are historical; since the birth of the WHO in 1948, there have been targets set at different time periods. One of the famous declarations was "Health for All by the Year 2000". With the recognition of fundamental human rights, the global target of achieving the highest standard of health for all by the year 2000 was launched in 1979. The global strategy was adopted by the World Health Assembly (WHA) by adopting Resolution WHA32.30. The global strategy represented a significant historic move by the Member States to ensure universal health coverage. It also signified the commitment of the world body to safeguarding its mandate of ensuring that a healthy world is achieved within a particular time frame. As previously mentioned, agenda setting is a way of guiding the energy and resources of stakeholders. A global target often comes with a global strategy, i.e., specific means of reaching the end. It also comes with different timelines and evaluation strategies to monitor progress in different parts of the world. The adoption of the WHA32.30 recognized that the target was achievable through the combined efforts of governments, individuals and partner organizations. "Health for All" (HFA) was the first global strategy: Ambitious and holistic.

Mahler (2016) expanded on the meaning of "Health for All", noting that it is multidimensional; it goes beyond the provision of health services to cover all conditions necessary to attain the highest standard of health. Mahler, who served as the Director-General of the WHO (1973–1983), observed that people need to have both socially and economically productive lives, in order to attain a state of good health. Invariably, "Health for All" means that all impediments (financial, cultural, political, etc.) to healthcare must be removed. Mahler (2016) noted that improvement in public health measures such as water and sanitation is sacrosanct to achieving these goals. Ensuring health goals involves the provision of health services by resolving medical problems (including inadequate health facilities and health workers) to stimulate demand by promoting the acceptability of modern healthcare. "Health for All" is only possible with an improved standard of living, making improvements in major industries (such as agriculture, education and communication) a prerequisite for the achievement of health goals (Mahler, 2016). Improving population health should not only be "formulated in purely technocratic terms—drugs, nurses, vaccines, hospitals, doctors, and X-ray equipment", but with the consideration of the fundamental determinants of health (Mahler, 2016).

One significant dimension of the global strategy of "Health For All" was the adoption of the Declaration of the International Conference on Primary Health Care (PHC), held in Alma-Ata, USSR, in 1978. The strategies required the formulation and implementation of national policies to achieve some health goals. The central deficient area noted by the then WHO Director-General was in health spending. Mahler (2016) explained the need for individual countries to increase their health budgets as a means of ensuring health for all. The poor health allocation in many low- and middle-income countries (LMICs) has always been a significant bottleneck in achieving universal healthcare. The former Director-General observed that most developing countries spend as low as 2%–3% of GNP (i.e., $4–6 per capita) on healthcare. Such spending is grossly inadequate and mitigated against the realization of most health goals. Improved health spending, among other factors, would have been a significant catalyst in achieving the global dream of health for all by the year 2000.

The primary basis of the "Health for All" strategy is primary healthcare meant for the delivery of countrywide health programs that reach the whole population (WHO, 1981). Primary Health Care (PHC) refers to

> essential health care based on scientifically sound and socially acceptable methods and technology, made universally accessible to individuals and families in the community through their full participation and at a cost that the community and the country can afford to maintain at every stage of their development in the spirit of self-reliance and self-determination (ICPHC, WHO and UNICEF, 1978: p. 16).

Cueto (2004) noted that several antecedents informed the development of PHC as a strategy. The first was the experience of missionaries, who, during the colonialism of developing nations, maintained relatively small health posts. The medical missionaries emphasized the training of lower-level healthcare workers who were meant to operate at the community levels with the necessary equipment. Cueto (2004) further noted that the development of PHC was also favored by the new political context characterized by the subsequent emergence of decolonized African nations. Another inspiration was the massive expansion of rural medical services with "barefoot doctors" in Communist China. The "barefoot doctors" were like auxiliary health workers with minimal basic medical and paramedical training, usually posted to rural villages in China. The goal of the PHC program is to improve health coverage in underserved areas. The barefoot doctor program effectively achieved this by reducing costs and providing timely treatment to rural people by providing essential services, including maternal and child care and simple surgical operations (Zhang and Unschuld, 2008). Ultimately, PHC is a way of maintaining local health facilities using minimal resources.

Despite some improvements, "Health for All" was not achieved by the year 2000, and significant gaps remain in the coverage of PHC in the Global South (Chatora and Tumusime, 2004; Ramírez et al., 2011; van Weel et al., 2016). A series of economic crises, political instability and the emergence of HIV/AIDS in the African region prevented many countries from providing adequate resources required to achieve health for all in sub-Saharan Africa (Chatora and Tumusime (2004). In South America, Ramírez et al. (2011) identified some major challenges in the implementation of the PHC, including difficulties in adopting a paradigm shift from hospital-based care to the community and preventative care; weak political will concerning social equity and health as a human right; and weak community participation, multidisciplinary and/or intersectoral action. The stories from South Asia are also similar, with low investment and poor planning as significant challenges to the implementation of PHC (van Weel et al., 2016). Overall, there is still a gross shortage of health facilities and health workers (including low-level health personal) in most communities of the Global South. Another major challenge that hindered achieving "Health for All by the Year 2000" was the inadequate preparation or anticipation of epidemiologic transitions, which manifested in a high burden of NCDs. Hence, rapid changes in health status and trends, demography, socio-economic trends and government priorities adversely affected the achievement of the health goal by the year 2000 (WHO, 2003).

The efforts toward health for all and the implementation of PHC lives on in the goal of universal healthcare coverage. Most countries continue with the provision of basic services to underserved regions, to achieve health for all. The approach and principles of PHC or health for all are still applicable in the drive toward the expansion of health coverage. The ambition only requires more political commitments in the form of increased funding and social investment that would improve the standard of living of the population. The PHC system should be rejuvenated in the developing world, especially in covering the healthcare needs of rural communities. Cueto (2004) pointed out that diseases in less-developed nations were largely a result of poor social determinants of health and that this needs a political response. The path of universal healthcare is still a valid response if it is appropriately re-engineered with profound political support. However, with the partial success recorded, there was the declaration of the Millennium Development Goals (MDGs) in the year 2000 with some health goals based on the priorities of that time, thereby setting a new direction for all nations.

10.2.2 From Health Targets of Millennium to Sustainable Development Goals

In the year 2000, new development goals were launched: The Millennium Development Goals (MDGs). The declaration was remarkable in that it set an agenda for national development programs with eight primary goals: The eradication of extreme poverty; achievement of universal primary education; promotion of gender equality and empowerment of women; reduction of child mortality; improvement in maternal health; combating of HIV, malaria and other diseases; ensuring environmental sustainability; and development of a global partnership for development (Amzat, 2009). The MDGs served as a global framework for development and a means for states to work together in securing a better future for all (UN, 2007). The goals were meant to be achieved by the year 2015. In 2015, UNECA observed that the MDGs had helped to mobilize various governments in addressing developmental issues on a global scale. The three public health-oriented goals of the MDGs helped draw attention to health issues as major developmental issues. Several global initiatives, such as Global Fund to Fight AIDS, Tuberculosis, and Malaria, GAVI and Education for All (EFA), worked at the frontlines to galvanize global action and resources around the development objectives (UNECA, 2015).

Most regions of the world made commendable progress in achieving the specific set of MDG goals. UNECA (2015) noted that Africa made impressive gains, including improved enrolment in schools, bridging the gender gap in school enrolment, improved representation of women in politics and reduction in child and maternal deaths, HIV/AIDS and malaria incidence and mortality. Stories from the Asia-Pacific Region also signified that the region achieved some remarkable improvements during the MDGs era; the goals helped to direct resources and policies of all the governments in the region toward common objectives (MDG Monitor, 2016). A remarkable achievement of the region included a nearly two-third reduction in the rate of poverty, surpassing the target to halve the burden of poverty. The second achievement came in the area of drinking water, with a reduction from 28% to 7% of those without access to clean water (MDG Monitor, 2016). The major areas of deficiency included maternal health services, sanitation and gender equality (MDG Monitor, 2016). ECLAC (2015) also reported substantial progress toward achieving the MDG health goals in Latin America and the Caribbean. The region achieved enormous progress in child health and curtailing infectious diseases (such as malaria, tuberculosis (TB) and HIV, although less so in the area of maternal health.

Despite the progress made, some lapses were still evident. In 2015, the United Nations General Assembly set the Sustainable Development Goals (SDGs): 17 development goals with 169 targets, with major health targets to be achieved within 15 years (from 2016–2030). Unlike the MDGs, the SDGs include only one health goal, but with nine specific targets, to "ensure healthy lives and promote well-being for all at all ages" (see Table 10.1). The WHO (2015) observed that the health goals were derived from the unfinished MDG agenda and World Health Assembly resolutions and related action plans. The sustainable development goals (SDGs) have a broader outlook, not only in terms of the number of goals but the depth expressed in the targets. The WHO (2015, p. 193) further observed that the SGDs use a holistic development framework that considers "the economic, environmental and social pillars of sustainable

Table 10.1 Sustainable Development Goal 3 with nine targets

3.1	By 2030, reduce the global maternal mortality ratio to less than 70 per 100,000 live births.
3.2	By 2030, end preventable deaths of newborns and children under five years of age, with all countries aiming to reduce neonatal mortality to at least as low as 12 per 1,000 live births and under-five mortality to at least as low as 25 per 1,000 live births.
3.3	By 2030, end the epidemics of AIDS, tuberculosis, malaria and neglected tropical diseases and combat hepatitis, waterborne diseases and other communicable diseases.
3.4	By 2030, reduce by one-third premature mortality from noncommunicable diseases through prevention and treatment and promote mental health and well-being.
3.5	Strengthen the prevention and treatment of substance abuse, including narcotic drug abuse and harmful use of alcohol.
3.6	By 2020, halve the number of global deaths and injuries from road traffic accidents.
3.7	By 2030, ensure universal access to sexual and reproductive healthcare services, including for family planning, information and education and the integration of reproductive health into national strategies and programs.
3.8	Achieve universal health coverage, including financial risk protection, access to quality essential healthcare services and access to safe, effective, quality and affordable essential medicines and vaccines for all.
3.9	By 2030, substantially reduce the number of deaths and illnesses from hazardous chemicals and air, water and soil pollution and contamination.

Source: WHO (2015, p. 8)

development with a strong focus on equity expressed frequently in the phrase, 'no one will be left behind'". The SDGs constitute a global development strategy focusing on how to bridge, to some extent, the gap between the Global North and South.

SDG 3 is the goal concerned with health (see Table 10.1). With nine sub-targets, the SDG 3 is more comprehensive than the three health goals of the MDGs. For instance, unlike in the MDGs, the SDGs earmark targets for NCDs and other conditions previously not targeted in the MDGs. One of the main strategies highlighted under the health goal is to strengthen the implementation of the framework for tobacco control. Tobacco use is a significant risk factor for many chronic diseases, including lung disease, heart disease, cancer, stroke and chronic obstructive pulmonary disease (COPD) (see Section 5.3.1). Another target deals with the prevention and treatment of substance abuse (including narcotic drug abuse and harmful use of alcohol) (WHO, 2015), which is another significant risk factor for NCDs (see Section 5.3.2). It is also important to note the inclusion of a target to halve the death burden from road accidents by 2030. While these have long been recognized as significant health risks, their inclusion on the global targets demonstrates acknowledgment that both NCDs and infectious diseases impact populations worldwide.

The target SDG 3 focuses on the prevention of child morbidity and mortality, a goal that was neglected in the MDGs in many countries of the Global South. The provision regarding access to medicines and vaccines for all prioritizes continuing the universal coverage of childhood vaccination to prevent childhood diseases. The list of vaccine-preventable diseases now includes malaria, which is a major health problem in sub-Saharan Africa (SSA). The development of vaccines against Ebola has also been recorded. The global efforts aim at promoting more research and development of vaccines and medicines for all. The target recognizes the deficient health financing and workforce in developing countries (WHO, 2015). One of the strategies of ensuring healthy lives includes how to improve both health financing and workforce in disadvantaged areas. The last strategy focuses more on infectious diseases of global significance such as Ebola, Zika, dengue, West Nile virus, Venezuelan Equine Encephalitis, Leptospirosis, Lassa fever, monkeypox and other neglected diseases. The priority of the strategy is about preparedness, early warnings and risk management.

SDG 3 should not be regarded as a standalone; it is connected to other SDG goals, the realization of which will significantly influence the actualization of SDG 3. Health is multidimensional (social, political, ecological and economic), with various social determinants (see Section 3.2.1) that are connected to other goals. Ensuring good health and well-being is undoubtedly and significantly connected to poverty (Goal 1); hunger (Goal 2); quality of education (Goal 4); gender equality (Goal 5); clean water and sanitation (Goal 6); affordable and clean energy (Goal 7); decent work and economic growth (Goal 8); industry, innovation and infrastructure (Goal 9); reduced inequality (Goal 10); sustainable cities and communities (Goal 11); responsible consumption and production (Goal 12); climate action (Goal 13); life below water (Goal 14); life on land (Goal 15); peace, justice and strong institutions (16); and partnerships to achieve the goals (Goal 17). Again, all other goals constitute a fundamental context that could fast-track the realization of healthy lives and well-being. Beyond the connectedness, as mentioned earlier with other goals, there are still critical issues within the health system of the Global South that need to be addressed toward the realization of health targets.

10.3 Critical Factors in the Healthcare Situation of the Global South

There are still fundamental issues with the situation of healthcare in most countries of the Global South that are responsible for the relatively poor healthcare indicators. Collins (2003) observed that globalization impacts health in different regions, with a notably higher burden of morbidity and mortality in the developing world. The prevailing socio-economic and political inequalities among and within countries negatively affect access to healthcare (Collins, 2003). Labonté et al. (2011) observed that the healthcare crisis in the different regions has inherently global causes and consequences. Global economic crises or situations influence healthcare financing and set apart the South from the North. The differential healthcare situation can only be adjudged as unfair, and tremendous improvement is required to curtail the disease burden in the Global South. It is just a few years into the 15-year dream of SDGs; there is the hope of reaching the goals if specific critical issues are given due consideration. A surprising aspect is that the impediments to health goals are known, but there has always been a slow pace in removing such impediments. It is often a matter of the same old stories and ineffectual actions. The world should be more determined to achieve the SDGs by instituting the required actions, developing institutions and monitoring progress. Health goals can often be practically demonstrated in the form of a reduced burden of morbidity and mortality and access to essential healthcare. The critical factors are not overwhelming but surmountable.

10.3.1 Access to Medicines and Vaccines

Access to healthcare has been previously explained as a social determinant of health (see Section 3.2.1.5). While the previous section focused more on the micro level, the focus here is at the macro level. The provision or availability of essential drugs and vaccines is crucial in improving healthcare delivery in any nation. Unfortunately, there are embedded politics involved in accessing medicines between the South and North. The argument hinges on the political economy of the pharmaceuticals in providing access to medicines, especially in the South. There are over two billion people without adequate access to essential medicines; a situation that exacerbates their health problems (WHO, 2017).

Despite the efforts made over the years, the major gaps are still observable in the lower wealth quantile of the world, with the Global South still carrying the burden of the suffering of limited access to medicines. The WHO (2017) observed that healthy living is impossible without access to pharmaceutical products. So also, the goal of universal health coverage cannot be achieved in the face of the non-availability of affordable health technologies. In the face of limited access to essential medicines, mortality from easily avertable situations becomes inevitable: People die from stings and bites, (maternal) bleeding, falls and uncomplicated medical emergencies, and preventable infections such as malaria, cholera and diarrhea. The high burden of preventable death is mainly a result of inadequate access to essential medicines and vaccines in the Global South (WHO, 2017). Despite the known cure for many preventable diseases, millions still die annually. The situation calls for some ethical concerns in the face of a global push to reduce the burden of such health problems. For instance, issues remain concerning access to insecticide-treated bednet (ITN) in malaria prevention and antiretroviral therapy for HIV in SSA. Several over-the-counter drugs can cure most childhood infections, yet child mortality remains high in the low-income regions. More so, billions of people (up to 80% of the world's population) live in places with minimal access to controlled drugs for relieving moderate to severe pain (WHO, 2017).

In creating access to medicine, pharmaceutical companies and various governments have a crucial responsibility to enhance the flow of medicines. The pharmaceutical companies, principally private-for-profit, are responsible for research and development, which often require high levels of funding. The pharmaceutical companies are huge multinational corporations, mostly in the Global North (especially North America and Europe). The WHO (2017, p. 15) viewed the companies as dominant economic operators with enormous political power, creating a polarizing tension between economic interests and public health concerns. The critical question is whether compelling ethical imperatives, based on life-saving or health-promoting actions, are enough to improve access to medicines and vaccines across the world (Ahmadiani and Nikfar, 2016; WHO, 2017). The ethical consideration is in the context of the right to health without any barrier; this right cannot be guaranteed without access to medicine and other medical technologies (including drugs, vaccines and diagnostic tools). The primary causes of inadequate access to medicine, such as economic and social causes, are unfair reasons, but pharmaceutical companies are not charity organizations. Hence, the polarizing tension presents an unresolved (ethical) contradiction.

Furthermore, Ahmadiani and Nikfar (2016) examined the problem of access to medicines from a legal perspective. The duo stressed that the global legal framework or structures (such as patent rights) contribute to the limited access to medicine in several countries. Name-brand medicine often comes with high prices because its production is often initiated within a period of monopoly (usually without low-priced generics) (Ahmadiani and Nikfar, 2016). In many LMICs, such medicines, if available at all, are usually out of reach for the high number of people living in poverty. The non-availability of low-priced generics increases the catastrophic costs of disease in terms of morbidity and mortality in low-income countries (Ahmadiani and Nikfar, 2016; Stevens and Huys, 2017). Patent rights exist under the Trade-Related Aspects of Intellectual Property Rights (TRIPS), a global legal treaty among all member nations of the World Trade Organization (WTO). Within the period of monopoly, any attempt to produce or import generics is a breach that can lead to a legal battle. Ahmadiani and Nikfar (2016) also described the development of TRIPS-plus, an initiative of the US with some TRIPS members to expand and deepen the TRIPS agreement by decreasing the flexibilities and increasing the duration of patents in some cases. The decrease in flexibilities further constrains developing nations. Ahmadiani and Nikfar (2016) and the WHO (2017) highlighted some other critical issues relating to access to medicine in the Global South, including:

1. The economic operators, in this case, the pharmaceutical companies, produce products that attract more profits. This explains the low concentration of the diseases of the Global South (i.e., diseases not common in the North). Hence, some diseases are neglected because

of low incentive to invest in research and development of medicines to treat those rare diseases.

2. The preceding argument implies that there is much attention to the diseases of the Global North, the primary constituency of the pharmaceuticals. Such attention implies a skewed focus on noncommunicable diseases. Medicines of chronic conditions yield more market value because such conditions are life-long; hence, medicines are used long term.

3. There is a concern about how to ensure uninterrupted supplies of medicines. Structural gaps in local health systems and infrastructures hamper the delivery of medicines to millions of people. For instance, the storage specifications of some medicines impede their delivery to hard-to-reach regions. The supply impediments, in some cases, also include administrative bottlenecks, such as tax/tariff policies and mark-ups along the supply chain.

4. Access to essential medicine is also jeopardized by the proliferation of counterfeit/fake or substandard drugs. In cases of an insecure supply chain, fake drugs are marketed, further exacerbating the disease burden in terms of morbidity and mortality. Thus the WHO often advocates for the strengthening of national drug regulatory authorities with a sound system for pharmacovigilance.

Both TRIPS and TRIP-plus were developed based on economic terms, with less consideration for both global health and health ethics. A significant dilemma in this respect is how to balance economic and ethical goals, as the production of medicine involves a big investment and returns are necessary to remain in business. It is commendable that some pharmaceutical companies are providing some off-price percentage to create access to several drugs (including antiretrovirals). However, more altruism is required to meet global health targets. Another big task is to increase the flexibilities in both TRIPS and TRIP-plus to create more access to medicine in LMICs. Some models involving stakeholders (governments, non-state actors and the pharmaceutical industry) have been used to ease access to medicine, including (1) product development partnerships (PDPs), which are a kind of public–private partnership (PPP) model; (2) flexible intellectual property rights (IPRs), i.e., with some exemptions in low-income regions, without compromising research and development; and (3) pricing models, sometimes involving tiered pricing with subsidies and lower prices in LMICs (Stevens and Huys, 2017). The LMICs must be proactive in pushing for what works best to improve access to medicines. It is also essential for the concerned countries to facilitate the flow of essential medicines and improve pharmacovigilance in order to enhance access to affordable and quality drugs.

10.3.2 Health Worker Migration

Inadequate health personnel remains a significant concern in low-income countries of the Global South. The global health goals and targets cannot be achieved without an adequate healthcare workforce. The health systems in most countries of the Global South are weak, with inadequate access to medicines (see Section 10.3.1). In many rural communities, health facilities are non-existent, which prompts reliance on traditional medicine. A primary symptom of the weak health system is the high burden of morbidity and mortality from both noncommunicable diseases (see Section 5.2) and infections (see Section 6.2). Most LMICs are still too far from achieving universal healthcare coverage. Therefore, the greatest challenge of healthcare provision or bridging the inequality gap exists within communities in the Global South. Many low-income countries of SSA are languishing in poor healthcare delivery—especially in rural areas. Preventable diseases such as malaria and diarrhea remain the top leading causes of morbidity and mortality, especially among children. The region also accounts for the highest maternal mortality rate. There are still millions of births occurring without any assistance from a skilled birth attendant. The weak healthcare system is compounded further by the emigration of domestic health workers.

Globalization is facilitating the exodus of health workers, especially nurses, physicians and pharmacists, from the Global South to the North. Mahler (2016) noted that the Global North is attracting health workers from LMICs—with a concentration of migrant physicians in Australia, Canada, Germany, the United Kingdom and the USA. Health worker migration is of a great benefit to the North but at a very huge cost to the South. It is a further catastrophe on already deficient health system. There are international conventions, soft agreements (such as the WHO Global Code of Practice on the International Recruitment of Health Personnel adopted in 2010 by all WHO Member States) and ethical principles to reduce migration of health workers from settings having acute shortages (of health workers), but these are often breached for the benefits of the North. Any unfavorable laws or codes to the North are often neglected, without any consequences. It is always a matter of lip-service without any drastic action.

Many middle-income countries also attract health workers from low-income countries. As of 2009, Naicker et al. (2009) observed that there were 57 countries with a critical shortage of health workers—amounting to a deficit of 2.4 million physicians and nurses. The study further noted that the situation in Africa is as low as 2.3 health workers per 1,000 of the population, while it is as high as 24.8 health workers per 1,000 of the population in the Americas. The WHO (2016) estimated the global need of health workers at 17.4 million (at least 2.6 million doctors and 9 million nurses and midwives, among others. Southeast Asia and Africa would require 6.9 million and 4.2 million, respectively. The shortage of healthcare workers is severe in SSA, with several countries (including Malawi, Mali, Senegal, Somalia, Zimbabwe, Uganda) having fewer than 2 physicians per 10,000 of the population. The shortage of nurses is less severe, but still far short of the required number. Unfortunately, the problem is only increasing, with a shortage of up to 7.2 million in 2017 and a projected global shortage of 12–14 million by 2035 (WHO, 2016; Miseda et al., 2017). Another dimension of the problem is the lack of various specialties of health workers. There is a massive gap in several health specialties, including cardio-surgeons, neurosurgeons, oncologists, nephrologists, cardiology nurses, forensic nurses, dental nurses, accident and emergency nurses and oncology nurses (Miseda et al., 2017).

Poor working conditions, characterized by poor salary and welfare packages, poor health budgets, underfunding of health facilities, and inadequate equipment are a crucial push factor that must be addressed to improve the retention of health workers in LMICs. The same poor conditions are preventing many Southern health professionals trained in the Global North from returning to LMICs. In most cases, the work conditions in the context of poor infrastructure might not support some professional practice. For instance, certain medical equipment and technologies require a constant source of power, which might not be available in many parts of LMICs. Globalization is encouraging freedom of movement of labor and opening up the labor market for health workers, leaving questions around ethical issues and individual rights to movement in its wake. In this scenario, the flow of health workers is not forced; it involves the individual quest for greener pastures in the context of push and pull factors. The pull factors are the favorable conditions in the destination countries (such as better working conditions and higher wages). Deliberate restriction of opportunities to seek a better life and advanced training would be tantamount to a violation of individual rights. However, the fact remains that the recruitment of health workers from low-income countries compromises the ability of such countries to meet their population's healthcare needs, which constitute a more serious human right or ethical concern.

With the projected growth in the shortage of health workers in many parts of the world, the situation constitutes an impediment to the achievement of the SDG health goals by 2030, and universal healthcare in general. One of the SDG strategies for achieving the health goal is recruitment, development, training and retention of the health workforce in LMICs. Both the costs and duration of training constitute challenges in turning out health workers. It is also challenging to facilitate the return of migrant health workers to their countries of origin. The countries with a severe shortage of health workers need to do more to avert or mitigate the push factors. Such efforts must also be situated in overall development efforts, including political and economic stability.

10.3.3 Healthcare Financing

One crucial indicator of the state of healthcare in different countries is the amount a country is willing to invest in healthcare. Health financing is reflected in the health budget: The amount and the percentage of the national budget earmarked for healthcare based on the population and health needs of a particular country. The budget alone does not tell the whole story; the amount spent relative to the population and disease burden of the country is decisive. Every nation must prioritize healthcare as instrumental in ensuring healthy lives and attracting the desired development. Unfortunately, despite the importance of healthcare, the reality in many countries of the Global South is that of inadequate funding relative to the burden of disease and population. Healthcare financing is in the realm of politics regarding the allocation and management of resources. Therefore, healthcare is regarded as a form of politics. Healthcare policies and allocation of resources require political intricacies and economic considerations. Healthcare requires considerable resources to procure medicines and vaccines, build health facilities, train and recruit health workers, among others. Therefore, healthcare spending is a significant public policy priority.

Ortiz-Ospina and Roser (2019) analyzed healthcare financing around the world and observed major gaps in average healthcare spending per capita in different countries. The duo recorded (expressed in US dollars as of 2011) the lowest figures in African countries (e.g., CAR: 24.96 and the Democratic Republic of Congo: 32.28), and the highest in the United States with 9,402.54. The data from some Global South countries (China: 731; India: 267 Pakistan: 129; Indonesia: 299.41; Philippines: 329; Cambodia: 182; Bolivia: 422.41; Guyana: 378; and Peru: 656) also show relatively low healthcare expenditure. While healthcare spending will increase in the next few years, the projected increase might still not meet the required need. For instance, per capita health spending in 2040 of low-income countries and middle-income countries is projected to range from only $40 (24–65) to $413 (263–668) and from $140 (90–200) to $1,699 (711–3,423), respectively (GBDHFCN, 2018). The only good news about healthcare spending is that it has been increasing gradually, although at a slow pace. However, the fastest growth in annual per capita health spending is expected in lower-middle-income and upper-middle-income countries up to 2050 with the lowest in SSA. Despite the growth, the gap between the North and South will remain similar (GBDHFCN, 2019). The continuous growth hinges on the greater prioritization of the health sector and increased government spending, and greater impact is expected in low-income countries (GBDHFCN, 2019).

Beyond government spending, approximately 90% of the population of LMICs still use the out-of-pocket health spending model (WHO, 2017, p. 15). Out-of-pocket payment for healthcare expenditure is the norm in the face of poor health insurance coverage. GBDHFCN (2019) has projected that out-of-pocket spending would remain substantially high in LMICs up until 2050. Out-of-pocket payment has the potential to further impoverish people already living in poverty, pushing them into an economic catastrophe of selling personal assets during a health crisis (WHO, 2017). The lack of functional insurance and social protection is a major problem militating against access to healthcare in most parts of the Global South (see also Section 3.2.1.5). Indirect costs of care (such as transportation costs) and even low-cost generic products (where available) are a heavy financial burden to households living in poverty (WHO, 2017).

Nearly all high-income countries have full health insurance coverage, some middle-income countries (including Argentina, Brazil, China and South Africa) also have very high levels of coverage (Ortiz-Ospina and Roser, 2019). Low or no insurance coverage is still the norm in several low-income countries except for in The Gambia, Ghana, Rwanda and Vanuatu (Ortiz-Ospina and Roser, 2019). For several countries in SSA, insurance coverage is less than 20%.

Health financial assistance is also a significant source of health funding, especially in LMICs. The Global Fund to fight malaria, TB and HIV is a typical example of global development aid flowing to the developing world. Many low-income countries are heavily dependent upon the availability of global aid to mitigate their health crises. It is worrisome that several low-income countries would continue to depend on the availability of this development assistance for an extended period (GBDHFCN, 2019). Above all, improved healthcare financing is a significant means of improving public healthcare, which is a requisite for achieving the global development agenda. There must also be a steady drive to reduce the burden of out-of-pocket payment systems through the provision of social protection schemes (especially health insurance).

10.3.4 *Urban Bias in Healthcare Services*

Urban bias in the provision of healthcare services is a major reality in most countries of the Global South, especially in Asia and Africa. Urban bias means that the concentration of services and amenities are found in the urban areas, at the expense of the rural areas. Lipton (1977) developed the concept of urban bias to explain the political economy of development in the developing world. The new category describes the urban class who, by their central location in urban areas, protect their interests by attracting or situating development projects in the urban centers, which invariably truncate opportunities and development in the rural areas. The urban class has enormous stake and power in both the public and private sectors to perpetuate such bias. While urban bias can also be applied to explain the differential development between the global North and South, the crux here is to focus on the primary application: Between urban and rural areas. Blomqvist and Lundahl (2002) observed that the most critical conflict in the developing world is not between labor and capital but urban and rural areas. Urban bias is a major indicator of unequal development between urban and rural areas.

One of the core indicators of the differences between rural and urban areas is in the area of health services. The defining features of rural areas in the developing world are poverty and acute shortage of infrastructures. While poverty and inadequate infrastructures are general features of a typical country of the Global South, the rural areas bear the more significant burden within a country. Beyond the inequalities between North and South, there exist fundamental inequalities within the country. Those localized inequalities are also of global concern because the idea of universal coverage should make everyone count, irrespective of location.

The worst health indicators in most countries of the Global South come from rural areas. A slightly higher percentage of the population in the Global South still lives in rural areas. Rural dwellers constitute more than 70% of the total population in many countries in SSA (including Burundi, Ethiopia, Malawi, Niger, Eritrea, Chad, Lesotho, Swaziland, Burkina Faso, South Sudan, Uganda) (Amzat and Razum, 2018). Despite increasing urbanization, most countries in SSA still have more rural settlements than urban centers (albeit densely populated). More than 83% and 54% of the population in rural areas in Africa and Asia, respectively, have very limited entitlement to healthcare (Scheil-Adlung/ILO, 2015).

Figure 10.1 shows that there are still large gaps in health coverage between the rural and urban areas in most regions of the Global South. Beyond the financial deficits, additional issues adversely affect access to healthcare in rural areas. Urban bias in the distribution of health facilities allows a greater concentration of health facilities in the urban centers. The spatial

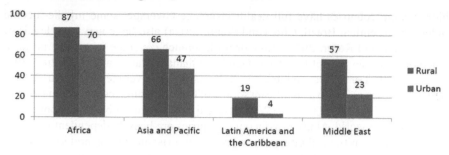

Figure 10.1 Estimated health coverage gap due to financial deficits in rural/urban areas, selected regions, 2015 (percentages) (Source: Scheil-Adlung/ILO, 2015)

inequality undermines the effort toward universal healthcare. In many instances, health facilities are non-existent in many rural communities, forcing them to rely on traditional medicine, which is limited in terms of service capacity, among other disadvantages. There is also the maldistribution of healthcare professionals, as most healthcare workers prefer urban postings to the rural ones, mainly due to the deficient infrastructure (such as transportation, communication and education) in rural settlements (Amzat and Razum, 2018). The added fact that rural areas may have poorer working conditions and lack basic needs (such as water, sanitation and power supplies) decreases the likelihood of attracting healthcare workers.

Within the ongoing efforts to meet healthcare goals, there must also be a focus on the rural areas. Rural dwellers are more vulnerable to all major social problems (food insecurity, inadequate education, unemployment and poverty), which incidentally are significant social determinants of health. Invariably, the rural areas constitute a converging of major health risks of infectious diseases due to inadequate public health measures. The rural area also bears a higher burden of neglected diseases. Therefore, the overall progress toward health goals should also be defined by efforts to narrow the health inequalities between the rural and urban areas of the Global South.

10.3.5 The Fall and Rise of Alternative Medicine

Traditional medicine was the mainstay in the control of disease before the advent of modern healthcare. The whole of medicines outside the (official) modern medicine is now regarded as complementary and alternative medicine (CAM). The enlightenment and scientific revolutions were essential landmarks in the development of modern medicine. With the advent of modern healthcare, there was a gradual decline in the use of alternative medicine. The entire discussion about the improvement of health services is focused on modern healthcare, which is the dominant healthcare system worldwide. Whether in the North or South, all governments prioritize the modern healthcare system as the most effective way of combating health crises. Despite the previous assertion, there is considerable use of alternative medicine both in the North and the South. Whether it is called ethnomedicine, traditional or folk medicine, or CAM, it has (re) gained some popularity in the face of inadequate modern health services. The use of traditional medicine is higher than 70% in many African countries, including Benin, Burundi and Ethiopia (WHO-Africa, 2013). It is notable that the scarcity of modern health services is not the only reason for the renewed popularity of alternative medicine; cultural orientation also plays an important role. Alternative medicine is traditional to the community.

It has been reported that some demographic characteristics, such as socio-economic status, education, religion and location, play essential roles in the use of traditional medicine (James et al. 2018), with lower education and economic status making the use of traditional medicine more likely. Concurrent treatment with the use of modern and traditional medicine is also prevalent in most developing societies (James et al., 2018). The utilization rate of traditional medicine also varies in Asia: Malaysia (56%), Singapore (43.7%), South Korea (44%), China (34%), Taiwan (34%) and Japan (27%) (Peltzer and Pengpid, 2015; Shim and Kim (2018) The utilization rate in Asia varies further by medical conditions, with utilization rates for chronic conditions (such as cancer, diabetes, asthma) between 20% and 84% (Peltzer and Pengpid, 2015). Many studies point to the increasing or sustained popularity of alternative medicine in many countries of the Global South. Despite their widespread use, Mpinga et al. (2013) observed that there are still concerns about rational use, safety, efficacy and regulation of alternative medicines. The efficacy of traditional medicine is not generally evidence-based. Most organized efforts regarding alternative medicine are meant to address the aforementioned concerns.

Mpinga et al. (2013) noted that the availability of CAM contributes to the realization of the right to health. Therefore, more efforts should be channeled toward its development and regulation. The WHO also acknowledges that traditional medicine will continue to be relevant in healthcare services for a very long time because it meets some healthcare needs (WHO, 2005, 2013). The WHO declared 2001–2010 and 2011–2020 as the first and second decades of traditional medicine. Perhaps the third decade will be declared to identify policy gaps and build on previous achievements. The general aim is to improve access to traditional medicine through sound policies that would improve safety, efficacy and rational use to achieve health for all (WHO, 2013). Improved investment in the development and regulation of CAM would help serve some primary care needs.

10.3.6 Health Governance and Political Will

There is a fundamental need to improve health governance and political will (see Section 8.2.4). Healthcare issues are highly political—there is a need for coordinated political action in order to achieve health targets, including universal healthcare. The first primary responsibility of accepting and working toward the achievement of these goals lies with the government. In other words, the government must take responsibility to pool resources and initiate public policies in line with the set targets. Savedoff et al. (2012) observed that political processes are ubiquitous, persistent and contingent on achieving health goals. Savedoff et al. (2012) highlighted three major political forces in the drive toward the achievement of universal healthcare, including 1) the creation of programs or regulations to improve access to care, improve equity and pool financial risks; 2) concomitant improvement in health spending to create more health services for the population; and 3) health policy to increase pooled financing rather than paying out-of-pocket. Beyond these three points, every government needs to invest in improving public health measures (i.e., access to water, sanitation and other related infrastructure). The government must also take steps to bring health information to people on a timely basis. Lastly, the government needs to ensure beneficial partnerships with other states and non-state actors to achieve the set goals.

Most governments in the developing world have been accused of not doing enough to achieve development goals. Sometimes, the allegation is about corruption and undue leakages in their political systems, and health systems, in particular. Health goals cannot be achieved in the face of weak political will (see Section 8.2.4). Every government, again, must accept the responsibility by instituting and implementing health policies and programs. Therefore, improving healthcare in a country requires a lot of political action, which reflects in decision-making, initiation of actions/programs, prioritization of needs and allocation of resources toward the achievement of the set health targets.

10.4 Summary

- Globalization influences inequalities in healthcare, especially between the Global South and North. Despite the inequality, universal healthcare is a global healthcare goal.
- This synching of health targets is a partial means of ensuring accountability in the management of the health sector. The primary collective efforts include the identification of the existing gaps and disadvantaged regions. The ultimate goal of the agenda setting is to bring nations together by establishing a legitimate direction for each nation. Therefore, global agenda setting in healthcare is also meant to promote local "responsibilization".
- This chapter examines the historical health targets from the "Health for All by the Year 2000", the health aspects of the millennium development goals and the third goal of sustainable development goals. All the goals are intricately connected to the realization of global health targets, which help to direct the focus and energy of global actors toward a common policy direction.
- This chapter also examines the situation of healthcare in the Global South through a macro analytic lens. It is noted that, despite the efforts made over the years, the major gaps are still observable in the lower wealth quantile of the world, with the Global South still carrying the burden of the suffering of limited access to medicines, with 80% of the world's population living in places with minimal access to controlled drugs.
- The main argument is that of unresolved polarizing tension: While limited access to medicine is unfair, pharmaceutical companies are not charity organizations. In creating access to medicine, pharmaceutical companies and various governments have a crucial responsibility to enhance the flow of medicines.
- Trade-Related Aspects of Intellectual Property Rights (TRIPS) and TRIP-plus were developed based on economic terms, with less consideration for both global health and health ethics. A significant dilemma in this respect is how to balance economic and ethical goals. The big task is to increase the flexibilities in both TRIPS and TRIP-plus to create more access to medicine in low- and middle-income countries.
- Health worker migration is also a major challenge. Globalization is facilitating the exodus of health workers, especially nurses, physicians and pharmacists, from the Global South to the Global North, thereby creating a critical shortage of highly skilled health workers.
- Health worker migration is of a great benefit to the North but at a very huge cost to the South. It is a further catastrophe on an already deficient health system in the South. There are international conventions, soft agreements and ethical principles to reduce migration of health workers from settings having acute shortages (of health workers), but these are often breached for the benefits of the North.
- Healthcare financing is generally poor in the Global South and most governments are not doing enough, concerning political will, to support population health. Urban bias in the provision of healthcare services is another reality in most countries of the Global South, especially in Asia and Africa. Urban bias means that the concentration of services and amenities is in urban areas at the expense of the rural areas.
- Most governments in the developing world have been accused of not investing enough to achieve development goals. Sometimes, the allegation is about corruption and undue leakages in their political and health systems. Improving healthcare in a country requires a lot of political action, which reflects in decision-making, initiation of actions/programs, prioritization of needs and allocation of resources toward the achievement of the set health targets.

Critical Thinking Questions

- How can the global agenda setting in healthcare promote local "responsibilization" to improve healthcare?
- The previous global health targets, "Health For All by the Year 2000" and health aspect of the millennium development goals, could not be achieved. Though there were some improvements, what could be done differently to actualize the SDG3 in the Global South?
- Discuss the impediments toward the realization of the SDG3 in the Global South. How can such impediments be mitigated through global measures?
- Highlight and discuss the critical factors responsible for the poor healthcare situation in the Global South.

Suggested Readings

- Amzat, J., and Razum, O. (2018). *Towards a sociology of health discourse in Africa.* Cham, Switzerland: Springer International Publishing. The book explains the health situation in Africa.
- Collin, J., and Lee, K. (2005). *Global change and health.* New York: McGraw Hill. The books discusses how global changes affect human health on a global scale.
- Labonté, R. and Arne Ruckert, A. (2019). Globalization as a "determinant of the determinants of health". In: *Health equity in a globalizing era: past challenges, future prospects.* Oxford: Oxford University Press. doi:10.1093/oso/9780198835356.003.0002. The chapter relies on two different frameworks to unpack globalization processes as meta-determinants of health inequities within and between nations.
- Lee, K. (2003). Health impacts of globalization: Towards global governance. London: Palgrave Macmillan. The book relies on specific case studies to discuss the impact of globalization on health.
- Stevens, H., and Huys, I. (2017). Innovative approaches to increase access to medicines in developing countries. *Frontiers in Medicine, 4,* 218. doi:10.3389/fmed.2017.00218. The article documents the problematic access to medicines in the developing world and how to improve it.

References

Ahmadiani, S., & Nikfar, S. (2016). Challenges of access to medicine and the responsibility of pharmaceutical companies: A legal perspective. *Daru: Journal of Faculty of Pharmacy, 24*(1), 13. doi: 10.1186/s40199-016-0151-z.

Amzat, J. (2009). Assessing the progress towards millennium development goals in Nigeria. In Olutayo, A. O., Ogundiya, I. S. & Amzat, J. (Eds.), *State and Civil Society Relations in Nigeria* (pp. 290–309). Ibadan: Hope Publications.

Amzat, J., & Razum, O. (2018). Rural health in Africa. In *Towards a Sociology of Health Discourse in Africa.* Cham, Switzerland: Springer International Publishing. doi: 10.1007/978-3-319-61672-8_8.

Blomqvist, H. C., & Lundahl M. (2002). *The Distorted Economy.* London: Palgrave Macmillan.

Brownell, K. D., & Yach, D. (2006). Lessons from a small country about the global obesity crisis. *Globalization and Health, 2,* 11. doi: 10.1186/1744-8603-2-11.

Chatora, R. R., & Tumusime, P. (2004). Primary health care: A review of its implementation in sub-Saharan Africa. *Primary Health Care Research and Development, 5,* 296–306.

Collins, T. (2003). Globalization, global health, and access to healthcare. *International Journal of Health Planning & Management, 18*(2), 97–104.

Cueto, M. (2004). The origins of primary health care and selective primary health care. *American Journal of Public Health, 94*(11), 1864–1874. doi: 10.2105/ajph.94.11.1864.

Economic Commission for Latin America and the Caribbean (ECLAC) (2015). Latin America and the Caribbean: Looking ahead after the millennium development goals. In *Regional Monitoring Report on the Millennium Development Goals in Latin America and the Caribbean*, 2015 (LC/G.2646), Santiago, Chile: ECLAC.

Global Burden of Disease Health Financing Collaborator Network (GBDHFCN) (2018). Trends in future health financing and coverage: Future health spending and universal health coverage in 188 countries, 2016–2040. *Lancet, 391*, 1783–98.

GBDHFCN (2019). Past, present, and future of global health financing: A review of development assistance, government, out-of-pocket, and other private spending on health for 195 countries, 1995–2050. *Lancet, 393*, 2233–2260.

International Conference on Primary Health Care (ICPHC) {[1978: Alma-Ata, USSR}], World Health Organization (WHO), & United Nations Children's Fund (UNICEF) ([1978)[. Primary health care: Report of the international conference on primary health care, Alma-Ata, USSR, 6-12 September 1978/jointly sponsored by the World Health Organization and the United Nations Children's Fund. Geneva: World Health Organization. https://apps.who.int/iris/handle/10665/39228. Accessed on October 24, 2019.

James, P. B., Wardle, J., Steel. A. & Adams, J. (2018). Traditional, complementary and alternative medicine use in Sub-Saharan Africa: A systematic review. *BMJ Global Health*, 3, e000895.

Labonté, R., Mohindra, K. & Schrecker, T. (2011). The growing impact of globalization for health and public health practice. *Annual Review of Public Health, 32*(1), 263–283.

Lipton, M. (1977). *Why Poor People Stay Poor: Urban Bias in World Development*. London: Temple Smith.

Lorenz, N. (2007). Effectiveness of global health partnerships: Will the past repeat itself? *Bulletin of the World Health Organization, 85*(7), 567–568.

Mahler, H. (2016). The meaning of "Health for All by the Year 2000". *American Journal of Public Health, 106*(1), 36–38. doi: 10.2105/AJPH.2016.106136.

MDG Monitor (2016). MDG progress report of Asia and the Pacific in 2015. www.mdgmonitor.org/mdg -progress-report-asia-the-pacific-2015/. Accessed on October 23, 2019.

Miseda, M. H., Were, S. O., Murianki, C. A., Mutuku, M. P. & Mutwiwa, S. N. (2017). The implication of the shortage of health workforce specialist on universal health coverage in Kenya. *Human Resources for Health, 15*(1), 80. doi: 10.1186/s12960-017-0253-9.

Mpinga, E. K., Kandolo, T., Verloo, H., Bukonda, N. K. Z., Kandala, N. & Chastonay, P. (2013). Traditional/alternative medicines and the right to health: Key elements for a convention on global health. *Health and Human Rights Journal, 15*(1), E44–57.

Naicker, S., Plange-Rhule, J., Tutt, R. C. & Eastwood, J. B. (2009). Shortage of healthcare workers in developing countries: Africa. *Ethnicity & Disease, 19*(Suppl 1), S1-60-4.

Nye, J. (2002). Globalism versus globalization. www.theglobalist.com/globalism-versus-globalization/ Accessed on July 17, 2019.

Ortiz-Ospina, E., & Roser, M. (2019). Financing healthcare. Published online at *OurWorldInData.org*. Retrieved from: https://ourworldindata.org/financing-healthcare. Accessed on October 28, 2019.

Peltzer, K., & Pengpid, S. (2015). Utilization and practice of traditional/complementary/alternative medicine (T/CAM) in Southeast Asian Nations (ASEAN) Member States. *Studies on Ethno-Medicine, 9*(2), 209–218. doi: 10.1080/09735070.2015.11905437.

Ramírez, N. A., Ruiz, J. P., Romero, R. V. & Labonté, R. (2011). Comprehensive primary health care in South America: Contexts, achievements and policy implications. *Cad. Saúde Pública, Rio de Janeiro, 27*(10), 1875–1890.

Ritzer, G. (2003). Rethinking globalization: Glocalization/grobalization and something/nothing. *Sociological Theory, 21*(3), 193–209.

Ritzer, G. (2018). *McDonaldization of Society: Into the Digital Age* (9th ed.). London: Sage.

Savedoff, W. D., de Ferranti, D., Smith, A. L. & Fan, V. (2012). Political and economic aspects of the transition to universal health coverage. *Lancet, 380*, 924–932.

Scheil-Adlung, X., & ILO (2015). *Global Evidence on Inequities in Rural Health Protection: New Data on Rural Deficits in Health Coverage for 174 Countries*. Extension of Social Security series; No 47. Geneva: International Labour Office, Social Protection Department.

Shim, J., & Kim, J. (2018). Cross-national differences in the holistic use of traditional East Asian medicine in East Asia. *Health Promotion International*, *33*(3), 536–544. doi: 10.1093/heapro/daw089.

Stevens, H., & Huys, I. (2017). Innovative approaches to increase access to medicines in developing countries. *Frontiers in Medicine*, *4*, 218. doi: 10.3389/fmed.2017.00218.

United Nations (UN) (2007). *Millennium Development Goals Report 2007*. New York: UN.

United Nations Economic Commission for Africa (UNECA) (2015). *Assessing Progress in Africa towards the Millennium Development Goals*. Addis Ababa: Economic Commission of Africa.

van Weel C., Kassai, R., Qidwai, W., Kumar, R., Bala, K., Gupta, P. P., Haniffa, R., Hewageegana, N. R., Ranasinghe, T., Kidd, M. & Howe, A. (2016). Primary healthcare policy implementation in South Asia. *BMJ Global Health*, *1*, e000057. doi: 10.1136/bmjgh-2016- 000057.

Wallerstein, I. M. (2004). *World-systems Analysis: An Introduction*. Durham, NC: Duke University Press.

World Health Organization (WHO) (1981). *Global Strategy for Health for All by the Year 2000*. Geneva: WHO.

WHO (2003). *A Global Review of Primary Health Care: Emerging Messages*. Geneva: WHO.

WHO (2005). *National Policy on Traditional Medicine and Regulation of Herbal Medicine: Report of a WHO Global Survey*. Geneva: WHO.

WHO (2013). *WHO Traditional Medicine Strategy: 2014–2023*. Geneva: WHO.

WHO (2015). *Health in 2015: From MDGs, Millennium Development Goals to SDGs, Sustainable Development Goals*. Geneva: WHO.

WHO (2016). *Health Workforce Requirements for Universal Health Coverage and the Sustainable Development Goals*. Geneva: WHO.

WHO (2017). *Ten Years in Public Health, 2007–2017: Report by D.r Margaret Chan, Director-General, World Health Organization*. Geneva: WHO.

WHO-Africa (2013). Enhancing the role of traditional medicine in health system: A strategy for the African Region. In Report of Secretariat on Regional Committee Meeting, Brazzaville, Republic of Congo, 2–6 September 2013. Brazzaville: WHO.

Zhang, D., & Unschuld, P. U. (2008). China's barefoot doctor: Past, present, and future. *Lancet*, *372*(9653), 1865–1867. doi: 10.1016/S0140- 6736(08)61355-0.

11 Global Health Initiatives in the Global South

11.1 Introduction

There are critical challenges to improving healthcare situations in low- and middle-income countries. Despite these challenges, there has been a gradual improvement in meeting the healthcare needs of people living in relatively poor settings. There is always a need to harness local knowledge and draw up strategies or initiatives that would be adaptable to settings in the developing world. While advanced technologies will help, most times, the solutions do not lie solely in sophisticated technologies. The essence of primary healthcare (PHC) is to use methods and techniques that are sustainable and adaptable within the socio-economic context of the concerned areas. Drawing up initiatives or innovations in resource-constrained societies might be challenging, but it requires a simple solution with a blend of adaptable technologies. Predominant rural communities bear the burden of infectious disease because they are underserved with health facilities and public health measures. Where there are health facilities, human resources and equipment might be inadequate. The general situation of healthcare only holds promise, but it is still inadequate in meeting the health needs of the general population in resource-constrained settings.

The African region bears the substantial brunt of morbidity and mortality from infectious diseases, which, unlike noncommunicable diseases, are curable. Malaria, tuberculosis (TB) and human immunodeficiency virus (HIV) continue to take their toll on the population health in low-income countries. The African region also bears the considerable burden of pneumonia, diarrhea and measles. The burden of child and maternal mortality is also relatively high. Even within Africa, sub-Saharan Africa bears more of a burden than other regions of Africa and the Global South, including inadequate access to medicines, limited health spending and urban bias in healthcare, among others. Increasing rates of NCDs in Africa present fundamental challenges to the health system. The Asian region also portends a similar health situation as Africa (see Chapters 5 and 6), but is perhaps slightly better off on some indicators. There are still pressing issues to improve the healthcare situation in Asia, particularly around TB, HIV and stroke. In general, middle-income countries are faring better than low-income countries. The differential burden (or health inequalities) within the Global South is not surprising since income itself is a significant determinant of health. The state of development also accounts for the situation of healthcare. The social determinants of health are better in high-income countries. Therefore, the state of development shapes the situation of healthcare.

In the last few years, some improvements have been recorded around the world in the situation of healthcare. There has been some reduction in the burden of morbidity and mortality through concerted efforts. The health goals of the SDGs have been set—all regions must collaborate to achieve the targets by 2030. There is still considerable optimism around meeting the targets, but considerable initiatives and innovation will be required to reduce health risks

DOI: 10.4324/9781003247975-11

and help people to meet their healthcare needs. Different initiatives have started, and some success is recorded. Consolidating on such an initiatives has the potential to improve the situation further. Stakeholders must move beyond wishful thinking and engage in practical initiatives in the delivery of healthcare. It is essential to examine some crucial initiatives that have had considerable health impacts or that hold some promise in improving healthcare in the Global South.

11.2 Understanding Global Health Initiatives

One primary aim of global health initiatives (GHIs) is to mobilize global stakeholders and communities to achieve set goals. While the community is at the macro level, it has great potentials for micro-mobilization, so that every individual will subscribe to the project or policy plan. The prevailing ideology or slogan is that "no one should be left out". When it comes to population health, every individual should count. The ideas of innovation in the Global South are, therefore, not about highly mechanized or sophisticated technologies, but actions that prove effective in addressing the common health needs and reaching the maximum number of people. It is not misplaced to conclude that most fundamental health needs are in the areas of controlling risk factors (for both infections and noncommunicable diseases). In recent years, most efforts have focused on maternal and child health (MCH), including immunization, HIV, TB, malaria, diarrhea and access to essential health services in general.

Global health initiatives constitute collaborative efforts to improve global health. Although often poorly conceived in terms of humanitarian activities, the initiatives hold promise in improving global health through the provision of essential resources (both material and nonmaterial), notably in resource-constrained settings. Provision of healthcare should not merely be conceived as a charity; perhaps an attempt to make it a responsibility will improve political commitment at the global level to extend initiatives on a global scale. Taking on such responsibility or not largely depends on the ideological orientation used in the global health policy of different nations (see Section 8.3). Despite the foregoing, global health initiatives are still viewed through the flowing of humanitarian aid, especially to low- and middle-income countries. GHIs are often conceived of in terms of development aid. Therefore, the success of an initiative is defined by the amount the development partners are willing to earmark for that initiative. It is in this realm that Mwisongo and Nabyonga-Orem (2016) observed that there had been some improvements in population health in LMICs in the last few decades, due to interventions from development partners.

Mwisongo and Nabyonga-Orem (2016) summarized the characteristics of GHIs, some of which are reflected in the definition of global health (see Section 2.2). The GHIs address health issues of global concern because they target several countries. Many health problems transcend national boundaries and are thus global health problems. They are of global significance not merely because of global vulnerabilities/risks, but in the interest of maintaining a healthy world. The broader geographical coverage is a significant attribute of global health initiatives. Many of their initiatives have been on the frontlines in ensuring that resources are available to reduce the burden of specific diseases around the globe. The GHIs link people, partners and organizations. Concerted efforts require pooling resources from all quarters to address health problems. The initiative must bring together all actors to achieve the set goals; there is power in working together. Therefore, GHI is a domain of state and non-state actors, including individuals and private organizations, with commitments in resolving global health issues.

Furthermore, while there are many health problems and issues, numerous initiatives are defined by a specialized focus on specific diseases or selected interventions, commodities or services (Mwisongo and Nabyonga-Orem, 2016). Most initiatives are specific to a particular area of intervention. The domain of global politics defines priority setting and determines which problem gets what amount of resources and why. Global politics define the frame in terms of the problem and identification of networks and actors willing to commit resources. For some organizations, child immunization is a priority, while for others, it might be family planning. The (global health) actors are usually with profound interests, which influence the strategies to be deployed in managing any health issue. For instance, GAVI is a major vaccine alliance dedicated to promoting the well-being of children through access to vaccinations. The International Planned Parenthood Federation (IPPF) is specifically committed to reproductive health services on a global scale. The IPPF also attracts grants from other global bodies and actors to pursue its missions. Mwisongo and Nabyonga-Orem (2016) observed that another significant characteristic of a global health initiative is the ability to generate resources. One of the hallmarks of health initiatives is that they require large amounts of material and non-material resources. It is thus an initiative as far as it attracts the required resources to address health problems around the globe with particular consideration for LMICs.

In essence, the GHIs have been a significant factor in the aid environment, with the mission to alleviate certain suffering across the globe (Crux and McPake, 2011). Inadequate material and non-material resources constitute a significant impediment in meeting the healthcare needs in various quarters, especially in low-income countries, with the opportunity to provide needed resources and engage state actors. The initiatives often function in the form of global public–private health partnerships, which have now become an essential means of financing and ameliorating disease burden (Buse and Harmer, 2007). Therefore, the initiatives are also considered to be institutionalized partnerships, also known as global health partnerships (GHPs). Buse and Harmer (2007) also acknowledged that partnerships bring concerned new actors, resources, business models and a sense of urgency to addressing health problems.

Buse and Harmer (2007) highlighted some of the critical value that GHIs add to the ever-continuing global health efforts. Initiatives help to project health issues onto the national and global agenda. Initiatives help to renew national interest in prioritizing health problems with the hope of gaining support from various partnerships. Buse and Harmer (2007) noted that GHIs have been able to raise the profile of specific diseases on policy agendas by concentrating on brand-building and public relations. Initiatives often attract attention to specific health problems through advocacy and solicitation of commitments from various partners. For instance, the Global Fund and Roll Back Malaria champion sustained efforts in the fight against malaria, with some remarkable results recorded. The significant implication is that the various initiatives help to influence health policy directions and healthcare resource allocations in various countries. The dominant argument is about priority setting, and in healthcare, choices must be made because of the countless health problems in the face of insufficient resources to tackle all simultaneously. The primary added value is the continuous argumentation of healthcare capacity in various settings—otherwise, some of those services and support might not be available.

Another major area of support has been in research and development (R&D). The availability of funds also stimulates research into various diseases. R&D is crucial in meeting future healthcare needs, primarily through the development of technologies, innovations and interventions or solutions. The development of medicines and vaccines is a significant area that requires continuous funding to meet global health needs. Beyond the development of medical technologies, there is also a continuous need to fund applied research needed to identify practices that improve outcomes and to learn how to implement effective practices, not only within the community but also in clinical care (Lieu and Platt, 2017). It is not enough to just develop the technologies; applied research in delivering the technologies and services to the communities is important as well. The overall goal is often to make health interventions and services reach the underserved (Buse and Harmer, 2007). The initiatives have, over the years, provided health interventions and services in remote places in very cost-effective manners. As such, many initiatives serve as models for bringing health to hard-to-reach regions or areas with limited ability to pay.

11.2.1 Roll Back Malaria (RBM)

The Roll Back Malaria (RBM), sometimes called RBM Partnership to End Malaria, is a global initiative devoted to the control of malaria, a primary infectious disease of underdevelopment or poverty. The initiative was launched in 1998 (in New York) to coordinate action against malaria, with the ultimate vision of ensuring a malaria-free world. As previously mentioned, one of the crucial strategies of a global initiative is to mobile support and resources. The RBM action started with in-country and cross-countries consultations. Since its inception, it has attracted over 500 partners, including community health workers, scientists and other private actors (RBM, 2019). Malaria is prevalent in many countries in Asia, the Pacific, the Americas, Middle East and Africa. Apart from sub-Saharan Africa (SSA), India, Indonesia, Myanmar, Pakistan and Papua New Guinea still account for a considerable burden of malaria (WHO and RBM, 2012). There has been increasing progress in most parts of the world; since its inception, the RBM (2019) claimed to have recorded remarkable progress against malaria with a reduction of malaria deaths by 60% and over 7 million lives saved. The RBM also reported that more countries are malaria-free than ever before, and 44 countries report less than 10,000 malaria cases. The ultimate effort is toward increased investment to ensure malaria elimination. The *World Malaria Report 2018*, drawing on data from 87 malaria-endemic countries, estimated about 219 million cases and 435,000 related deaths in 2017 (with children under-5 years old accounting for 61%). The African region accounts for 92%, Southeast Asia region 5% and the Eastern Mediterranean Region 2% (WHO, 2018). The Malaria burden is heaviest (80%) in 5 countries, including Nigeria (25%), Congo DR (11%), Mozambique (5%), India (4%) and Uganda (4%) (WHO, 2018).

Malaria parasites are transmitted to humans by the bite of Anopheles mosquitoes. While the disease is preventable and curable, the emergence of drug resistance to previously effective drugs was a significant turning point in malaria control. Simply put, malaria drug resistance is a situation whereby certain drugs previously used in the treatment of malaria become ineffective or inefficacious in curing the disease. Such has been the case with chloroquine (CQ) in the treatment of malaria, especially *falciparum* malaria. The first report of failures of CQ to cure *falciparum* malaria came out of Venezuela in 1960 (Wernsdorfer and Payne, 1991), and in Africa (Kenya) in 1977 (Fogh et al., 1979). By 1989, CQ resistance had been reported in most sub-Saharan countries. Due to growing chloroquine resistance, the world has had to switch to artemisinin-based combination treatment (ACT) in the first-line treatment of malaria (Laxminarayan, 2004). Although ACT is highly effective, partial drug resistance has also been reported (WHO, 2018). The primary preventive measure is the use of insecticide-treated bed nets (ITN), first unveiled in Nigeria in the year 2000. Preventive health management advocates self-responsibility in health management, whereby people are expected to accept and use prevention means.

Most malaria-endemic African countries were incorporated into the Roll Back Malaria initiative in the year 2000, following a RBM summit in Abuja, Nigeria, at which April 25 was declared Africa Malaria Day. As of 2008, April 25 is now World Malaria Day. Participants at the summit reported that the burden of malaria had slowed economic growth in Africa. Africa leaders resolved to halve the burden of malaria by 2010 by pursuing RBM objectives through the implementation of its six critical elements. The WHO (2000) highlighted the critical elements, including: (i) Evidence-based decisions using surveillance-appropriate responses and building community awareness; (ii) rapid diagnosis and treatment close to, or at, home; (iii) multiple forms of prevention, using insecticide-treatment mosquito nets and making pregnancy safer; (iv) focused research to develop new medicines, vaccines and insecticides, and to help epidemiological, operational activities and social science research on how to influence the behavior of those requiring treatments; (v) well-coordinated actions for strengthening existing health services and policies and providing technical support; and (v) harmonize actions to build a dynamic global movement.

Again, the RBM initiative has made marked progress, with a considerable reduction in death rates between 2010 and 2017 occurring in Southeast Asia (54%), Africa (40%) and the Eastern Mediterranean (10%) (WHO, 2018). Also, Southeast Asia has made up to a 59% reduction in malaria incidence between 2010 and 2017. The Americas, on the other hand, recorded an increase, especially in three countries (Brazil, Nicaragua and Venezuela); and in the African region, after initial progress, the prevalence remained stable at 219 cases per 1,000 of the population in 2017. The RBM also subscribed to the SDGs goals concerning malaria control. In 2015, the RBM launched a new initiative called Action and Investment for a Malaria-free world (AIM) to defeat Malaria by 2030 (RBM, 2019). Between AIM and the SDGs, the targets are to: (i) Reduce malaria incidence and mortality rates globally by at least 90% compared with 2015 levels; (ii) eliminate malaria in 35 countries; and (iii) prevent re-establishment of malaria in all malaria-free countries. Achieving the set goals requires the RMB to reverse the dwindling funding to fight malaria, especially in high-burden countries. Remarkable success has been made in the development of vaccines. With vaccines and more funding, there is great potential to achieve the set goals within the time limit.

11.2.2 Global Fund to Fight AIDS, TB and Malaria (GFATM)

The Global Fund to Fight AIDS, Tuberculosis (TB) and Malaria (also known as the Global Fund), founded in 2002, has been a frontline global health initiative. As the name implies, it is committed to accelerating the end of three infectious diseases: AIDS, TB and Malaria. Unlike RBM, the Global Fund is a funding mechanism, i.e., a financier of health projects across the globe. Its method is to support partners working to improve health conditions across the globe. As of mid-2019, the initiative has expended over US$40 billion (Global Fund, 2019). The initiative now mobilizes more than US$4 billion annually to support over 100 local partners and initiatives. The initiative began at a challenging moment in global health history, in which the trio of AIDS, TB and malaria were devastating populations worldwide. The dawn of the millennium was the terminal period for the global movement for "Health for All", which could not be met due to some challenges, including an inadequate coordinated pool of funds to pursue the vision, among other issues. The period also marked the inception of the millennium development goals (MDGs), including three primary health goals.

The health devastation (caused by AIDS, TB and malaria) was overwhelming. For instance, in the early 2000s, malaria was responsible for up to a million deaths and an estimated 300–500 million cases every year (Bloland et al., 2000; Nuwaha, 2001; Amzat and Omololu, 2009; Amzat, 2011). The Global Fund is also focused on ending the HIV pandemic, another global health problem. Roser and Ritchie (2019) observed a drastic increase in HIV incidence and deaths in the 1990s—with a peak of around 3.5 million new cases in 1997, followed by a gradual decline to less than 2 million in 2017. HIV mortality also increased throughout the 1990s, with a peak at an average of 1.95 million deaths in 2006. The number of deaths is around 950,000 as of 2017. The heaviest burden of HIV (among 15–49 years old) is in Southern Africa: 23.8% in Lesotho, 22.8% in Botswana, 18.8% in South Africa, 13.3% in Zimbabwe, 12.5% in Mozambique, 12.1% in Namibia and 11.5% in Zambia (Roser and Ritchie, 2019). The significant global investment in

HIV/AIDS focuses on HIV prevention and access to treatment. HIV prevention, especially the use of condoms during sexual intercourse, has substantially improved but remains a significant challenge in many regions. Access to treatment has also improved substantially and helped to avert millions of deaths. As in the case of malaria, more resources are still urgently required to end the HIV pandemic.

The Global Fund also focuses on TB control. The incidence of TB had also reached a critical level in the early 2000s in every part of the world. Dollin et al. (1994) forecasted a rapid global rise in tuberculosis-related morbidity and mortality between 1990 and 1999, with about 88 million new cases of TB (about 10% of which would be attributable to HIV infection) and 30 million deaths. This forecast worked out to over eight million cases and three million deaths every year within that period. Corbett et al. (2003) confirmed the new incidence of about 8.3 million in the year 2000, but the reported mortality was "only" about 1.8 million. Corbett et al. (2003) also reported that the HIV pandemic exacerbated the global TB control efforts because of co-infection. Therefore, the control of HIV-related TB in areas of high HIV prevalence is of vital importance. As in the case of malaria, the emergence of drug resistance also posed a major challenge to the global efforts in TB control. The pace of progress in the control of TB has been very slow, with an annual decrease of 2% in TB incidence (WHO, 2019a). While some drops in morbidity and mortality have been recorded, greater effort is required to end the scourge of TB. For instance, as of 2016, there were still up to 1.7 million deaths, with the Africa region accounting for up to 25% and about 2.5 million new cases in Africa (WHO, 2019a). It is further reported that eight countries (namely, India, Indonesia, China, the Philippines, Pakistan, Bangladesh, Nigeria and South Africa) accounted for two-thirds of new cases in 2018—44% of new cases in Southeast Asia, 24% in Africa, 18% in Western Pacific and the remaining 14% occurred in the rest of the world in 2015 (WHO, 2019b). In total, the Global South accounts for over 90% of TB cases and deaths. Despite the slow pace in the control efforts, some considerable achievements have also been made, with about 53 million lives saved between 2000 and 2015. One of the health targets of the SGDs is to end the TB epidemics by 2030.

Despite the prevailing challenges, The Global Fund deserves credit for the considerable progress made thus far in the control of AIDS, TB and malaria. The disbursement of funds has, remarkably, focused on low-income countries; between 2017 and mid-2019: 72% in SSA, 3% in the Middle East and North Africa, 3% in Eastern Europe and Central Asia, 20% in Asia and the Pacific, and 2% in Latin America and the Caribbean (Global Fund, 2019). The Global Fund prides itself on three major principles: Partnerships, country ownership and performance-based funding. The global initiative is about supporting local initiatives (of government and non-state actors, including civil societies and technical partners) to respond to the challenges. Disbursement of the fund is based on the effectiveness and outcomes of programs and strategies, which sometimes support home-grown solutions.

11.2.3 Global Alliance for Vaccines and Immunizations

The Global Alliance for Vaccines and Immunizations (GAVI, also officially known as Gavi) is a major public–private health initiative focusing on vaccination of children against common childhood diseases. Gavi was launched in the year 2000 as a replacement for the Children's Vaccines Initiative previously established in 1990. GAVI attracts both material and non-material resources from various global health partners and state actors to promote vaccination, especially in countries with limited resources (Gavi, 2018). There have always been challenges relating to the immunization of children in low-income countries. The situation has left several million children uncovered by essential infant immunizations. The primary mission is to make vaccines more available, accessible and affordable, and coordinate efforts to achieve the mission. Common vaccine-preventable diseases of children include diphtheria, pertussis (whooping cough), polio, hepatitis B and measles, among others. It is highly recommended that every child receives the shots in order to fortify their immune system against common childhood diseases. The promise of vaccination is that diseases can be eradicated (once such diseases are vaccine-preventable) through global coverage of the immunization program. Success is possible; smallpox was eradicated globally in (May 8) 1980 (Tognotti, 2010), and the world is currently at the tail-end of eradicating poliomyelitis (Razum et al., 2019).

There are still up to 1.5 million vaccine-preventable deaths (VPDs) every year, although this does represent a decline from 5.1 million in 1990 (Vanderslott and Roser, 2019). There has been a remarkable decline in measles-related deaths from 2.7 million annually (before 1963) to 95,000 deaths in 2017 (Vanderslott and Roser, 2019). The same level of success has been recorded against other VPDs such as pertussis and tetanus. Despite the achievements, there are still up to 19.5 million infants at risk of VPDs because of a lack of or limited access to essential vaccines. Incomplete dosage or missed schedules of immunization, often considered as under-vaccination, are global concerns. Vaccine hesitancy—delay in acceptance or refusal of vaccination despite the availability of vaccination services—is also of global concern (MacDonald and SageVH, 2015). Apart from other determinants of vaccination such as limited supply and political issues, there is (re)emerging deliberate withdrawal from vaccines due to specific fears (including perceived risk), beliefs, ignorance or poor public understanding, mistrust or skepticism, rumors and other speculative reasons (Ogundele et al., 2020).

Global inequalities exist in childhood immunizations between the Global North and South—also within the Global South (low- and middle-income countries)—and between the urban and rural areas in low-income countries (see WHO, 2016; Vanderslott and Roser, 2019). Over the years, although the inequality gap has been closing, challenges remain. There continue to be countries in SSA (e.g., Chad, Central African Republic, South Sudan, Guinea and Somalia) with less than 50% childhood vaccination coverage. Children in difficult circumstances, such as disasters and conflicts, are often not adequately covered. There are global concerns about vaccine coverage in many conflict-ridden regions of Venezuela, Colombia, Syria, Afghanistan, Iraq, Somalia, Cameroun, Nigeria, South Sudan and Libya, among others. There is also some mistrust and skepticism regarding vaccination across the world including Liberia (28%), France (18%), Nigeria (16%), Namibia (16%), Peru (15%), Uganda (14%), Indonesia (12%), Togo (12%) and Gabon (12%) (Vanderslott and Roser, 2019). Depending on the population of each of the countries, the percentage translates to millions of individuals who might (potentially) widen the vaccination gaps. Public campaigns and information could be effective to ward off the skepticism.

The success recorded so far is also a result of concerted efforts. As previously mentioned, immunization gaps still exist, with millions of children unvaccinated or under-vaccinated, especially in LMICs. The challenge is also surmountable as the global initiative to improve vaccination is getting more robust within the global health context. Gavi continues to promise (and might likely achieve) greater vaccine coverage by 2030. Vaccination coverage was 80% as of 2017 in Gavi-supported countries, with the hope of getting to 84% in 2020 (Gavi, 2018). With the progression toward 2030 in the context of SDGs, there is a strong possibility of reaching up to 90% (or more) of vaccination coverage at the national level and 80% at all districts to keep the VPDs to the barest minimum. The critical area in the global vaccination efforts is about the vulnerability of the existing gains. There are constant threats of complacency—skepticism and mistrust about the effectiveness of vaccines, and new waves of vaccine hesitancy in both the Global South and North.

11.2.4 Global Alliance for Improved Nutrition (GAIN)

The Global Alliance for Improved Nutrition (GAIN), founded in 2002, is a major initiative working to eradicate malnutrition in poor settings, especially among children. The initiative is a platform that coordinates actions and brings together major players in the area of nutrition. The initiative also attracts funding for other stakeholders with interest in bridging nutrition inequalities around the world. "No child should go to bed hungry" was an earlier slogan developed as the objective of the World Food Conference of 1974. Malnutrition constitutes a significant problem around the world, especially in low-income countries. Food production is depleting in the face of population growth. Unfortunately, the regions with a relatively higher population growth bear the brunt of malnutrition. The population figures of those countries become a burden in the face of the low carrying capacity of those countries. Population growth becomes a problem when there is no commensurate economic progress. In line with the Malthusian perspective, when the population outgrows the food production, it leads to crises such as pestilence and famine. Children are often the worst hit by a food crisis; while adults have some capacity to fend for food, children are highly dependent on the adult population for food. Even those still taking breastmilk can only get the required nutrients when the adult mother is adequately fed. Before venturing into some of the gains of GAIN, it is important to assess the world food crisis.

The world food crisis is a global reality, adversely affecting global health. Poverty prevents many households from accessing adequate food. Most households in the low-income region are primarily agrarian, on a low-scale, usually with outdated equipment. Most farmers are affected by seasonal changes since there are often limited technologies to support agricultural production during the dry season. The result is sometimes that of seasonal famine or poverty. Ritchie (1986) predicted that by the year 2000, there would be a shortage of land and water in 64 countries, thereby requiring food aid. At the same time, improved maternal and child health would lead to an increase in child survival and, subsequently, an increase in the world population, especially in low-income countries.

By the year 2000, the dawn of the launch of the MDGs, over 800 million people were chronically undernourished, 95% of whom were living in the Global South (FOA, 2000). One of the MGDs aimed to halve the burden of hunger between the years 2000 and 2015. By 2010, an estimated 926 million were still undernourished, constituting about 16% of the population of developing countries (FAO, 2010). While there was an improvement in the real percentage, population growth meant that a higher absolute number of people were living with hunger. Global undernourishment as of 2010 showed global inequalities, with Asia and the Pacific accounting for 578 million, SSA 239 million, Latin and the Caribbean 53 million, and the Near East and North Africa 37 million, while the developed world accounted for 19 million (FAO, 2010). The prevalence of hunger declined from 20% in the early 1990s to 16% in 2010.

At the end of the MDG timeline (the end of 2015), about 793 million people were undernourished (FAO, IFAD and WFP, 2015), which represented a decline of 133 million, despite population growth. There have been some improvements in the developing world, but conflict and economic crises in some states have adversely affected progress. More than 60 countries were unable to halve the burden of hunger (FAO et al., 2015). Following the realization of the extent of world hunger and the potential for its rise in the next few decades, the world has been making efforts to end hunger by 2030. Currently, poor nutrition is responsible for nearly half of child mortality, amounting to over three million deaths each year. As of 2018, over 149 million children under-5 years old were chronically undernourished (UN, 2019).

It is not just about access to food, but about required micronutrients for healthy living. Hence, GAIN launched a global fortification program in 2003 and, within a decade, reached 610 million people with nutritionally enhanced food (Moench-Pfanner and Ameringen, 2012).

Micronutrient malnutrition (of iodine, vitamin A, iron and B vitamins, among others) accounts for up to 7.3% of the global burden of disease (WHO and FAO, 2006). It has been estimated that more than 2 billion people suffer from micronutrient deficiencies. Food fortification with micronutrients is a valid technology for reducing micronutrient malnutrition (WHO and FAO, 2006). GAIN focuses on two separate but related areas—improving access to food and to required micronutrients. The initiative aims at reaching one billion people with improved nutritious food by 2022 (GAIN, 2019). The goal is attainable by continually improving the availability and affordability of nutritious food, while simultaneously stimulating consumer demand. GAIN also works to improve market incentives and regulations that will enhance the production and consumption of required nutritious food (GAIN, 2019). GAIN is a frontline initiative working with other global agencies (including FAO and the World Food Program, among others) to ensure a world without hunger by 2030.

11.2.5 Global Health Council

The Global Health Council (GHC), formerly called the National Council of International Health, founded in 1972, is a private non-profit US-based organization involved in alleviating global health problems. The council has a relatively broad vision, from advocacy to policy. It aims to improve healthcare management by focusing on several health issues and the coordination of various stakeholders to improve health investment and global health outcomes. Specifically, it aims to advocate within the US and multilateral forums for improved and sustainable global health policies and resources; organize and mobilize stakeholders across all sectors and regions to advance support for global health programs; and intensify concern for global health to improve global well-being (GHC, 2019). The council's vision requires more efforts and coordination across an extensive range of concerns within global health. The priority areas of the council, however, include child health, women's health, HIV/AIDS, infectious diseases, emerging health threats and health systems.

In most developing countries, health systems are too weak to accommodate the burden of disease (Orach, 2009). This is primarily due to problems of availability and affordability; inequalities in access to healthcare explain the inequalities in morbidity and mortality. Strong advocacy is needed to ensure fairness and equity in the provision of healthcare, especially in the Global South. The state of the health system is a social determinant of health reflected in the implementation and effectiveness of health policies across various regions (Orach, 2009). The GHC works in the area of health system strengthening, to ensure equitable distribution of healthcare. The focus on women's health also supports global concerns about the gender dimension in healthcare and outcomes. The artificial character of risk distribution in the name of gender norms, among other social determinants, is a global concern (Amzat and Grandi, 2011; Amzat, 2015). In most regions of the South, women's healthcare needs and expectations are underprioritized.

For the GHC, the starting point is looking inward at the US government and agencies to prioritize global health issues. The primary focus of their advocacy is to stimulate the US government to provide leadership in global health through the allocation of resources to address global health concerns. It is important to generate some local voices to influence US foreign policy to fill some global health voids, especially in developing countries. The US is a global leader in health initiatives around the world. The primary hope or projection is that the US could use its powerful position to take more responsibilities in ensuring global health equity. The priorities of GHC significantly reflect the priorities of the US global health initiatives focusing on HIV/AIDS, maternal and child health, sexual and reproductive health, and emerging global health threats. Most of the mentioned health issues have embedded gender dimensions; hence, the women-centered approach is a core principle in US-led global health initiatives across the Global South. The USAID is often in the lead in addressing global health concerns, for example, through Child Survival Call to Action. The President's Emergency Plan for AIDS Relief (PEPFAR) and the Presidential Malaria Initiative (PMI) have also made some remarkable achievements in reducing the burden of HIV and malaria, respectively. The initiatives are in addition to contributions to other global health bodies (such as GAVI). One important initiative in the US is the InterAction, an umbrella network of international non-government organizations working to alleviate global suffering in all spheres of life. With over 200 members, InterAction mobilizes toward collective efforts to addressing global challenges (InterAction, 2013).

The GHC is also interested in closing the gaps between policy and practice in global health. There are known best practices, woven into various policies, that, if implemented, would improve population health both at the community and the global level. The observable loop-holes lie in the implementation of those policies. The GHC is a platform advocating for "voice for action", stepping beyond the policy to the actual implementation of actions on global health issues. The strategy is toward community engagement in delivering global healthcare. The various communities of the grassroots, professional, vulnerable groups, political leaders and faith-based leaders, among other actors, must be fully engaged in the efforts to deliver global health goods. The notion of engagement also brings to the forefront the notion of accountability within the global health campaign. There should be accountability in global health considera-tion; accountability involves multipolar relationships, responsibility, transparency, participa-tion and fairness (Bruen et al., 2014). In the context of the goals of GHC, the US must be accountable and stimulate cooperation from partners in ensuring a healthy world.

11.3 Major Challenges of Global Health Initiatives

The previous section (11.2) has only examined five of the major global health initiatives, but there are many more. In the wake of the MDGs, the year 1999–2002 marked the beginning of many global health initiatives. The Multi-country HIV/AIDS Program (MAP), established in 1999, is an initiative of the World Bank, devoted to the fight against HIV/AIDS, especially in SSA. The WHO and the World Bank support the International Health Partnerships (IHPs) devoted to achieving universal health coverage by 2030. These and other initiatives aim to bridge gaps in the global efforts by strengthening global strategies for disease control and devel-oping structures for monitoring progress. In general, the initiatives are laudable and commend-able in the spirit of solidarity espoused by the notion of global health, but with some crucial challenges within their modes of operation.

Despite the ongoing collaborations and achievements so far, the burden of disease is still unacceptably high, and weak health systems still exist in some regions. There are still billions of people with limited or no effective health services. The threats of emerging and re-emerg-ing diseases are constant. Preventable diseases such as malaria, diarrhea and pneumonia still account for millions of deaths annually (Amzat and Shehu, 2020). The healthcare situation in many countries of the Global South is still relatively poor.

Figure 11.1 shows the challenges facing global health initiatives. Global health inequalities still exist in all ramifications—developing and developed nations, majority and minorities, peo-ple living in poverty and riches, and rural and urban dwellers, among other defining characteris-tics (including the source of health funding). The most significant sources of funding and other resources for global health programs come from the Global North. The countries of the North with their agents (and initiatives) enter into global agreements and programs with a dominant stance, which often impacts negatively on other nations. Such agreements and programs are

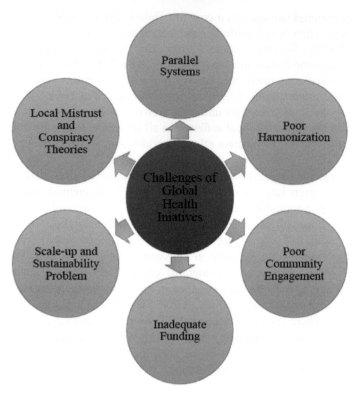

Figure 11.1 Challenges of global health initiatives

laden with definite interests to be protected. The current global health situation is still unacceptable; hence a call for healthy lives and universal healthcare by 2030 and beyond. The initiatives were designed to alleviate the global disease burden drastically, but they faced several challenges, briefly examined in the next section (see Figure 11.1).

11.3.1 Improved but Inadequate Funding

Health financing has been at the top of the list of resources required to initiate, implement, sustain and scale-up global health strategies. Funding is the core gap that most initiatives aim to bridge. It is first necessary to acknowledge the initiation of the various partnerships, which created a global forum to pool resources in addressing various global health challenges. The last goal of the MDGs was to harness resources through sustainable partnerships. The initiatives and MDGs attracted increased funding for global health projects (McCoy et al., 2009). Reports indicated an increase in development assistance for health (DAH) from US$2.5 billion in 1990 to approximately US$14 billion in 2005, with donors accounting for up to 50%. Donations from the new global health initiatives GFATM, GAVI and the Gates Foundation accounted for 13% (of DAH) (World Bank, 2007). The World Bank also assisted over 100 countries, with US$12 billion from 1997–2006. In the early 2000s, official development assistance grew by nearly 40%, with donor funding for global health reaching US$14 billion in 2004 (Kates et al., 2006). In 2006, health spending in developing countries grew from 4.1% to 5.7% of developing-country GDP (World Bank, 2007).

Kates et al. (2006) concluded that there must be a continuous increase in global health funding to facilitate various projects, including the scaling up of essential interventions, health system development, and R&D concerning diseases of people living in poverty. Since 2006, there has been an upward movement in the global flow of health financing in the form of DAH, estimated at around US$38.9 billion in 2018 (IHME, 2019). The Global South regions (especially SSA, North Africa and the Middle East and South Asia) are the most prioritized in the aid allocation. Unlike Shiffman's (2017) argument that child health was not adequately prioritized compared to maternal health, there has been a dramatic shift in the allocation of DAH with a very high percentage focusing on child and newborn health (IHME, 2019). For 2018, HIV, child and newborn health, and reproductive and maternal health top the disease focus in aid allocation, but NCDs are still not adequately prioritized.

The continuous increase in health financing is partly due to a considerable increase in the number of global health actors and initiatives transforming the global health landscape. Despite the increase, the consensus is that health funding still falls far short of the global need (see Marco et al., 2019; Ortiz-Ospina and Roser, 2019). The main reasons are that domestic spending (by the respective governments, especially in the Global South) on health remains low and inefficient, high level of out-of-pocket spending to finance healthcare in the absence of pooled funds, and insufficient DAH. Marco et al. (2019) observed that the current state of funding is a significant obstacle to the achievement of SDG 3 because it is still grossly inadequate. As of 2016, in low-income countries, the per head spending, including donor funding, was $19, which was not up to half of what was required (Marco et al., 2019). The UN also lamented that the available finance (within the global financial system) is not channeled at the scale required to achieve global development needs. Therefore, finance still constitutes to be a major challenge in achieving all the SDGs.

11.3.2 Parallel Systems

Global health initiatives or partnerships are organized structures or systems with vital missions. Sometimes, such initiative missions are overwhelming, and therefore, override some other considerations in terms of national strategies of the host countries or communities. The GHIs have emerged with dominant structures coercive of the national structures. The context of power and resources, emerging from the Global North, generate some forms of power play. First, it is like a charity gesture and not a responsibility. A proverb says that "he who pays the piper calls the tune". The initiators have enormous power to dictate the targets and health goals. What constitutes a health problem, and what financial amount gets allocated is at the discretion of the donors or initiators. For instance, some diseases are considered as neglected diseases because of inadequate attention. Impliedly, such diseases are not on the priority lists of global health problems; hence, meager resources are dedicated to tackling such health problems. The contestable assumption is often that every country owns its systems. The funder often comes with the idea of what should work or what has worked elsewhere; perhaps not a bad idea, but sometimes it fails because of the questions of ownership and sustainability. Biesma et al. (2009, p. 239) noted that most GHIs often operate by "establishing parallel bodies and processes that are poorly coordinated and aligned with national systems".

On the foregoing arguments, Mwisongo and Nabyonga-Orem (2016) observed that GHIs often operate vertically with less consideration for the country systems. The vertical approach is usually a disease-specific and top-down approach. In the vertical approach, it is easier to earmark funds for HIV, develop or select strategies to be funded and measure the health outcomes in terms of HIV prevalence rates yearly. The Global Fund uses a vertical approach in targeting three major infectious diseases highly prevalent in low-income countries. On the other hand, the horizontal approach is broader, with some consideration of some correlates of diseases within the population. Each approach has its strengths and weaknesses, but the prevailing funding regime is more vertical, and hence, with a defining stance regarding its strategies. The vertical manner is a product of the international health regime, in tune with the provision of purposive assistance. It is also a product of the ideology and interest driving the foreign policy of the powerful nations (see Ng and Ruger, 2011). Most initiatives are still significantly connected to the world powers, thereby not as independent or private as they may seem. The initiatives have, either consciously or unconsciously, muddled some powerful interests or values. The value-laden stance of government agencies (such as USAID, GIZ and DFID) might be excusable as instruments of foreign policies, but for "private" initiatives, there are fundamental concerns.

Ng and Ruger (2011) observed that it is hard to delineate a clear boundary between the global health players (especially between state and non-state actors) in terms of approach and roles—a question of multiple functions as sources of funding, as originators of initiatives, and as implementers, monitors and evaluators. The influence of the frame of mere foreign policy is also buttressed by the fact that the powerful nations are the biggest donors to most of the initiatives. Hence, there are "rumbles in the ring" of global health governance because of the lack of definite architecture of global health. However, Ng and Ruger (2011) noted the advantageous multiagency play of the UN, WB, IMF, WHO, UN organizations, multinational corporations and some influential international NGOs. However, the concern is about structural and operational chaos. As earlier observed, rumbles of interests and significantly, "funding and initiatives often bypass governments, which complicates national planning, and donor requirements (e.g., for accountability) often lead to duplication and waste". In short, bypassing the governments and parallel systems constitute significant concerns because the states, irrespective of DAH, still carry the substantial responsibilities (including funding) in the deployment of resources and management of healthcare systems.

11.3.3 Poor Harmonization of Health Strategies

A previous section discussed the globalization of health indicators and targets (see Section 2.3.5) and the importance of health goals in setting policy directions. However, there are still concerns regarding diverse health strategies. The first major issue highlighted in the last subsection on the disease-specific approach also implies that global health can be unbundled into global-specific disease strategies—then the list is endless. The different initiatives also focus on different diseases, which necessitates numerous disease-specific strategies. For instance, the integrative community case management (iCCM) strategies focusing on malaria, diarrhea and pneumonia are gaining popularity in many parts of developing countries (Amzat and Shehu, 2020). These are the three deadliest childhood infectious diseases, but most funding initiative focuses on malaria only, leaving diarrhea and pneumonia inadequately prioritized in global health initiatives. The iCCM evolved as a strategy to train, supply, and supervise lower-level health workers (such as the community health workers [CHWs]) to manage diarrhea, malaria and pneumonia in communities with poor access to health services (Oliphant et al., 2014). In 2016, 26 malaria-affected countries had iCCM policies in place, of which 24 had started implementing those policies (WHO, 2017, p. XV). Through the harmonization of strategies, there could be more funding to cover the iCCM.

In general, global initiatives influence country policies and strategies, sometimes to force harmonization with some specific donors, sometimes at odds with other donors (Mwisongo and Nabyonga-Orem, 2016). A case study of Uganda showed a conflict of strategies between the government and GHI, as the Ugandan government preferred the sector-wide approach (SWAp) to the donors' disease-specific approach (Cruz and McPake, 2011). The main accusation was that the GHIs often skew or dislodge national policies for the interest of the funders. Biesma et al. (2009) reviewed the activities of the Global Fund to Fight AIDS, TB, and Malaria, the World Bank Multi-Country AIDS Program (MAP) and the US President's Emergency Plan for AIDS Relief (PEPFAR) in HIV/AIDS control, typically in resource-poor countries. The researchers reported the distortion of recipient countries' national policies with some adverse effects on the general health systems. The donor agencies come with different priorities, areas and interests, thereby putting pressures, through the multiplication of (planning) structure, on the recipient countries to deliver on specific parameters. This external gaze, in terms of priorities and solutions, is most times not consistent with the prevailing local circumstances. Therefore, harmonization of the different selective strategies and alignment with countries' epidemiologic profiles would strengthen the policy direction and yield more global health returns (Mwisongo and Nabyonga-Orem, 2016). The challenges, as mentioned earlier, are not new; hence, "the 2005 Paris Declaration on Aid Effectiveness" recommends alignment or synchronization with national strategies and priorities (Buse and Harmer, 2007). The GHIs have been encouraged to endorse and implement the six principles of best practice (ownership, alignment, harmonization, managing for results, accountability and governance) (Buse and Harmer, 2007). However, poor harmonization is still a common challenge. It is in light of this poor harmonization that sector-wide approaches (SWAp) (although developed in the 1990s) have been gradually gaining popularity. The SWAp holds an excellent potential to promote

> health sector coordination, stronger national leadership and ownership, and strengthened countrywide management and delivery systems ... reduce duplication, lower transaction costs, increase equity and sustainability, and improve aid effectiveness and health sector efficiency (Hutton, 2004).

Therefore, SWAp will, in the long run, help to reduce the fragmentation of strategies and enhance harmonized and coherent health strategies. Another option is a centralized inter-action agency in every country to coordinate and harmonize strategies, but also with SWAp.

11.3.4 Poor Community Engagement

Grassroots participation is the bedrock of health programs or interventions, whether at the national, international or global level. Community resources must be harnessed to support the implementation of health programs. The initiative involves the community members in the identification of existing gaps and resources. The top-down approach, where the community is passive, often adversely affects the principle of ownership, which most of the initiatives aim to promote. The moment there is a more considerable influence of power, the nation is indirectly arm-twisted to own or accept a strategy that might not be effective. Global health cooperation or partnership is a multilateral flow of action and participation in every stage of the process. In several circumstances, global health actors are "expatriates" with the technical know-how to design and teleguide how program or intervention should be implemented, with less consideration of local stakeholders, including the communities and local scientists. In most cases, local actors only act as rubber-stamps to pre-designed programs or actions. In the circumstances of limited participation, it is challenging to promote ownership. While the principle of local participation is recognized, the determination for quick results is often responsible for its boycott or scrappy arrangements.

The process of participation also comes with some challenges (Buse and Harmer, 2007), but not enough to outrightly override the gains. Participations yield more gains if considered in priority setting, decision-making and oversight. The main challenges are about the form and extent such participation should take, "whether representative, delegated or direct, who should be involved, through what processes, as well as the feasibility of implementation at a global level" (Buse and Harmer, 2007). Bruen et al. (2014) noted that the Global Fund, for instance, considered vertical models more convenient than multi-stakeholder participatory models, which could yield more gains. The Global Fund often uses a combination of the models in its activities. The goal of accountability, however, favors a participatory approach, which makes the stakeholders answerable to local communities. The implication is that participatory models offer more transformative potentials than other models (Bruen et al., 2014).

Community engagement (CE) is all about community consultation at all levels of the intervention process. The CE process involves the development of genuine partnerships, collaborative initiative, mutual respect, inclusive participation, power-sharing and equity (Tindana et al., 2007). One critical area is that CE involves two-way learning: Both the initiators and host communities learn in the process of the collaboration. This requires a great deal of humility on the part of the initiators (Garnett et al., 2009). The argument, so far, implies that more participation of stakeholders from the Global South is fundamental to the success of the GHIs. A participatory model is a need-driven approach; the host nations will help in the prioritization of needs. Participation in the implementation of the initiative also helps to unlock or build national capacities. The lack of participation has been implicated in the earlier resistance to immunization programs in many countries of the Global South. It is not always enough to just identify a solution without proper consultation or participation of the recipient nations. Besides capacity building, participatory models are also crucial in getting value for money measured using the three Es (economy, efficiency and effectiveness). Community participation enhances ownership and effectiveness. The economic cost of the program or project is usually minimized because of the utilization of some community resources (both tangibles and intangibles) (Amzat, 2020). The preceding argument implies that there is a tension between globalization and glocalization (see Section 1.2.2). Glocalization can only triumph through the participation of various stakeholders, especially the recipient countries. At the country level, districts and communities also need to be incorporated into the implementation process. Beyond the gains of the intervention, the participatory model is a significant way of building mutual trust—built from the global to the community and vice-versa.

11.3.5 Local Mistrust and Conspiracy Theories

Some suspicions and mistrust surround global health initiatives. In this context, mistrust and medical conspiracies are about suspecting malevolent goals, either intended or unintended, of global health initiatives. The argument is not solely about issues unheard or fabricated but some significant social concerns. Global health is a domain of inequalities, and this generates tension. The unequal power relations and handed-down interventions with limited participation can create suspicion. The global health domain is also a space of controversies and dissidence, which should be examined for their merits or not. Besides inequalities in power relations, the limited participation of recipient countries and local communities have often tainted the health initiatives or partnerships as a space of secrecies, which might undermine the values or lives of the recipient communities. Such mistrust sometimes starts with unconfirmed or unclarified issues, then rumors spread around the communities. Some mistrust is also a result of cultural beliefs and lay conceptions of health interventions that are at variance with standard cultural practices. The lack of or limited cultural competencies could generate mistrust and dissidence, which could take time to control.

Mistrust and conspiracies are historical, and they must be understood in that context. The historical relations, which first manifest in the name of colonial medicine in many countries of the Global South, still adversely affect modern healthcare (see Keller, 2006). The initial historical trajectory was that modern medicine is an arm of colonial structures, used to perpetrate all forms of atrocities against the locals. The historical romance of colonialism and (colonial) medicine sustains some mistrust, suspicion or conspiracies, even in the global era (see Keller, 2006). Keller (2006) argued that despite the ideology of global "healing", there is a constant recollection of past malevolent antecedents in contemporary global encounters that reflect on contemporary global health. The global biomedicine's expansion reflects "a powerful legacy of mistrust that tightly links economic, cultural, and political globalization to the new imperialism of the late nineteenth century" (Keller, 2006, p. 26). Keller noted another contemporary reality, which is the militarization of medicine and aid in conflict zones—military intervention comes with health posts to treat victims of the same intervention.

At least with the constant threats of neo-imperialism, it can be observed that such historical mistrust is not over. Notably, globalization is sometimes considered to be an extension of historical exploitation. Also, globalization as an un-equalizing process buttresses the tendency to re-examine some embedded exploitations, and hence, some valid concerns; past unethical practices and research have significantly generated mistrusts. Historically, modern medicine or healthcare has been used in most instances to benefit the powerful at the expense of underprivileged groups around the world. A substantial number of Black Americans still hold many AIDS conspiracies because of their historical experience of exploitation and unethical medical experiments in the US (see Oliver and Wood, 2014). The aggressiveness and energies used to ensure saturation of interventions is often interpreted in the light of historical antecedents (politics and ethics). In the face of limited community input, the results are cautious acceptability. Whether valid or not, conspiracies are founded on historical experiences, prevailing unequal power relations and global alienation, with the Global South on the receiving end. Historically, some conspiracy theories turned out to be true, while the vast majority have been false (see van Prooijen and Douglas, 2018; Andrade, 2020). For instance, the historical use of humans (especially, minority and vulnerable groups) as experimental guinea pigs was once a conspiracy theory before generating ethical concerns and apologies (see Ford, 1968 for specific examples).

Mistrust and conspiracies, usually known and endorsed across various groups (both North and South), have adverse effects on the acceptance of interventions, and in particular, affect health behavior (van Prooijen and Douglas, 2018). Generally, van Prooijen and Douglas (2018) observed that conspiracy theories are consequential, universal, emotional and social. Within global health, the consequences are felt in the sometimes cordial and uncordial interaction and suspicion in the development projects. Even in terms of policy-lines, there has been suspicion of deliberate mis-prioritization and malevolent political twisting, which generate some negative results. For instance, the structural adjustment programs (SAP) promoted by the World Bank in many LMICs have been described as a deliberate malignant economic and political policy. The World Bank (WB) and International Monetary Fund (IMF) promote strangulating loan conditionalities with attendant adverse effects on vital institutions in LMICs. Unfortunately, the same institutions propagate health interventions to mitigate the adverse effects of limited finance and health infrastructures. Institutions like the WB and IMF are seen as the faces of neo-colonialism, and when they come with health programs, then it is suspected that it is neo-colonial healthcare, which requires some precautions.

Mistrust has significantly affected global health initiatives concerning AIDS, vaccination, family planning, global health emergencies, medical research and development, climate control and terrorism, among others. Some structures (e.g., facilities of Doctors without Borders and Red Cross) of GHIs are sometimes soft targets for militants (Keller, 2006). Trust issues, bordering on safety concerns, reflect in the resurgence of measles in many countries (Editorial, 2019). Vaccine hesitancy, as a result of fears and mistrust, is a global health threat (Editorial,

2019). Such mistrust tends to spread faster in the age of social media. Unfortunately, there are no vaccines against mistrust except transparency, inclusive participation, rumor surveillance, counter-narratives and the constant efforts to promote more benevolent goals in the spirit of global health. In empirical studies of 337 partners in 40 health promotion partnerships using a postal survey, Jones and Barry (2018, p. 16) observed mistrust. However, they concluded that "power-sharing and trust-building mechanisms need to be built into partnerships from the beginning and sustained throughout the collaborative process". Community participation and transparency in the planning and implementation phases can also significantly help to build trust.

11.3.6 Scale-Up and Sustainability Problem

There have been several implementation research and best practices, which have worked to alleviate different health problems in different contexts in the Global South. There has also been the development of innovative technologies (such as rapid diagnostic tools, and general advances in digital health). The main challenge has always been the ability to scale-up and sustain the solution in the face of other challenges, such as funding and health system issues. Milat et al. (2016) observed that the wide-scale implementation of effective intervention is vital in population health. Such interventions need only be tailored to the peculiarities of the new setting. Scale-up refers to the wide-scale implementation of effective strategies to reach a broader population or multiple settings. The main goal is to improve the impacts of successful interventions after considerations of their political, institutional and fiscal context. Scaling-up intervention is a significant challenge in implementation research because the initial implementation might only cover a relatively small setting, and the primary goal is often to maximize the benefits of the intervention. Milat et al. (2016) explained that scaling up is a systematic process involving four stages: Scalability assessment, development of a scale-up plan, preparation for scale-up and scaling up the intervention. At that point, an intervention can move from the community to the district to the national, and even the global level. Scaling up an intervention is easier when the relevant political authorities and other stakeholders take ownership to further the intervention. Scaling up can be attained by providing more political support or increased funding to continue a particular innovation.

In light of the political and economic considerations, it is clear why scaling up might constitute a problem. Zomahoun et al. (2019) observed that many issues hamper the motive to scale-up evidence-based interventions, including contextual, ethical and cost issues, among others. Most health interventions are not usually composite solutions that would fit all, but are vulnerable to contextual factors that could constrain the scope of implementation. Sometimes it is not at all cost-effective to provide some interventions on a large scale. Ethical issues include differential priorities from one community or country to another. A qualitative study involving experts of implementation science in LMICs revealed some other pitfalls in scale-up efforts, including limited human resources, low health systems capacity, inadequate engagement of local implementers and the adopting community and inadequate integration of research into scale-up efforts (Zomahoun et al., 2019).

Another vital implementation issue connected to scale-up is sustainability. Intervention must be designed in such a way that they ensure sustainability. In other words, health intervention must be built to last, without which, the problem will soon resurge. Sustainability can be described in two ways. Sustainability is about the delivery of interventions over an extended period after the termination of external support (Rabin and Brownson, 2017). The other way is what is described as sustainment, creating and sustaining structure and processes that would support the maintenance of a particular intervention within the system (Aarons et al., 2016).

Community participation or engagement and investment in health systems, or simply SWAp, is critical to enhancing sustainability or sustainment. Hailemariam et al. (2019) reviewed several studies relating to the sustainment of health interventions and observed that limited efforts toward sustainment were due to limited funding. Predictably, some evidence-based interventions might be short-lived after external support or when the implementers turn away from recipient communities. Therefore, encouraging sustainable global health interventions by addressing relevant pitfalls would enhance scale-up and eventually improve healthcare in LMICs (see Zomahoun et al., 2019; Hailemariam et al., 2019). Improved and sustained global health efforts will pay off toward healthy lives on a global scale.

11.4 Summary

- Global health initiatives or global health partnerships constitute collaborative efforts to improve global health. Although often poorly conceived in terms of humanitarian activities, the initiatives hold promise in improving global health through the provision of essential resources (both material and non-material), most notably in resource-constrained settings.
- The chapter examines some major global health initiatives, including Roll Back Malaria, the Global Fund to Fight AIDS, TB and Malaria, the Global Alliance for Vaccines and Immunizations, the Global Alliance for Improved Nutrition and the Global Health Council.
- Despite the ongoing collaborations and achievements, the burden of disease is still unacceptably high in the Global South, which is the primary focus of the Initiatives. Several challenges embedded in the initiatives' modes of operation stymie the achievement global health goals.
- Health financing has been at the top of the list of resources required to initiate, implement, sustain and scale-up global health strategies. Funding is the core gap that most initiatives aim to bridge. Despite the increase in funding over the years, health funding still falls far short of the global need.
- Global health initiatives or partnerships are organized structures or systems with vital missions. Sometimes, such initiative missions are overwhelming, and therefore override some other considerations in terms of national strategies of the host countries or communities. The GHIs have emerged with dominant structures coercive of the national structures.
- There are often the problems of poor harmonization of strategies with the host countries and donor-driven prioritization which limits transparency and participatory approach. A lack of transparency fosters mistrust and development of medical conspiracy theories.
- A participatory model and sector-wide approach seem promising to reduce the fragmentation of strategies and enhance harmonized and coherent health strategies in the Global South.

Critical Thinking Questions

- To what extent are the global health initiatives coercive of the national health structures and thereby counter-productive?
- How supportive and adequate is development assistance for health (DAH) to propel universal healthcare irrespective of regions?
- What global health strategies work or not in improving healthcare situation in the Global Health?
- Critically identify and examine some mistrusts or conspiracy theories concerning global health initiatives. How valid are the mistrusts and conspiracy theories?

Suggested Readings

- Jones, J., and Barry, M. M. (2018). Factors influencing trust and mistrust in health promotion partnerships. *Global Health Promotion, 25*(2),16–24. The article examines mistrust in global health partnerships.
- Mwisongo, A., and Nabyonga-Orem, J. (2016). Global health initiatives in Africa – governance, priorities, harmonisation and alignment. *BMC Health Services Research, 16*(Suppl 4), 212. doi:10.1186/s12913-016-1448-9. The article focuses on why the coordination of global health partnership is still problematic in Africa.
- Shiffman, J. (2017). Four challenges that global health networks face. *International Journal of Health Policy Management, 6*(4), 183–189. doi:10.15171/ijhpm.2017.14. The article discusses the impediments of global health networks.
- Malagón de Salazar, Ligia, Luján, Roberto Carlos (Eds.) (2018). Globalization and Health Inequities in Latin America. Cham, Switzerland: Springer International Publishing. This book critically analyses the influence of international policies and guidelines on the performance of interventions aimed at reducing health inequities in Latin America.
- Murphy, J., Neufeld, V. R., Habte, D., Aseffa, A., Afsana, K., Kumar, A., Larrea, M. and Hatfield, J. (2012). Ethical considerations of global health partnerships. In Andrew Pinto, A., and Upshur, R. (eds.), *An introduction to global health ethics*. New York: Routledge. The chapter provides examples of collaboration and partnership for global health, and how principles such as social justice and solidarity are realized through such relationships.

References

Aarons, G. A., Green, A. E., Trott, E., Willging, C. E., Torres, E. M., Ehrhart, M. G. & Roesch, S. C. (2016). The roles of system and organizational leadership in system-wide evidence-based intervention sustainment: A mixed-method study. *Administration and Policy in Mental Health and Mental Health Services Research, 43*(6), 991–1008.

Amzat, J. (2011). Assessing the progress of malaria control in Nigeria. *World Health and Population, 12*(3), 42–51.

Amzat, J. (2015). The question of autonomy in maternal health: A rights-based consideration. *Journal of Bioethical Inquiry, 15*(2), 283–293. doi: 10.1007/s11673-015-9607-y.

Amzat, J. (2020). Beyond wishful thinking: The promise of science engagement at a community level in Africa. *Journal of Developing Societies, 36*(2), 206–228. doi: 10.1177/0169796X20910600.

Amzat, J., & Grandi, G. (2011). Gender context of personalism in bioethics. *Developing World Bioethics, 11*(3), 136–145.

Amzat, J., & Omololu, O. F. (2009). Towards a community model for malaria control in sub-Sahara Africa. *Africana Bulletin, 57*, 166–183.

Amzat, J., & Sheu, S. (2020). The deadly trio of malaria, pneumonia and diarrhea: Assessing community knowledge gaps and beliefs within integrated community case management (iCCM) practice in a Nigerian State. *The Nigerian Journal of Sociology and Anthropology, 18*(1), 13–31. doi: 10.36108/NJSA/0202/81(0120).

Andrade, G. (2020). Medical conspiracy theories: cognitive science and implications for ethics. *Medicine, Health Care and Philosophy*, 1–14. Advance online publication. doi: 10.1007/s11019-020-09951-6.

Biesma, R. G., Brugha, R., Harmer, A., Walsh, A., Spicer, N. & Walt, G. (2009). The effects of global health initiatives on country health systems: A review of the evidence from HIV/AIDS control. *Health Policy and Planning, 24*(4), 239–252.

Bloland, P. B., Ettling, M. & Meek, S. 2000. Combination therapy for malaria in Africa: Hype or hope? *Bulletin of the World Health Organization, 78*, 1378–1388.

Bruen, C., Brugha, R., Kageni, A. & Wafula, F. (2014). A concept in flux: questioning accountability in the context of global health cooperation. *Globalization and Health, 10*, 73. doi: 10.1186/s12992-014-0073-9.

Buse, K., & Harmer, A. M. (2007). Seven habits of highly effective global public–private health partnerships: Practice and potential. *Social Science and Medicine, 64*(2), 259–71.

Corbett, E. L, Watt, C. J, Walker, N., Maher, D., Williams, B. G., Raviglione, M. C. & Dye, C. (2003). The growing burden of tuberculosis: Global trends and interactions with the HIV epidemic. *Archives of Internal Medicine, 163*(9), 1009–1021. doi: 10.1001/archinte.163.9.1009.

Cruz, V. O., & McPake, B. (2011). Global health initiatives and aid effectiveness: Insights from a Ugandan case study. *Global Health, 4*(7), 20. doi: 10.1186/1744-8603-7-20.

Dollin, J. P., Raviglione, M. C. & Kochi, A. (1994). Global tuberculosis incidence and mortality during 1990–2000. *Bulletin of the World Health Organization, 72*(2), 213–20.

Editorial (2019). Trust issues. *The Lancet Infectious Diseases, 17,* 1099. doi: 10.1016/S1473-3099(19)30128-8.

Fogh, S., Jepsen, S. & Effersoe, P. (1979). Chloroquine-resistant malaria in Kenya. *Transactions of the Royal Society of Tropical Medicine and Hygiene, 73,* 228–229.

Food and Agriculture Organization (FAO) (2000). *The State of Food and Agriculture 2000.* Rome: FAO.

FAO (2010). *The State of Food Insecurity in the World: Addressing Food Insecurity in Protracted Crises.* Rome: FAO.

FAO, International Fund for Agricultural Development (IFAD), & World Food Programme (WFP) (2015). *The State of Food Insecurity in the World 2015. Meeting the 2015 international hunger targets: taking stock of uneven progress.* FAO.

Ford, A. B. (1968). Human guinea pigs: Experimentation on man. *JAMA,* 204(6), 552. doi: 10.1001/jama.1968.03140190134023.

Garnett, S. T., Crowley, G. M., Hunter-Xenie, H., Kozanayi, W., Sithole, B., Palmer, C., Southgate, R. & Zander, K. K. (2009). Transformative knowledge transfer through empowering and paying community researchers. *Biotropica, 41*(5), 571–577. doi: 10.1111/j.1744-7429.2009.00558.x.

Global Alliance for Improved Nutrition (GAIN) (2019). Achieving impacts at GAIN: Better nutrition for all. www.gainhealth.org/sites/default/files/impact/achieving-impact-at-gain.pdf. Accessed on November 12, 2019.

Global Alliance for Vaccines and Immunizations (GAVI) (2018). *2017 Annual Progress Report.* Geneva: GAVI.

Global Fund (2019). Global Fund overview. www.theglobalfund.org/en/overview/. Accessed on November 8, 2019.

Global Health Council (GHC) (2019). A guide to US investment in global health: transforming communities worldwide. https://ghbb.globalhealth.org. Accessed on November 13, 2019.

Hailemariam, M., Bustos, T., Montgomery, B., Barajas, R., Evans, L. B. & Drahota, A. (2019). Evidence-based intervention sustainability strategies: A systematic review. *Implementation Science, 14,* 57. doi: 10.1186/s13012-019-0910-6.

Hutton, T. (2004). The sector-wide approach: A blessing for public health? *Bulletin of the World Health Organization, 82*(12), 893–894.

Institute for Health Metrics and Evaluation (IHME) (2019). *Financing Global Health Visualization.* Seattle, WA: IHME, University of Washington. http://vizhub.healthdata.org/fgh/. Accessed on November 14, 2019.

InterAction (2013). Global health: Investing in our future. In *Global Health Briefing Book 62.* Washington, DC: InterAction.

Jones, J., & Barry, M. M. (2018). Factors influencing trust and mistrust in health promotion partnerships. *Global Health Promotion, 25*(2),16–24.

Kates, J., Morrison, S. & Lief, E. (2006). Global health funding: A glass half full? *Lancet, 368*(9531), 187–188.

Keller, R. C. (2006). Geographies of power, legacies of Mistrust: Colonial medicine in the global present. *Historical Geography, 34,* 26–48.

Laxminarayan, R. (2004). Act now or later? Economics of malaria resistance. *American Journal of Tropical Medicine and Hygiene, 71*(Suppl. 2), 187–195.

Lieu, T. A., & Platt, R. (2017). Applied research and development in health care: Time for a frameshift. *The New England Journal of Medicine, 376,* 710–713. doi: 10.1056/NEJMp1611611.

MacDonald, N. E., & The Sage Working Group on Vaccine Hesitancy (SageVH) (2015). Vaccine hesitancy: Definition, scope and determinants. *Vaccine, 33*(34), 4161–4164.

Marco, S., Sebastian, M., Osondu, O., Lewis, S. M., & Gavin. Y. (2019). Trends in global health financing. *BMJ, 365*, l2185.

McCoy, D., Chand, S. & Sridhar, D. (2009). Global health funding: How much, where it comes from and where it goes. *Health Policy and Planning, 24*(6), 407–417. doi: 10.1093/heapol/czp026.

Milat, A. J., Newson, R., King, L., Rissel, C., Wolfenden, L., Bauman, A., Redman, S. & Giffin, M. (2016). A guide to scaling up population health interventions. *Public Health Research and Practice, 26*(1), e2611604.

Moench-Pfanner, R., & Ameringen, M. V. (2012). The global alliance for improved nutrition (GAIN): A decade of partnerships to increase access to and affordability of nutritious foods for the poor. *Food and Nutrition Bulletin, 33*(4, suppl3), S373–S380.

Mwisongo, A., & Nabyonga-Orem, J. (2016). Global health initiatives in Africa: Governance, priorities, harmonisation and alignment. *BMC Health Services Research, 16*(Suppl 4), 212. doi: 10.1186/s12913-016-1448-9.

Ng, N. Y., & Ruger, J. P. (2011). Global health governance at a crossroads. *Global Health Governance, 3*(2), 1–37.

Nuwaha, F. (2001). The challenge of chloroquine-resistant malaria in sub-Saharan Africa. *Health Policy and Planning, 16*(1), 1–12.

Ogundele, O. A., Ogundele, T. & Beloved, O. (2020). Vaccine hesitancy in Nigeria: Contributing factors – way forward. *Nigerian Journal of General Practice, 18*, 1–4.

Oliphant, N. P., Muñiz, M., Guenther, T., Diaz, T., Laínez, Y. B., Counihan, H. & Pratt, A. (2014). Multi-country analysis of routine data from integrated community case management (iCCM) programs in sub-Saharan Africa. *Journal of Global Health, 4*(2), 020408. doi: 10.7189/jogh.04.020408.

Oliver, J. E., & Wood, T. (2014). Medical conspiracy theories and health behaviors in the United States. *JAMA Internal Medicine, 174*(5), 817–818.

Orach, C. G. (2009). Health equity: Challenges in low-income countries. *African Health Sciences, 9*(Suppl 2), S49–S51.

Ortiz-Ospina, E., & Roser, M. (2019). Financing healthcare. Published online at *OurWorldInData.org*. https://ourworldindata.org/financing-healthcare [Online Resource]. Accessed on November 14, 2019.

Rabin, B. A., & Brownson, R. C. (2017). Terminology for dissemination and implementation research. In Brownson, R. C., Colditz, G. A. & Proctor, E. K. (Eds.), *Dissemination and Implementation Research in Health: Translating Science to Practice*. Volume 2 (pp. 19–45). Oxford: Oxford University Press.

Razum, O., Sridhar, D., Jahn, A., Zaidi, S., Ooms, G. & Müller, O. (2019). Polio: From eradication to systematic, sustained control. *BMJ Global Health, 4*, e001633.

Ritchie, J. A. S. (1986). Towards better nutrition: Lip service or a realistic fight? *Nutrition and Health, 4*(2), 113–123.

Roll Back Malaria (RMB) (2019). RBM partnership to end malaria. https://endmalaria.org/about-us/vision. Accessed on November 7, 2019.

Roser, M., & Ritchie, H. (2019). HIV/AIDS. Published online at *OurWorldInData.org*. Retrieved from: https://ourworldindata.org/hiv-aids [Online Resource]. Accessed on November 8, 2019.

Shiffman, J. (2017). Four challenges that global health networks face. *International Journal of Health Policy Management, 6*(4), 183–189. doi: 10.15171/ijhpm.2017.14.

Tindana, P. O., Singh, J. A., Tracy, C. S., Upshur, R. E., Daar, A. S., Singer, P. A., Frohlich, J. & Lavery, J. V. (2007). Grand challenges in global health: Community engagement in research in developing countries. *PLoS Medicine, 4*(9), e273. doi: 10.1371/journal.pmed.0040273.

Tognotti, E (2010). The eradication of smallpox, a success story for modern medicine and public health: What lessons for the future? *Journal of Infection in Developing Countries, 4*(5), 264–266. doi: 10.1016/0196-6553(82)90003-7.

United Nations (UN) (2019). Sustainable development goals: Goal 2: Zero hunger. www.un.org/sustainabledevelopment/hunger/.

van Prooijen, J. W., & Douglas, K. M. (2018). Belief in conspiracy theories: Basic principles of an emerging research domain. *European Journal of Social Psychology, 48*(7), 897–908. doi: 10.1002/ejsp.2530.

Vanderslott, S., & Roser, M. (2019). Vaccination. Published online at *OurWorldInData.org*. Retrieved from: https://ourworldindata.org/vaccination [Online Resource]. Accessed on November 8, 2019.

Wernsdorfer, W. H., & Payne, D. (1991). The dynamics of drug resistance in P. falciparum. *Pharmacology and Therapeutics*, *50*, 95–125.

World Health Organization (WHO) (2016). *State of Inequality: Childhood Immunization*. Geneva: WHO.

WHO (2019a). Tuberculosis. www.afro.who.int/health-topics/tuberculosis-tb. Accessed on November 8, 2019.

WHO (2019b). Tuberculosis. www.who.int/news-room/fact-sheets/detail/tuberculosis. Accessed on November 8, 2019.

WHO. (2000). *Roll Back Malaria: Advocacy Guide*. Geneva. WHO/CDS/RBM/2000.26.

WHO (2017). *World Malaria Report 2017*. Geneva: WHO.

WHO (2018). *World Malaria Report 2018*. Geneva: WHO.

World Health Organization (WHO) & Food and Agriculture Organization (FAO) (2006). *Guidelines on Food Fortification with Micronutrients*, Allen, L., de Benoist, B., Dary, O. & Hurrell, R. (Eds.). Geneva: World Health Organization.

WHO, & Roll Back Malaria (RMB). (2012). *Defeating Malaria in Asia, the Pacific, Americas, Middle East and Europe*. Geneva: WHO.

World Bank (2007). *Healthy Development*: *The World Bank Strategy for Health, Nutrition, and Population Results* 2007. Washington, DC: World Bank.

Zomahoun, H., Ben Charif, A., Freitas, A., Garvelink, M. M., Menear, M., Dugas, M., Adekpedjou, R. & Légaré, F. (2019). The pitfalls of scaling up evidence-based interventions in health. *Global Health Action*, *12*(1), 1670449. doi: 10.1080/16549716.2019.1670449.

Index

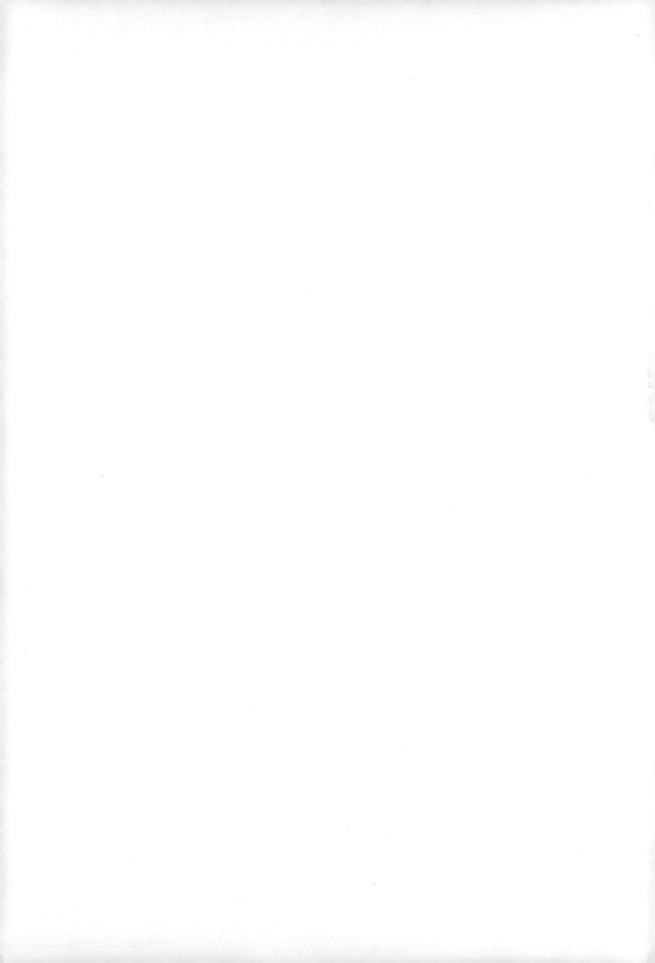